Evidence-Based Women's Oral Health

Editors

LESLIE R. HALPERN
LINDA M. KASTE

DENTAL CLINICS OF NORTH AMERICA

www.dental.theclinics.com

April 2013 • Volume 57 • Number 2

ELSEVIER

1600 John F. Kennedy Boulevard • Suite 1800 • Philadelphia, Pennsylvania, 19103-2899

http://www.dental.theclinics.com

DENTAL CLINICS OF NORTH AMERICA Volume 57, Number 2
April 2013 ISSN 0011-8532, ISBN 978-1-4557-7080-9

Editor: Yonah Korngold; y.korngold@elsevier.com

Dental Clinics of North America (ISSN 0011-8532) is published quarterly by Elsevier Inc., 360 Park Avenue South, New York, NY 10010-1710. Months of issue are January, April, July, and October. Business and Editorial Offices: 1600 John F. Kennedy Boulevard, Suite 1800, Philadelphia, PA 19103-2899. Periodicals postage paid at New York, NY and additional mailing offices. Subscription prices are $269.00 per year (domestic individuals), $474.00 per year (domestic institutions), $127.00 per year (domestic students/residents), $322.00 per year (Canadian individuals), $595.00 per year (Canadian institutions), $390.00 per year (international individuals), $595.00 per year (international institutions), and $192.00 per year (international and Canadian students/residents). International air speed delivery is included in all *Clinics* subscription prices. All prices are subject to change without notice. **POSTMASTER:** Send address changes to *Dental Clinics of North America*, Elsevier Health Sciences Division, Subscription Customer Service, 3251 Riverport Lane, Maryland Heights, MO 63043. **Customer Service (orders, claims, online, change of address): Elsevier Health Sciences Division, Subscription Customer Service, 3251 Riverport Lane, Maryland Heights, MO 63043. Tel: 1-800-654-2452 (U.S. and Canada). Fax: 314-447-8029. E-mail: journalscustomer service-usa@elsevier.com (for print support); journalsonlinesupport-usa@elsevier.com (for online support).**

Reprints. For copies of 100 or more, of articles in this publication, please contact the Commercial Reprints Department, Elsevier Inc., 360 Park Avenue South, New York, NY 10010-1710. Tel.: 212-633-3812; Fax: 212-462-1935; E-mail: reprints@elsevier.com.

The *Dental Clinics of North America* is covered in *MEDLINE/PubMed (Index Medicus), Current Contents/Clinical Medicine, ISI/BIOMED* and *Clinahl*.

Printed and bound by CPI Group (UK) Ltd, Croydon, CR0 4YY

Transferred to digital print 2012

Contributors

EDITORS

LESLIE R. HALPERN, MD, DDD, PhD, MPH
Associate Professor, Program Director, Oral and Maxillofacial Surgery, Meharry Medical College, School of Dentistry, Nashville, Tennessee

LINDA M. KASTE, DDS, MS, PhD
Diplomate, American Board of Dental Public Health; Associate Professor, Department of Pediatric Dentistry, College of Dentistry; Division of Epidemiology and Biostatistics, School of Public Health, University of Illinois at Chicago, Chicago, Illinois

AUTHORS

KRISTINA CHRISTOPH, DMD
DMD Candidate, Harvard School of Dental Medicine; Department of Orthopedic Surgery, Brigham and Women's Hospital, Boston, Massachusetts

ELLEN DALEY, PhD, MPH
Associate Professor, Department of Community and Family Health; Co-Director, Center for Transdisciplinary Research in Women's Health, College of Public Health, University of South Florida, Florida

RITA DIGIOACCHINO DEBATE, PhD, MPH, FAED
Associate Professor, Department of Community and Family Health; Co-Director, Center for Transdisciplinary Research in Women's Health, College of Public Health, University of South Florida, Florida

THERESE A. DOLECEK, PhD
Division of Epidemiology and Biostatistics, School of Public Health, Institute for Health Research and Policy, University of Illinois at Chicago, Chicago, Illinois

DAPHNE FERGUSON-YOUNG, DDS, MSPH
Associate Professor, Program Director, General Practice Residency, Meharry Medical College, School of Dentistry, Nashville, Tennessee

GRETCHEN GIBSON, DDS, MPH
Diplomate of the American Board of Special Care Dentistry; Director, Oral Health Quality Group, VA Office of Dentistry, Washington, DC; Veterans Health Care System of the Ozarks, Fayetteville, Arkansas

JULIE GLOWACKI, PhD
Professor of Orthopedic Surgery, Department of Orthopedic Surgery, Harvard Medical School; Professor of Oral and Maxillofacial Surgery, Department of Oral and Maxillofacial Surgery, Harvard School of Dental Medicine; Director of Skeletal Biology, Department of Orthopedic Surgery, Brigham and Women's Hospital, Boston, Massachusetts

SARA GORDON, DDS, MSc, FRCD(C), FDS-RCSEd
Diplomate, American Board of Oral and Maxillofacial Pathology; Associate Professor,
Department of Oral Medicine and Diagnostic Sciences, University of Illinois at Chicago,
Chicago, Illinois

LESLIE R. HALPERN, MD, DDD, PhD, MPH
Associate Professor, Program Director, Oral and Maxillofacial Surgery, Meharry Medical
College, School of Dentistry, Nashville, Tennessee

IRENE V. HILTON, DDS, MPH
Dentist, San Francisco Department of Public Health; Clinical Instructor, Department of
Family and Community Medicine, School of Medicine; Clinical Instructor, Division of Oral
Epidemiology and Dental Public Health, School of Dentistry, University of California,
San Francisco, California

NICOLE HOLLAND, DDS, MS
OMFS Orofacial Pain Fellow, Massachusetts General Hospital, Boston, Massachusetts

HIROKO IADA, DDS, MPH
Diplomate, American Board of Dental Public Health; Assistant Professor, University of
North Carolina School of Dentistry, Chapel Hill, North Carolina

MARITA R. INGLEHART, Dr. phil. habil.
Associate Professor of Dentistry, Department of Periodontics and Oral Medicine,
University of Michigan – School of Dentistry, Ann Arbor, Michigan

LINDA M. KASTE, DDS, MS, PhD
Diplomate, American Board of Dental Public Health; Associate Professor,
Department of Pediatric Dentistry, College of Dentistry; Division of Epidemiology and
Biostatistics, School of Public Health, University of Illinois at Chicago, Chicago, Illinois

JUHEE KIM, MS, ScD
Associate Professor, Department of Public Health, Center for Health Disparities,
Brody School of Medicine, East Carolina University, Greenville, North Carolina

TARU H. KINNUNEN, MA, PhD
Associate Professor, Department of Epidemiology and Oral Health Policy, Harvard School
of Dental Medicine, Boston, Massachusetts

JOHN R. LUKACS, PhD
Professor Emeritus, Department of Anthropology, University of Oregon, Eugene, Oregon

ESPERANZA ANGELES MARTINEZ-MIER, DDS, MSD, PhD
Director, Fluoride Research Program, Indiana University School of Dentistry; Associate
Professor, Department of Preventive and Community Dentistry; Director, Binational/
Cross-Cultural Health Enhancement Center, Oral Health Research Institute,
Indiana University School of Dentistry, Indianapolis, Indiana

LINDA C. NIESSEN, DMD, MPH
Diplomate of the American Board of Dental Public Health, Diplomate of the American
Board of Special Care Dentistry, Clinical Professor, Department of Restorative Dentistry,
Baylor College of Dentistry, Texas A&M University, Dallas, Texas; Vice President,
Chief Clinical Officer, Dentsply International, York, Pennsylvania

ORRETT OGLE, DDS
Hempstead, New York

STEFANIE L. RUSSELL, DDS, MPH, PhD
Clinical Associate Professor, Department of Epidemiology and Health Promotion,
NYU College of Dentistry, New York, New York

RENEE SAMELSON, MD, MPH, FACOG
Professor, Department of Obstetrics and Gynecology, Albany Medical College,
Albany, New York

JEFFRY R. SHAEFER, DDS, MS, MPH
Assistant Professor, Department of Oral and Maxillofacial Surgery, Harvard
School of Dental Medicine, Boston, Massachusetts

PRIYAA SHANMUGAM, BDS, MS, DSc
Instructor in Oral Health Policy and Epidemiology, Department of Oral Health Policy and
Epidemiology, Harvard School of Dental Medicine, Boston, Massachusetts

DEEPTHI SHETTY, BDS, MPH
Resident in Dental Public Health, Division of Oral Epidemiology and Biostatistics,
Columbia University College of Dental Medicine, New York, New York

BARBARA J. STEINBERG, DDS
Diplomate, American Board of Oral Medicine, Clinical Professor of Surgery,
Drexel University College of Medicine; Adjunct Associate Professor of Oral Medicine,
University of Pennsylvania School of Dental Medicine, Philadelphia, Pennsylvania

MARY TAVARES, DMD, MPH
Program Director, Dental Public Health Residency, Oral Health Policy and Epidemiology,
Harvard School of Dental Medicine, Boston, Massachusetts

LISA A. THOMPSON, DMD
Program Director, Geriatric Dental Fellowship, Oral Health Policy and Epidemiology,
Harvard School of Dental Medicine, Boston, Massachusetts

ANA MIRIAM VELLY, DDS, MS, PhD
Assistant Professor, Faculty of Dentistry; Investigator, Division of Clinical Epidemiology,
Department of Dentistry, Jewish General Hospital, McGill University, Montreal,
Quebec, Canada

JULIA S. WHELAN, MS
Reference and Education Services Librarian, Countway Library of Medicine, Harvard
Medical School, Boston, Massachusetts

JOCELYN R. WILDER, MPH, MS
Doctoral Student, Division of Epidemiology and Biostatistics, School of Public Health,
University of Illinois at Chicago, Chicago, Illinois

ANDREA FERREIRA ZANDONA, DDS, MSD, PhD
Director, Graduate MSD/MS Preventive Dentistry Program; Director, Early Caries
Research Program; Associate Professor, Department of Preventive and Community
Dentistry, Oral Health Research Institute, Indiana University School of Dentistry,
Indianapolis, Indiana

ATHANASIOS I. ZAVRAS, DMD, DDS, MS, Dr MedSc
Associate Professor and Head, Division of Oral Epidemiology and Biostatistics,
Columbia University College of Dental Medicine, New York, New York; Adjunct Associate
Professor of Epidemiology, Department of Epidemiology, Harvard School of Public
Health, Boston, Massachusetts

Contents

Women's health, including oral health, is an evolving science with foundation knowledge from many disciplines. Key milestones, particularly in the last decade, provide a roadmap towards the necessary inclusion of gender into dental practice. Such focus is especially important for the evolving role of oral health care providers as primary health care providers. Continued progress of the vibrant incorporation of evidence-based women's oral health into the standard practice of oral health care is encouraged. This expanded preface provides an introduction to this DCNA issue, a brief history and timeline of major women's oral health events, and resources for further consideration.

This article examines the differences and interaction between sex and gender, and how they affect women's oral and general health. The authors provide a definition of women's health, and examples of how this definition can be used to describe various oral health conditions and diseases in women. The article reviews the research on sex and gender and provides examples of their interactions. Examples of oral diseases that affect primarily women are reviewed. Advice for clinicians on the diagnosis, management, and prevention of these conditions is provided.

Current research shows that women tend to receive less dental care than usual when they are pregnant. In 2012, the first national consensus statement on oral health care during pregnancy was issued, emphasizing both the importance and safety of routine dental care for pregnant women. This article reviews the current recommendations for perinatal oral health care and common oral manifestations during pregnancy. Periodontal disease and its association with preterm birth and low birth weight are also discussed, as is the role played by dental intervention in these adverse outcomes.

The impact of dietary behaviors and food consumption and their relation to oral health are significant public health issues. Women and men exhibit different dietary behaviors. Understanding the influences of dietary behaviors on oral health from the perspective of gender disparities, however, is limited. This article provides the intersections of dietary factors and oral-systemic health for which women are at greater risk than men. Topics include the effect of dietary choices on oral health disparities seen in female patients.

Interventional strategies at the local and community level that are designed to influence the balance between dietary habits and oral-systemic health are discussed.

Gender is the biggest risk factor in the development of temporomandibular disorders (TMD) and orofacial pain. Gender differences in pain thresholds, temporal summation, pain expectations, and somatic awareness exist in patients with chronic TMD or orofacial pain. There are gender differences in pharmacokenetics and pharmacodynamics of medications used to treat pain. A better understanding of the mechanisms that contribute to the increased incidence and persistence of chronic pain in females is needed. Future research will elucidate the sex effects on factors that protect against developing pain or prevent debilitating pain. Gender-based treatments for TMD and orofacial pain treatment will evolve from the translational research stimulated by this knowledge.

Despite wide variations in the size and shape of the human face, head, and body, there is remarkable consistency for quantifiable gender-specific facial traits. The relationships between the growing jaws and tooth eruption are complex, but they show gender-specific trajectories in children and adolescents. Disturbances in genetic, endocrine, and nutritional regulatory controls result in gender-specific and nonspecific disorders. Gender-specific differences are also apparent in the aging jaw, with the acceleration of jawbone atrophy upon loss of teeth, especially in women.

Violence and abuse (V/A) is recognized as a significant public health problem, especially in females. Injuries to the head, neck, and/or mouth are clearly visible to the dental team during examination. This article provides compelling evidence that supports the pivotal position occupied by oral health care professionals within the arena of detection, intervention, and prevention of V/A. This article reviews the epidemiology of orofacial risk factors for V/A, diagnostic tools and surveys for identifying victims of all ages, and suggests interdisciplinary educational curricula/specific algorithms to provide the necessary core competencies for identifying victims in the oral health care environment.

Dental caries remains a common disease worldwide. There is evidence indicating that many caries risk factors provide a gender bias, placing women at a higher caries risk. Generally, dental caries disproportionally affects the poor and racial or ethnic minorities worldwide, with women suffering more from the disease. Differences in access to care as reflected by untreated caries rates also reflect gender disparities. There is a lack of evidence in regard to gender differences and dental caries. Therefore, there is an urgent need to develop the evidence necessary to meet the oral health needs of both women and men worldwide.

This review highlights what is known regarding differences in tooth loss by sex/gender, and describes: gender-related tooth ablation (the deliberate removal of anterior teeth during life) found in skulls from history and prehistory; potential mediators of the relationship between sex/gender and tooth loss; the current epidemiology of gender differences in tooth loss (limited to North America); and risk factors for tooth loss in the general population and in women.

Although in the United States the incidence of oral and pharyngeal cancer (OPC) has been significantly higher in men than in women, the identification of human papilloma virus as a risk factor for OPC has focused new scrutiny on who may develop OPC. One surprising element is that non-Hispanic white women have a higher incidence of OPC than of cervical cancer. OPC is thus a woman's disease, and diligence is needed to ensure that the occurrence of OPC in women does not go undetected by their oral health care providers.

Research findings concerning the role of gender in patient-physician interactions can inform considerations about the role of gender in patient-dental care provider interactions. Medical research showed that gender differences in verbal and nonverbal communication in medical settings exist and that they affect the outcomes of these interactions. The process of communication is shaped by gender identities, gender stereotypes, and attitudes. Future research needs to consider the cultural complexity and diversity in which gender issues are embedded and the degree to which ongoing value change will shape gender roles and in turn interactions between dental patients and their providers.

Modifications of the traditional dental workforce have been proposed. The focus of this article is on expanding the role of the dentist as a primary health care provider, and includes topics that are emerging in the realm of general dentistry for further integration into primary health care and women's health. The evidence base for the clinical application of these topics in dentistry is under development. In the near future, dentistry will have core competencies involving the topics discussed in this article as well as other new interdisciplinary health care aspects to enhance the overall health and well-being of patients.

DENTAL CLINICS OF NORTH AMERICA

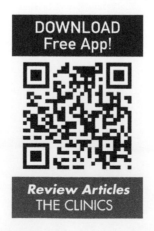

Erratum

Errors were made in the January 2013 issue of *Dental Clinics* on pages 107 and 113 in "Temporomandibular Joint Disorders in Children" by James A. Howard. On page 107, the third to last sentence should read, "Biological plausibility for an occlusal etiology is difficult to establish..." On page 113, the legend for Figure 6 should read, "Fig. 6. Lateral cephalometric (A) and panoramic (B) images of a 15-year-old boy with JIA demonstrating condylar resorption (blue)..."

Dent Clin N Am 57 (2013) xiii
http://dx.doi.org/10.1016/j.cden.2013.03.001
0011-8532/13/$ – see front matter © 2013 Elsevier Inc. All rights reserved.

dental.theclinics.com

Erratum

Errors were made in the January 2013 issue of Seminars on pages 107 and 113 in "Temporomandibular Joint Disorders in Children" by James A. [review] On page 107, the mid to last sentence should read, "Endured durability for an occlusal etiology is difficult to establish." On page 113, the legend for Figure 6 should read "Fig. 6 Lateral cephalometric (A) and panoramic (B) images of a 15-year-old boy with TMJ demonstrating condylar resorption [blue]."

Semin Orthod 2013;19:16
http://dx.doi.org/10.1053/j.sodo.2013.03.001
1073-8746/13/$ – see front matter © 2013 Elsevier Inc. All rights reserved.

dental.theclinics.com

Preface

Women's Oral Health: Growing Evidence for Enhancing Perspectives

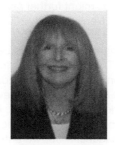 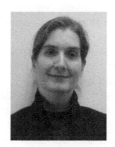

Leslie R. Halpern, MD, DDD, PhD, MPH   Linda M. Kaste, DDS, MS, PhD
Editors

With Preface Co-Authors:

Charlotte Briggs, PhD, Bay Path College, Longmeadow, MA, USA

Luisa A. DiPietro, DDS, PhD, University of Illinois at Chicago, Chicago, IL, USA

Katherine Erwin, DDS, MPA, MSCR, Community Health/Preventive Medicine, Morehouse School of Medicine, Atlanta, GA, USA

Julie Frantsve-Hawley, RDH, PhD, Center for Evidence-based Dentistry, American Dental Association, Chicago, IL, USA

Sara Gordon, DDS, MS, Department of Oral Medicine and Diagnostic Sciences, College of Dentistry, University of Illinois at Chicago, Chicago, IL, USA

Brenda Heaton, PhD, MPH, Department of Health Policy and Health Services Research, Boston University, Henry M. Goldman School of Dental Medicine, Boston, MA, USA

Michelle M. Henshaw, DDS, MPH, Department of Health Policy and Health Services Research, Boston University, Henry M. Goldman School of Dental Medicine, Boston, MA, USA

Renée Joskow, DDS, MPH, Health Resources and Services Administration, U.S. Department of Health and Human Services, Rockville, MD, USA; Captain, U.S. Public Health Service, Washington, DC, USA

Susan T. Reisine, PhD, University of Connecticut, School of Dental Medicine, Farmington, CT, USA

Jeanne C. Sinkford, DDS, PhD, Dean Emeritus Howard University College of Dentistry and American Dental Education Association, Washington, DC, USA

Dent Clin N Am 57 (2013) xv–xxviii
http://dx.doi.org/10.1016/j.cden.2013.02.007
0011-8532/13/$ – see front matter © 2013 Published by Elsevier Inc.

dental.theclinics.com

KEYWORDS

- Women's health • Oral health • Evidence-based dentistry • Dental education
- Dental research

"Another issue on women's health?" you might ask. You are right; *Dental Clinics of North America (DCNA)* has previously provided the platform for dissemination of information on women and oral health. "Has much changed?" you might further ask. It has been more than a decade since the full issue "Women's Oral Health" in July 2001,[1] and in that time, yes, a lot has changed.

Certainly our understanding of women's health has changed, but there has been an even deeper change in our expectations as clinicians. These days, we clinicians demand increased depth and veracity of the information forming the foundations from which we work, for making our decisions evidence based. Not only have our expectations changed, the contexts in which we are working have changed. As we further integrate into comprehensive health care for our patients, it behooves us to be on a level playing field with our other health care colleagues. Also, we anticipate that our patients and communities have different expectations of us.

The question "Does sex matter?" has been discussed for years. The Institute of Medicine (IOM) report entitled *Exploring the Biologic Contributions to Human Health: Does Sex Matter?*,[2] like the *DCNA* on women's oral health, was published in 2001. Its preface concludes: "Sex does matter. It matters in ways we did not expect. And it matters in ways we have not yet begun to imagine."[2]

A decade ago, the previous *DCNA* on women's health[1] drew attention to the complex interrelationships among sex, gender, and systemic and oral health. The issue moved dentistry into the "emerging field of women's health,"[1] recognizing the need and value of "gender-specific evaluation and treatment considerations for dental patients who are women."[1]

This introduction provides a brief history, and encourages continued progress on the vibrant incorporation of evidence-based women's oral health into the standard practice of oral health care. It includes a review of the definitions of sex, gender, and evidence-based dentistry; a timeline of major women's oral health events; and resources for further research and curricular development.

SEX AND GENDER

A recently published article by Springer and colleagues[3] provides insight into the complexities of defining sex and gender. Sex is not a clearly dichotomous variable (male/female) that is solely a function of hormones and anatomy. Instead, social and environmental influences (gender) are inextricably interwoven with biologic ones whenever sex-related health issues are considered.[3] Biology has an impact on gender, but environmental factors in turn have an impact on biology.[3] In short, sex and gender are entangled concepts and not separate domains.

In 2011, the IOM held a workshop that led to the report "Sex-specific Reporting of Scientific Research: A Workshop Summary."[4] This report suggested that issues of sex/gender need to be included more often in scientific publications. Suggestions included identifying the sex of the individuals in journal populations, sharing of sex-identified raw data, giving extra credit in reviews of articles that include sex-specific information, and requiring sex-stratified analysis where applicable."[4]

A dental perspective on these nuances can be seen in an article published in the United Kingdom. Doyal and Naidoo[5] discuss the experience of pain and the causation of dental caries as examples of where sex and gender interact.

EVIDENCE-BASED ORAL HEALTH

Medicine and dentistry have recently embraced evidence-based clinical decisions to optimize oral health outcomes for their patient populations. Individual decisions incorporate the best available scientific evidence, the clinician's expertise, and the patient's health care needs and personal preferences. A previous volume of the *DCNA* was dedicated to evidence-based dentistry (EBD).[6]

Although most agree that it is good to apply current scientific evidence to clinical decision making, the translation of research into health care practice usually lags by several years. Barriers to EBD include lack of time, obstacles to accessing studies, lack of understanding the significance of results, and lack of user-friendly resources.

Strategies to identify the best available scientific evidence for treatment decisions include using evidence-based guidelines, systematic reviews, and accessing the primary scientific literature. **Box 1** contains examples of resources for online information on EBD.

The American Dental Association (ADA) is a leader in EBD, but the evidence base for women's oral health care is still evolving. **Box 2** gives brief examples of topics related to women's oral health captured in the ADA database on systematic reviews. "Women's Health" is an article in the 2012 *The ADA Practical Guide to Patients with Medical Conditions*.[7] Perhaps a wider perspective of women's health is warranted given the broadening view by medicine and health research.

AN OVERVIEW OF MILESTONES

The timeline (**Fig. 1**) on women's oral health in the United States formally starts only 30 years ago (1983), when the Department of Health and Human Services (DHHS) Coordinating Committee on Women's Health provided a report to Congress seeking improvement of women's health in the United States. Great progress has subsequently occurred. The work shows how challenging the consideration of sex and gender continues to be.

From a bird's-eye view, the major US players in the timeline (see **Fig. 1**) who have promoted research and clinical practice on women's oral health are the National

Box 1	
Selected Web site resources for online information on EBD	
Resource	**Web Site Address**
American Dental Association EBD Web site	http://ebd.ada.org
Searchable database of systematic reviews in oral health	http://ebd.ada.org/SystematicReviews.aspx
PubMed	http://www.ncbi.nlm.nih.gov/pubmed/
Cochrane Oral Health Group	http://ohg.cochrane.org
TRIP	http://www.tripdatabase.com/
American Congress of Obstetricians and Gynecologists	www.acog.org
American Medical Association	http://www.ama-assn.org/
National Guideline Clearinghouse	http://guideline.gov

Box 2
Examples of women's oral health topics found in the ADA systematic review database

General Areas	Example Topics
Pregnancy	Smoking cessation
	Oral health during pregnancy
	Periodontal disease and adverse pregnancy outcomes
	Prenatal cleft lip and palate detection
Bone dynamics	Bisphosphonates/osteonecrosis of the jaw
	Osteoporosis and bone mineral density
	Gender effects on unilateral condylar hyperplasia
	Sex differences in periodontal disease
	Sex differences in temporomandibular disorders
Cardiovascular disease	Cleft palate and risk of cardiovascular events
	CVD and osteoporosis among women with physical disability
Other topics	Oral and perioral piercings
	Oral human papillomavirus infection
	Menopause and oral health
	Human immunodeficiency virus–related oral disease among women

Institutes of Health (NIH), particularly the Office of Research on Women's Health (ORWH) and the National Institute of Dental and Craniofacial Research (NIDCR); Health Resources and Services Administration (HRSA); IOM; ADA; and the American Dental Education Association (ADEA).

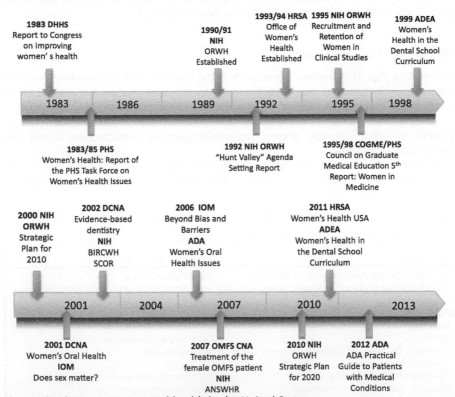

Fig. 1. Timeline on women's oral health in the United States.

NIH/ORWH

For a health condition to be considered as a women's issue, it should be unique, more prevalent, or more serious among women than among men, or it should have risk factors or interventions that are different for women. These criteria were defined in the 1985 report "Women's Health: Report of the Public Health Service Task Force on Women's Health Issues,"[8] chaired by Dr Ruth Kirschstein. It provides the foundation for contemporary thinking, policies, and programs involving women's health and sex/gender differences research.

The NIH/ORWH was established in 1990 as part of a congressional mandate to include women as subjects and investigators in scientific research. Its agenda-setting 1993 report, *Report of the National Institutes of Health: Opportunities for Research on Women's Health* (known as the Hunt Valley report)[9] included broad public participation in the process of priority setting. This model has been used subsequently for both professional and public commentary regarding women's health issues and women's health research.

An extensive national effort that included researchers, scientists and other stakeholders resulted in the *Agenda for Research on Women's Health for the 21st Century*.[10] This document boosted the collaborative multidisciplinary research efforts of the NIH/ORWH with regard to women's health research.

The most recent strategic plan from the NIH/ORWH was developed through town hall meetings held around the country between March 2009 and February 2010. *Moving Into the Future with New Dimensions and Strategies: A Vision for 2020 for Women's Health Research*[11] aims to increase understanding of major diseases and conditions that disproportionately affect the overall quality of life for women. Both women and men should benefit from the increased understanding of sex/gender in disease risk, vulnerability, progression, and outcomes.

Oral Health Strategic Plan Component of the ORWH

In September 2009, the Working Group on Oral Health and Systemic Conditions was convened under the direction of the NIH/ORWH. Its goals were to identify gaps in the current knowledge, the specific impact of oral health on women's health, and future research needs. It made 12 recommendations of topics for future research areas and specific research activities. **Box 3** lists the basic recommendations.[12]

Two overall themes emerged from the working group: oral health is integral to general health, so the two should not be evaluated in isolation; and oral-systemic relationships are bidirectional and complex. They noted that regular reviews of the current evidence base should occur, and updates to the recommendations should be made accordingly.

NIDCR

The NIDCR (www.nidcr.nih.gov) includes "oral and craniofacial diseases that disproportionately or solely affect women" within its mission "to promote the general health of the American people by improving craniofacial, oral, and dental health through research." NIH biannual reports[13] reveal that these efforts cover the spectrum from cellular to human populations; animal models to dental practice-based research networks; biometrics to longitudinal cohorts; genomics to health disparities; pregnancy to menopause. The most recent report, 2009 to 2010, highlights accomplishments in chronic pain and temporomandibular disorders, osteoporosis and basic bone biology, bisphosphonate-associated osteonecrosis of the jaw, oral health of

---

Box 3
Research recommendation areas on women's oral health from the 2010 ORWH strategic plan

1. Salivary diagnostics
2. Pregnancy and oral health
3. Chronic disease and oral health
4. Impact of systemic disease treatments on oral health
5. Oral cancer
6. Caries prevention across the life span
7. Pain
8. Hormones across the life span
9. Longitudinal studies
10. Update women's health in medical and dental curriculum and other health profession studies
11. Provide leadership training
12. Mentored training programs

Data from Garcia R, Heaton B, Henshaw MM. Oral health and systemic conditions. In: U.S. Department of Health and Human Services, Public Health Service, National Institutes of Health, Office of Research on Women's Health. Moving Into the Future With New Dimensions and Strategies: A Vision for 2020 for Women's Health Research, Volume II — Regional Scientific Reports. Bethesda, MD: National Institutes of Health; 2010. p. 180–7. NIH Publication No. 10-7606-B.

---

pregnant women, oral health disparities, Sjögren syndrome, human immunodeficiency virus (HIV) infection, and craniofacial anomalies related to the health of women.

HRSA

HRSA, the access-to-care agency (www.hrsa.gov), supports women's health in several ways. The HRSA Office of Women's Health was created in 1994 to "ensure that women's health is given the highest priority through HRSA programs in training, research, treatment and service." In addition, HRSA's Maternal and Child Health Bureau oversees most of the programs specifically targeting women's health issues (eg, perinatal oral health).

HRSA provides an annual report on the health status, health behaviors, and use of health by US women. New topics in 2011 include secondhand tobacco smoke exposure, Alzheimer disease, preconception health, unintended pregnancy, oral health care use, and barriers to health care.[14] The section on oral health care utilization detailed cost as a significant barrier to dental care. From 2007 to 2009, more than 15% of women reported that they did not obtain needed dental care in the past year because they could not afford it. Health insurance helps to reduce cost as a barrier; only about 10% of women with health insurance, compared with 42.6% of women without health insurance, reported that they did not obtain needed dental care in the past year because of cost. **Box 4** shows HRSA resources pertinent to women's oral health.

IOM

The IOM, the health arm of the National Academies of Science, aims to provide unbiased scientific evidence for health policy and decision making in health care. In 2001, the IOM reported on biologic differences between the sexes, offering strong evidence to support gender-related research as a significant emerging resource for medical

---

Box 4

Examples of HRSA resources pertinent to women's oral health (www.hrsa.gov)

National Maternal and Child Oral Health Resource Center

Oral Health Care During Pregnancy: A National Consensus Statement Summary of an Expert Workgroup Meeting

The Multiple Roles of Oral Health Providers: Domestic Violence Screening and Connection to Care

---

health education. They specifically recommended that medical school curricula should evaluate evidence-based outcomes affecting both genders.[2]

The Committee on Maximizing the Potential of Women in Academic Science and Engineering of the National Academy of Sciences, National Academy of Engineering, and the IOM released in 2007 the report *Beyond Bias and Barriers: Fulfilling the Potential of Women in Academic Science and Engineering*.[15] This report explored why women do not remain in careers of academic science and engineering at the same rates they are represented as undergraduates, even though a significant proportion of educational resources are being devoted toward women. The good news from the report is that there are ways to intervene, but it takes unified, deliberate efforts to make improvements in challenges at both institutional and societal levels. Dentistry has not yet undertaken such a workforce evaluation. A summary of the report findings is listed in **Box 5**.

The Workshop on The US Oral Health Workforce in the Coming Decade[16] found that health care careers of women and men differ in many respects. Women are more likely than men to work fewer hours when there are young children in the home, but compensate with more hours later in their careers. Women are more likely to work in practice settings that provide more access for vulnerable populations. Women also have considerable influence on the oral health care utilization of their families.

Advancing Oral Health in America[17] observes that mothers are more likely than fathers to take time off work during the "51 million hours of school… missed by school-age children for dental visits or problems." Pregnant women and mothers are among specific populations that merit further discussion, because their oral health status may influence pregnancy outcomes and dental care use of their children.

Box 5

Findings of the *Beyond Bias* report

1. Women have the ability and drive to succeed in science and engineering

2. Women who are interested in science and engineering careers are lost at every educational transition

3. The problem is not simply the pipeline

4. Women are likely to face discrimination in every field of science and engineering

5. A substantial body of evidence establishes that most people (men and women) hold implicit biases

6. Evaluation criteria contain arbitrary and subjective components that disadvantage women

7. Academic organizational structures and rules contribute significantly to the underuse of women in academic science and engineering

8. The consequences of not acting will be detrimental to the nation's competitiveness

ADA and ADEA

Between 1998 and 2006, the ranks of professionally active female dentists increased by 50%, whereas the numbers of professionally active male dentists stayed the same.[18] Assessments of work hours[19] and scope of practice[20] show that practice patterns differ when stratified by male and female dentists. Women may be more likely to have reduced work hours during childbearing ages, whereas men may be more likely to reduce hours circa retirement age.[19] Via The Dental Practice-based Research Network, women seem to be more prevention oriented in their treatment approaches.[20]

The past decade shows an increase in the percentage of women among dental school applications, first-year enrollment, total enrollment, and graduation rates.[21] More than a third (37.5%) of the 2001 dental school graduates were female, whereas nearly half (45.3%) of the 2010 graduates were female.[21]

The ADEA has provided much insight into representation of women in dental education. The recent curricular review[22] provides historical perspectives on curricular and workforce representation. These ADA and ADEA findings suggest that women are inclined to choose dentistry as a career, but there is a need to actively recruit, support, and retain more women to reach parity across all aspects of the dental profession.

RESOURCES FOR RESEARCH AND LEADERSHIP TRAINING RELATED TO WOMEN'S ORAL HEALTH

Several mechanisms exist to help develop research as well as the researchers to contribute to the ongoing development of the evidence base on women's oral health. Some mechanisms are specific to women's health and some are more general mechanisms that could be applied to this area.

Building Interdisciplinary Research Careers in Women's Health, Specialized Centers of Research, and Advancing Novel Science in Women's Health Research

Three funding mechanisms from NIH are specifically aimed at increasing research on women's health. A mentored career development program Building Interdisciplinary Research Careers in Women's Health (BIRCWH) is a trans-NIH collaboration with ORWH programmatic oversight (http://orwh.od.nih.gov/interdisciplinary/bircwh/index.asp). The research focus of these individuals must be relevant to women's health, whether the research is basic, translational, behavioral, clinical, and/or health services. Dental faculty members can access these programs because half of the currently funded institutions have dental schools.

Another mechanism is the Specialized Centers of Research (SCOR) on Sex Differences (http://orwh.od.nih.gov/interdisciplinary/scor/index.asp). This program is also aimed at development of interdisciplinary research focusing on sex differences and major medical conditions affecting women. Similar to BIRCWH, the SCORs involve multiple components of NIH, including the ORWH. More than half of the currently funded institutions have dental schools.

The Advancing Novel Science in Women's Health Research (ANSWHR) program was established in 2007 (http://orwh.od.nih.gov/research/answhr.asp). This program is aimed at stimulating new approaches to women's health research. Prevention research is one of the areas of special emphasis for the ANSWHR program.

NIH Career Development Awards: K Awards

A more general mechanism, NIH Career Development Awards, or K Awards, help investigators establish research programs, become independent, and develop successful academic careers (http://grants.nih.gov/training/careerdevelopmentawards.htm). NIH has distributed more than $8 billion to more than 19,000 awardees since the program began.[23]

Men are twice as likely as women to apply for awards, and this rate has been consistent since 1990.[23] Female applications and success rates, at least for subsets of K-award types, have been constant since 1998, at about 30%.[24] A recent study[25] of gender differences in career trajectories of career development award recipients confirms that there are several significant demographic differences between male and female awardees.

It is clear that mentored career development awards can help women to initiate research careers and become independent investigators. The good news is that there are no gender differences in rates of success in these applications: the percentage of funded awards is proportional to the number of applications for both men and women. The bad news is that men are more than twice as likely as women to apply for such awards, and women with K awards are far less successful in subsequent NIH funding. These career outcomes may be related to inadequate mentoring of female junior faculty members.[26] More data are needed to evaluate these career development awards and their relationships to career outcomes.

Leadership Training for Women in Academia

There are many opportunities for leadership training in dentistry. The emphasis here is on training related to academic careers to consider the projection of influence on research and students, hence the future of the profession. **Box 6** provides examples of such programs. The Executive Leadership in Academic Medicine (ELAM) program has been evaluated by dental deans.[27]

Leadership workshops at large professional meetings are an alternative. For example, both ADEA and the American Association for Dental Research (AADR) regularly hold workshops related to leadership and mentoring at their annual meetings. Women Executives in Science and Healthcare (WESH) offers annual meetings that focus on leadership skills for women in academic medical centers.

Leadership training and opportunities exist outside academia as well. The National Association of Women Business Owners, the Interagency Institute for Federal Health Care Executives, and the Commissioned Officers Foundation are a few examples of resources for different career settings.

EMERGING STRATEGIES OF WOMEN'S ORAL HEALTH IN DENTAL EDUCATION

The quest to advance women's health education in North American dental schools faces challenges common to other fields of study. Previous investigators within the

Box 6 Examples of leadership training available	
ELAM	www.drexelmed.edu/ELAM/ Note: currently, 6 of the 9 female deans of US dental schools are ELAM graduates
HERS Summer Institutes Higher Education Resource Services	www.hersnet.org/
ADEA Leadership Institute	www.adea.org/
ADEA Summer Program for Emerging Academic Leaders	www.adea.org
Enid Neidle Fellowship of ADEA	www.adea.org

educational arena have introduced concepts and values that challenged the traditional role of students as uncritical recipients of knowledge. Scholars are now called on to disclose the influence on their scholarship of their own experience, culture, and social position. In addition, students are encouraged to draw on their own experiences, and to reflect on the diversity of experiences held by classmates to nuance their evolving understandings of the world.

Despite a long history of women's health activism,[28] women's health education[29] has been slow to develop outside of obstetric and gynecologic specialties. To bridge this gap, women's health advocates have embraced self-education and peer-education as essential to improvements in women's health, while simultaneously calling for increased research and for cultural changes within the health professions to better serve women. In organized medicine and public health, committees and women's professional groups have pushed for women's health research and advocacy, and have led associated efforts to incorporate these topics into curricula.

The American Medical Association (AMA) partnered with the Medical College of Pennsylvania and Hahnemann University (MCPHU) to form the National Academy of Women's Health Medical Education (NAWHME). The NAWHME guide[29] defines women's health in terms of preservation of wellness; prevention of illness; and screening, diagnosis, and management of conditions that are unique to, more common, more serious, or different in women. They state that women's health "recognizes the importance of the study of gender differences, recognizes multidisciplinary team approaches, includes the values and knowledge of women and experiences of health and illness, recognizes the diversity of women's health needs over the life cycle, and how these needs reflect differences in race, class, ethnicity, culture, sexual preference and levels of education and access to medical care, and includes the empowerment of women, as for all patients, to be informed participants in their own health care."[29] Women's own experiences are validated as a source of knowledge alongside physicians' evidence and expertise. Women's health is contextualized within a diverse set of social and economic factors. Genuine partnership between physician and patient is favored rather than paternalistic hierarchy based on expert authority.

ADEA has advocated the integration of women's health issues into the dental curriculum, stressing that all health professionals, regardless of specialization, need a full understanding of women's health issues, as well as the knowledge and skills to provide competent and optimal care to women of all ages. The most recent curricular report identified the need to include normal and abnormal female biology and pathology, gender-specific history taking, and a life-span approach.[21] Analyses by Sinkford and colleagues[30] indicated that dental education is making progress, but limited curricular time and institutional resources are devoted to women's oral health.

New standards from the Council on Dental Accreditation[31] require evidence of multicultural competence among graduates and commitment to diversity in the dental school environment. However, in dental education there is a focus on curricular content, summarized as hours of curricular time. Because curricular time is finite, dental educators view the expansion of oral health information as an intractable problem that must inevitably have winners and losers.

Although dental education is making progress on several related fronts, dental educators have yet to present a vision of the future that ultimately connects curricular reform to the broader goal of a more inclusive culture in the professions of oral health research, dental education, and dental practice. It is our hope that collaborative efforts in the women's oral health community, including this set of articles, will contribute to the development of that vision.

These documents, and other national reports cited in this special issue of *DCNA*, stress the continuing need to build and disseminate a body of evidence concerning women's oral health and oral health care. They suggest that oral health, as a field of research and study, is still in an early phase of acknowledging women's experience and of understanding sex differences. In many instances, women's oral health remains a special addition or exception to what is otherwise taught as normal and essential.

SUMMARY

This article provides a guide to this issue of *DCNA*, discusses the status of evidence-based women's oral health and the questions that remain to be answered. The articles discuss (1) gender-specific oral health and overall health and well-being; (2) oral health and reproductive health; (3) oral cancer in women; (4) caries risk assessment for women; (5) tooth loss in women as a health consequence or preventive measure; (6) dietary behaviors and oral health; (7) core competencies for recognition of victims of violence and abuse, who are disproportionately female; (8) temporomandibular disorders and pain; (9) the gender-specific criteria for evaluation of the aging jaw; (10) approaches for competencies in patient-doctor concordance in communication; and (11) emerging topics relating to the role of the dental practitioner as a primary health care provider.

We wish to extend our thanks to Yonah Korngold, Editor of *DCNA* for his support of this project. The authors have been fortunate to have experienced the educational riches, expertise, and creative insight brought by the many investigators of this issue. A multidisciplinary and interdisciplinary endeavor, this issue was made possible by the uniting of unique skills brought from backgrounds that not only include clinical excellence but also leaders in basic, clinical, and translational research on gender-related issues in oral health care. It is our hope that this issue will provide motivation for the further incorporation of evidence-based approaches of oral health and wellness for sex and gender into mainstream practice and in innovative strategies for advancement of lifelong learning for the dynamic field of women's oral health.

Leslie R. Halpern, MD, DDD, PhD, MPH
Associate Professor, Program Director, Oral and Maxillofacial Surgery
Meharry Medical College, School of Dentistry
1005 DB Todd Jr. Boulevard
Nashville, TN 37208, USA

Linda M. Kaste, DDS, MS, PhD
Department of Pediatric Dentistry
College of Dentistry
University of Illinois at Chicago
Chicago, IL 60612, USA

Division of Epidemiology and Biostatistics
School of Public Health
University of Illinois at Chicago
801 S. Paulina Street, MC 850, Room 563A
Chicago, IL 60612, USA

E-mail addresses:
leslie.halpern@yahoo.com (L.R. Halpern)
kaste@uic.edu (L.M. Kaste)

REFERENCES

1. Studen-Pavlovich D, Ranalli DN, guest editors. Women's Oral Health. Dent Clin 2001;45(3):i–xii, 433–617.
2. Wizemann TM, Pardue ML, Institute of Medicine Report. Exploring the biological contributions to human health: does sex matter? Washington, DC: National Academy Press; 2001.
3. Springer KW, Stellman JM, Jordan-Young RM. Beyond a catalogue of differences: a theoretical frame and good practice guidelines for researching sex/gender in human health. Soc Sci Med 2012;74:1817–24.
4. IOM (Institute of Medicine). Sex-specific reporting of scientific research: a workshop summary. Washington, DC: The National Academies Press; 2012.
5. Doyal L, Naidoo S. Why dentists should take a greater interest in sex and gender. Br Dent J 2010;209(7):335–7.
6. Goldstein GR, guest editor. Evidence based dentistry. Dent Clin 2002;46(1):i–xi, 1–169.
7. Niessen LC. Women's health. In: Patton LL, editor. The ADA practical guide to patients with medical conditions. Ames (IA): American Dental Association and Wiley-Blackwell; 2012. p. 399–417.
8. Women's Health. Report of the Public Health Service Task Force on Women's Health Issues. Public Health Rep 1985;100(1):73–106.
9. Office of Research on Women's Health, National Institutes of Health. Report of the National Institutes of Health: opportunities for research on women's health. Washington, DC: US Government Printing Office; 1993. NIH Pub. No. 92-3457.
10. NIH Office of the Director, US Department of Health and Human Services, Public Health Service, National Institutes of Health. Agenda for research on women's health for the 21st century. A report of the task force on the NIH women's health research agenda for the 21st century. Sex and gender perspectives for women's health research, vol. 5. Bethesda (MD): NIH; 1999. Publication No. 99-4389.
11. USDHHS Office of Research on Women's Health, National Institutes of Health. Moving into the future with new dimensions and strategies: a vision for 2020 for women's health research, vol. I. Washington, DC: US Government Printing Office; 2010. NIH Pub. No. 10-7606.
12. Garcia R, Heaton B, Henshaw MM. Oral health and systemic conditions. In: U.S. Department of Health and Human Services, Public Health Service, National Institutes of Health, Office of Research on Women's Health, editors. Moving Into the Future With New Dimensions and Strategies: A Vision for 2020 for Women's Health Research, Volume II — Regional Scientific Reports. Bethesda, MD: National Institutes of Health; 2010. p. 180–7. NIH Publication No. 10-7606-B.
13. Office of Research on Women's Health. Report of the Advisory Committee on Research on Women's Health, Fiscal Years 2009–2010: Office of Research on Women's Health and NIH Support for Research on Women's Health. Bethesda, MD: U.S. Department of Health and Human Services, Public Health Service, National Institutes of Health; 2011. http://orwh.od.nih.gov/about/acrwh/pdf/Report-of-the-ACRWH-FY-2009-2010.pdf. Accessed March 10, 2013.
14. US Department of Health and Human Services, Health Resources and Services Administration, Maternal and Child Health Bureau. Women's health USA 2011. Rockville (MD): US Department of Health and Human Services; 2011.
15. National Research Council. Beyond bias and barriers: fulfilling the potential of women in academic science and engineering. Washington, DC: The National Academies Press; 2007.

16. National Research Council. The US oral health workforce in the coming decade: workshop summary. Washington, DC: The National Academies Press; 2009.
17. National Research Council. Advancing oral health in America. Washington, DC: The National Academies Press; 2011.
18. American Dental Association. Distribution of dentists in the US, historical report, from 1998 to 2006. Chicago: American Dental Association; 2009.
19. Walton SM, Byck GR, Cooksey JA, et al. Assessing differences in hours worked between male and female dentists: an analysis of cross-sectional national survey data from 1979 through 1999. J Am Dent Assoc 2004;135:637–45.
20. Riley JL, Gordan VV, Rouisse KM, et al. Differences in male and female dentists' practice patterns regarding diagnosis and treatment of dental caries: findings from the dental practice-based research network. J Am Dent Assoc 2011;142:429–40.
21. American Dental Association. 2010-11 survey of dental education academic programs, enrollment, and graduates, vol. 1. Chicago: American Dental Association; 2012.
22. American Dental Education Association (ADEA). Women's health in the dental school curriculum: survey report and recommendations. Bethesda (MD): National Institutes of Health and American Dental Education Association; 2011.
23. National Institutes of Health Individual Mentored Career Development Awards Program. 2011. Available at: http://report.nih.gov/UploadDocs/K_Awards_Evaluation_FinalReport_20110901.pdf. Accessed March 10, 2013.
24. National Institutes of Health Office of Extramural Research, Women in Research: The Involvement of Women in Career Development, Ruth L Kirschstein NRSA Training and Fellowship Programs and NIH Extramural Research, 2008. http://report.nih.gov/NIH_Investment/PPT_sectionwise/NIH_Extramural_Data_Book/NEDB SPECIAL TOPIC-WOMEN IN RESEARCH.ppt. Accessed March 10, 2013.
25. Jagsi R, DeCastro R, Griffith KA, et al. Similarities and differences in the career trajectories of male and female career development award recipients. Acad Med 2011;11:1415–21.
26. Riska E. Gender and medical careers. Maturitas 2011;68:264–7.
27. Dannels SA, McLaughlin JM, Gleason KA, et al. Dental school deans' perceptions of the organizational culture and impact of the ELAM program on the Culture and Advancement of Women faculty. J Dent Educ 2009;73(6):676–88.
28. Seaman B, Eldridge L, editors. Voices of the women's health movement, vol. 1. New York: Seven Stories Press; 2012.
29. Donoghue GA, editor. Women's health in the curriculum resource guide for faculty. Philadelphia: National Academy on Women's Health (NAWHME); 1996. Available at: http://www.drexelmed.edu/portal/0/NAWHME_Guide.pdf. Accessed February 9, 2013.
30. Sinkford JC, Valachovic RW, Harrison SG. Women's oral health: the evolving science. J Dent Educ 2008;72(2):131–4.
31. Commission on Dental Accreditation. Accreditation standards for dental education programs. 2010. July 2013 adoption. Available at: http://www.ada.org/sections/educationAndCareers/pdfs/predoc.pdf. Accessed March 10, 2013.

FURTHER READINGS

American Dental Education Association (ADEA). Women's health in the dental school curriculum: report of a survey and recommendations. Bethesda (MD): US Department of Health and Human Services; Health Resources and Services Administration; National Institutes of Health; 1999.

Council on Graduate Medical Education (COGME). Fifth report: women and medicine. Bethesda (MD): Department of Health and Human Services; 1995.

Halpern LR, August MA, guest editors. Treatment of the female oral and maxillofacial surgery patient. Oral Maxillofacial Clinics North America 2007;19(2):i–xii, 141–286.

NIH ORWH. Recruitment and retention of women in clinical studies: a report of the workshop sponsored by the Office of Research on Women's Health. Bethesda (MD): NIH; 1995. Publication No. 95-3756.

Women's Oral Health
Why Sex and Gender Matter

Linda C. Niessen, DMD, MPH[a,b,*], Gretchen Gibson, DDS, MPH[c,d],
Taru H. Kinnunen, MA, PhD[e]

KEYWORDS

- Women • Oral health • Sex • Gender

KEY POINTS

- Understand the differences and interactions between sex and gender.
- List how sex and gender can affect health in women.
- Identify oral health issues that predominately affect women.
- Discuss systemic health issues that have different presentation, management, and treatment in women compared with men.
- Describe long-term care issues affecting women's oral health.

INTRODUCTION

Sex and gender, separately and together, serve as important determinants of health and play a role in cause or pathophysiology of certain illnesses. The relative importance of them varies depending on the chronologic and contextual life stage, and social and cultural contexts.[1]

In 2009, there were more female (155.6 million) than male (151.4 million) residents in the United States.[2] Women today are more likely to participate in the healthcare system, and the issues facing them are often different from those of men. Women also comprise disproportionally higher numbers of other social and cultural groups that are at risk for poor health outcomes (low income, ethnic minority, low education).[3] It has been recognized in science by the Institute of Medicine's Report "Exploring the biologic contributions to human health: does sex matter?"[3] and in society and policy with the 1994 change in the National Institutes of Health policy recommending

[a] Department of Restorative Dentistry, Baylor College of Dentistry, Texas A&M University, 3302 Gaston Avenue, Dallas, TX 75246, USA; [b] Dentsply International, 221 W. Philadelphia Avenue, Suite 60, York, PA 17401, USA; [c] Oral Health Quality Group, VA Office of Dentistry, 810 Vermont Avenue, Washington, DC 20420, USA; [d] Veterans Health Care System of the Ozarks, Dental Service, 1100 N. College Avenue, Fayetteville, AR 72703, USA; [e] Department of Epidemiology and Oral Health Policy, Harvard School of Dental Medicine, 188 Longwood Avenue, Boston, MA 02115, USA
* Corresponding author.
E-mail address: lniessen@bcd.tamhsc.edu

Dent Clin N Am 57 (2013) 181–194
http://dx.doi.org/10.1016/j.cden.2013.02.004
0011-8532/13/$ – see front matter © 2013 Elsevier Inc. All rights reserved.
dental.theclinics.com

inclusion of women and minorities as subjects in clinical research that sex and gender do matter in health. How to conceptualize and operationalize the sex and gender aspects in health, however, remains complex.

This article provides a framework for sex and gender considerations as they affect the unique oral health needs that women face throughout their lives. The article addresses hormonal changes during a woman's life that affect oral health and disease; certain chronic diseases, such as cardiovascular disease (CVD) and diabetes, which may present differently in women; and diseases that affect primarily women, such as Sjögren syndrome (SS) and breast cancer. Practical considerations are provided to assist oral health practitioners in caring for their patients.

Sex and Gender in Human Health

The Institute of Medicine defines sex as "The classification of living things, generally as male or female according to their reproductive organs and functions assigned by chromosomal complement." Gender is defined as "A person's self representation as male or female, or how that person is responded to by social institutions based on the individual's gender presentation. Gender is rooted in biology and shaped by environment and experience."[3] Recent research and subsequent guidelines have suggested that basic biomedical reductionist framework (ie, sex as a dichotomous variable) is insufficient to understand these issues. This argument stems from the notion that sex is frequently used as a proxy for biologic factors, even for those that do not involve reproductive issues. Recently Springer and colleagues[4] in 2012 suggested that "the vast majority of male-female health differences are due to the effects of the irreducibly entangled phenomenon of 'sex/gender' and therefore this entanglement should be theorized, modeled, and assumed until proven otherwise." They point out that the notion where sex (biologic) and gender (social) overlap is outdated, and one should construe sex and gender as simultaneously biologic and social without preconceived notions about causality to either direction. Furthermore, one should focus more on understanding the biologic mechanisms and impact of social status as drivers of male-female health differences.[4]

CVD, which is the leading cause of death among women, provides an example. Historically it was considered to be a "male-disease" until it was found that CVD also affects women significantly, although later in life and with different presentation, progression, and response to treatments.[5] How sex and gender are interwoven can be illustrated in an example where psychosocial stress among women, often a result of complex social and cultural roles (ie, gender), induces ovarian dysfunction, which in turn is considered as biologic, and hence, sex-related. Social and cultural issues can have a great impact on what presents itself biologically. Tobacco use, a leading preventable cause of mortality, provides an example of how current health policies may not be as effective in women as men. The adverse health consequences of the global tobacco use manifest themselves uniquely among women. Smoking is a causal risk factor for cervical cancer and increases risk for breast cancer and maternal smoking impacts fetuses. Unfortunately, many of the tobacco control policies and cessation programs have been found to be more effective in men than women.[6]

Arain and colleagues[5] reviewed the complexity of sex and gender at a physiologic level. Biologically driven sex dimorphisms have to be understood even at the intracellular level where the sex of the cell and its hormonal environment may affect the etiology, progression, and efficacy of medications.

The role of sex and gender must be conceptualized, researched, and reported as an interactive, interdisciplinary, and intersectional approach to health.[4,7] As scientific understanding increases around these issues, translational research will remain a critical determinant of human well-being.

Women's Health

Women's health spans multiple health disciplines including medicine, public health, pharmacy, nursing, social work, psychology, and oral health.[8] Women's health is defined as diseases or conditions unique to, more prevalent in, or more severe in women, including those for which manifestations, risk factors, and interventions differ in women.[9] CVD with its risk factors, such as hypertension, obesity, diabetes, tobacco use, and lipoprotein disorders, has received increased attention in the scientific literature during the past 10 years.[10] Tobacco use is an illustration of how a given risk factor disproportionately impacts women. Women's tobacco use confers a 25% greater relative risk compared with men for CVDs. Women are also more likely to be exposed to second-hand tobacco smoke, which has been shown to be a causal risk factor for CVD.[6]

In addition to CVD and breast cancer, there are numerous conditions and diseases that affect women in disproportionate degrees and across the life span. Examples include cervical dysplasia and cancer; lung cancer; temporomandibular joint disorders; sexually transmitted diseases; migraine headache; bone and joint disorders; and autoimmune disorders, such as SS, rheumatoid arthritis, scleroderma, and systemic lupus erythematosis. In addition, behavior and mental health issues (eg, depression), interpersonal violence, and HIV-AIDS also affect women in greater proportion than men. In preventive medicine, human papilloma virus vaccination, pap smears, mammograms, and colon cancer screenings are of critical importance for women's health.

Women's Health Across the Lifespan

There are many ways to construe health and its determinants. Koh and colleagues[1] suggested a model where determinants could be construed by population (ethnicity, sex); by disease (CVD, cancer); by risk factor (immunization status, drug use); or by geography (urban vs rural). Chronologic age, hormonal cycle (puberty, menopausal status), and life stages (pregnancy and motherhood) make understanding sex and gender differences across the lifespan more intuitive. However, women's health issues need to be considered also from the perspective of social status and other social determinants of health and within cultural contexts.

The social determinants of health include individual demographics and environmental concerns (urban vs rural; living conditions), whereas cultural considerations focus on women's health by exploring the intersection of social status, such as race and ethnicity, income, parenthood, and sexual orientation.[1] **Fig. 1** illustrates women's health issues with examples within three perspectives in health (life span, social determinants, and cultural context). These three approaches are overlapping but also individually may shape health trajectories. For example, a postmenopausal African American woman living in a poor inner-city neighborhood with limited access to care has a higher risk for CVD than a premenopausal highly educated white woman with good access to care.[10]

Interactions of Sex and Gender

Although it is not clear how to dissect sex and gender, one's biologic sex remains an important issue in health and wellness. However, it is critical to understand the specific biologic processes and mechanisms that drive the observed sex differences. One must consider data regarding sex and gender differences and similarities within the

CONSIDERATIONS FOR WOMEN'S HEALTH										
Broad Categories										
Reproductive Health	Hormonal Lifecycle	Autoimmune Diseases	Cancers	Joint & Bone Disorders	Breast Diseases	Systemic Health	Behavioral & Mental Health	Social & Environmental Health	Urogynecological Conditions	Wellness Prevention Access to Care
Examples of conditions affecting women										
Prenatal care	*Menopause*	*Lupus*	*Colon cancer*	*TMJ & Osteoporosis*	*Mastitis*	*CVD Diabetes*	*Depression Eating disorders*	*Exposure to toxins (e.g., hair dyes)*	*Urinary incontinence*	*Weight management HPV vaccination Community health*
LIFE SPAN APPROACH										
SOCIAL DETERMINANTS OF HEALTH										
CULTURAL CONSIDERATIONS										

Fig. 1. Examples of women's health issues across the life span. CVD, cardiovascular disease; HPV, human papilloma virus; TMJ, temporomandibular joint.

context of social and cultural aspects across the lifespan. The goal is to translate these findings to improve health outcomes for women and men. To promote a greater understanding of the complexity of sex and gender issues in women's oral health, the term "sex and gender" is used throughout this article.

WOMEN'S ORAL HEALTH
Puberty

At puberty, girls experience an increase in levels of estrogen and progesterone. These hormonal changes increase blood flow to the gingival tissues.[11] This can cause a greater reaction to any irritation caused by plaque or food particles. During this time, the gums may become edematous, erythematous, and feel tender. Microbial changes in oral flora have also been reported during puberty.[11] These changes have clear implications for young female patients. For the 11-year-old girl who has not yet gone through puberty, she may not experience gingivitis even though she does not her brush her teeth frequently or well. However, several months later when this young woman experiences puberty, she may find that the plaque and debris on her teeth as a result of her poor tooth brushing habits now cause red, swollen, and bleeding gums. Changes in the oral microflora and the inflammatory response as a result of puberty can result in an altered gingival tissue response.

Dental practitioners caring for girls about to experience puberty should provide oral hygiene education. Girls should understand that the hormonal changes they are about to undergo also can affect their oral health. Mild cases of gingivitis respond well to scaling and improved daily oral hygiene care. Severe cases of gingivitis may require more aggressive care (scaling, antimicrobial therapy, and possibly surgery). These patients may require more frequent recalls until the condition improves or resolves.

A caries risk assessment should be conducted to identify the patient's potential risk for dental caries. Risk studies have shown that the best predictor for future caries is present caries.[12] Good oral hygiene and plaque control is especially important because the increase in hormones results in an exaggerated inflammatory response to local irritants. Education in proper oral self-care techniques is a critical component of the preventive treatment plan. Scaling and root planing may be performed when needed to treat any periodontal infection.

Menses

Oral changes have been reported during menses and vary considerably among women. Although evidence-based reports on the epidemiology of oral changes with menses are lacking, anecdotal reports of oral changes include red, swollen gingival tissues, activation of herpes labialis, oral apthous ulcers, or halitosis. A good medical and clinical history is essential to understanding oral changes a woman may experience during menstruation.

Pregnancy

Dental professionals today can still hear a pregnant woman state that she believes that you "lose a tooth for each pregnancy." This misconception arose from the belief that the calcium needed for the developing fetal bones was available from the teeth. Calcium in the teeth does not serve as a reservoir for the calcium needed for fetal development.

The relationship between caries and pregnancy is not well defined. Very little epidemiologic data exist on the caries incidence rates of pregnant women. Because pregnant women often have food cravings, if the food she craves is cariogenic, it may increase her risk of caries. A clinical study on the effect of prenatal fluoride on the caries rates of the pregnant woman's offspring showed no differences in caries rates of the mothers who took the prenatal fluoride and the children of the mothers who did not take the prenatal fluoride.[13] As a result, prenatal fluoride vitamins are not recommended for pregnant women.

Bleeding gums or gingivitis is the most common oral condition experienced during pregnancy. It can range from mild inflammation to severe gingivitis, localized or generalized, and occurs in 60% to 75% of pregnant women.[11] As with puberty and menses, the increase in hormones exaggerates the gum tissue's response to bacterial plaque. The gingival tissue is usually red, swollen, and bleeds easily. It often occurs in the anterior part of the mouth. Patients can notice these changes at any time during the pregnancy.

A localized area of severe inflammation can also be called a "pregnancy tumor" or pyogenic granuloma. If the granuloma becomes large and interferes with functioning, such as speaking or chewing, it may require treatment and removal before the birth of the baby. Pregnancy granulomas excised before delivery may recur and patients should be warned of such occurrences.

Premature Births

In the United States, each year approximately 500,000 babies are born prematurely.[14] A preterm low-birth-weight baby is defined as a baby born before 37 weeks and weighing less than 2500 g (5 lb, 8 oz). Prematurity is a major risk for newborn death, chronic health problems, and developmental disabilities.

Periodontal disease has been investigated as a potential risk factor for preterm low-birth-weight babies.[15] The mechanism of action suggests that throughout pregnancy, cytokines and prostaglandins increase until a critical threshold is reached that induces labor and delivery. The bacteria associated with periodontal infection can stimulate excessive production of the mediators, which then induce labor and delivery prematurely. Although the scientific evidence on the effect of treatment of maternal periodontal disease is still unclear, dental professionals can provide advice and counsel on the importance of good oral health and periodontal disease prevention to their patients who are pregnant or considering becoming pregnant.

Women with periodontal disease who are considering becoming pregnant should seek treatment of their periodontal infection as a matter of good health. Eliminating infection in the body allows the body's immune system to function more efficiently. Good periodontal health should be considered as part of a healthy approach to pregnancy. An example is folic acid. Women considering or trying to become pregnant are recommended to start taking folic acid before they become pregnant to prevent neural tube defects.

Evaluation of the pregnant woman begins with a thorough medical history, including a review of systemic illnesses, particularly hypertension, previous miscarriages, recent cramping, or bleeding. A recent clinical trial demonstrated the safety of providing dental care to pregnant women.[16] Providing oral health for the pregnant woman is discussed elsewhere in this issue.

HEALTH ISSUES IN ADULT WOMEN

In general, as people age, they demonstrate greater variability in health, disease, and social attitudes. As a result, the differences between women and men vary considerably across adulthood. With age come an increasing number of medical diagnoses and number of medications, which can affect the oral health of patients. **Table 1** compares women and men with respect to cause of death. Both share the top four causes of death, with CVD being number one in men and women.

Table 1	
Top 10 causes of mortality in men and women age 65+ in 2009	
Women	**Men**
Major cardiovascular diseases	Major cardiovascular diseases
Heart disease	Heart disease
All malignant neoplasms (cancer)	All malignant neoplasms (cancer)
Ischemic heart disease	Ischemic heart disease
Stroke	Trachea, bronchus, and lung cancer
Chronic lower respiratory diseases	Chronic lower respiratory disease
Trachea, bronchus, and lung cancers	Myocardial infarction
Heart attack	Stroke
Alzheimer disease	Prostate cancer
Heart failure	Alzheimer's disease

Data from CDC Health Data Interactive. Mortality by underlying cause, ages 18+: US, state, 2001–2009 (Source: NVSS).

Cardiovascular Disease

Gender differences have been highlighted in research looking at CVD epidemiology, treatment, and mortality. Data support that women with CVD are more likely to present with atypical symptoms, such as pain more centered in the jaw and neck area, and more generalized symptoms of fatigue and dyspnea, compared with men.[17] Women have been shown to be more preventive oriented or proactive than men,[17] but there is also evidence showing women are less likely to receive specific acute and long-term treatments associated with CVD.[18,19] Various hypotheses have been suggested to account for this, including an historical opinion that CVD is primarily a disease diagnosed in men and did not affect women. In addition, women's roles as caregiver affected their care-seeking behavior when they experienced symptoms.[17,20]

A recent large cohort longitudinal study highlights some of the unanswered issues regarding gender differences in care and outcomes. Follow-up found that among a population of people with clinically identified atherosclerosis, women had better long-term prognosis than men after similar interventions and treatment, even after adjusting for age, smoking, and various other risk factors and health-related issues.[21] This is despite the fact that women were more likely to be current smokers and have a less favorable risk profile.[21] Another study looked at intensive care unit care and outcomes. Although women were less likely to receive various treatment options including invasive options, after adjustment, they were similar in outcomes.[22]

Data on use of dental services by Delta Dental Insurance reported that women seek dental care more than men and are more likely to seek preventive dental care.[23] Women are also more likely to heed and possibly follow-up prevention beyond dental interventions, such as blood pressure monitoring, diet, and other risk counseling. However, it seems that as a cohort, women are more likely to carry higher risk profiles regarding lipids or hypertension even during treatment; thus, attention to monitoring during dental procedures is especially important.[21]

Tobacco use remains a key risk factor for women. Oral health providers can easily identify this risk factor during regular examination and encourage women to quit and monitor their success. Research has shown that women smokers have a more difficult time quitting permanently than men.[6] Smoking cessation rates are low in women, even after invasive cardiovascular procedures.[24]

Several disease processes themselves are risks factors for CVD, which may occur with greater frequency in women. Obesity is one such risk factor, and has been increasing in developed countries. One study showed that obesity in women is slightly higher than in men.[25] This study also showed that for women, there is a large socio-economic gradient that shows a definite inverse relationship between socioeconomic status and obesity.[25] Women carry a heavier burden of poverty and these women are more likely to be obese.[25]

Research has shown that women experience a first time myocardial infarction about 9 years later than men. Most estimates show women suffer from coronary heart disease, on average, about 10 years later than men.[21,26] Anand and colleagues[26] showed that men carried a higher burden of modifiable risk factors, such as smoking, obesity, high-risk diet, and inactivity at a younger age than women. Research suggests that estrogen could play a beneficial effect that is lost to women later in life, at which time women catch up with men in terms of mortality and even surpass them in some aspects.[27] Various studies have espoused the possibility of hormonal protection for women regarding CVD as seen in women with depression or diabetes. However, this is not consistent with the use of hormone-replacement therapy, although timing of the treatment may be an issue.[27,28]

Depression

Depression is another disease that many are reluctant to acknowledge in their lives, especially among the elderly. Depression is a recurring and relapsing condition that when diagnosed can be treated. It is the most common psychiatric illness with a higher prevalence in women than men. It can be a risk factor for CVD[29] and lower bone mineral density.[30] In older populations symptoms of depression, such as cognitive impairment, are often misdiagnosed as signs of aging. Although the depression rates do not generally increase among the elderly, they can be as high as 15% to 25% in nursing home residents. Teng and colleagues[28] found that in older women, unlike men, chronic depression conferred an increased risk of mortality. Episodic depression seemed to be more of a risk for mortality in men.[28]

Dental professionals often note changes in their older patient's demeanor and behavior, and can discuss this with them regarding late-life depression. **Box 1** shows the two brief questions used as a screening tool for depression, the Patient Health Questionnaire 2.[31] These questions are easily woven into a conversation in the dental clinic setting. As health professionals, dentists are not necessarily called on to diagnose depression, but are capable of screening for this condition and referring a patient as needed. Depression has dental and systemic sequelae beyond the disease itself. Teng and colleagues[28] found that subjects with remitted depression enjoyed an improvement in survival over those with chronic depression.

Box 1
Patient health questionnaire 2

Over the past 2 weeks, how often have you been bothered by any of the following problems?

• Little interest or pleasure in doing things

• Feeling down, depressed, or hopeless

An answer of yes to either question for several days or more should prompt you to suggest a referral for a more detailed screening or work-up for depression.
Data from Thibault J, Steiner RW. Efficient identification of adults with depression and dementia. Am Fam Physician 2004;70(6):1101–11.

Diabetes Mellitus

Diabetes mellitus underlies a considerable amount of the morbidity in the United States. The growing level of obesity is thought to contribute to the increase in type II diabetes in the United States.[32] Diabetes is estimated to be found in 10.8% of women older than 20 years of age.[32] Because older women outnumber men older than age 65, older women are more likely to have diabetes than men in this age group. Such complications as heart disease, kidney disease, stroke, and blindness are accelerated in older adults.[33] Kramer and colleagues[34] found that among a group of diabetics, those women who were poorly controlled were older than poorly controlled men. They were more likely to have depression, and as in other studies, older women were more likely to live alone, which is associated with depression. In another study, young and middle-aged diabetic women were found to have lower perceived quality of life and mental well-being compared with men.[35] However, women who were poorly controlled were more likely to seek care and take more medications.[34] Care-seeking habits may have as much to do with gender and perceptions as they do with outcomes. Like other diseases, the contradictory findings in women compared with men speak to the need for more research.

For oral health professionals, it is important to recognize that an estimated quarter of women with diabetes are unaware of their diagnosis.[33] This highlights the important role dental professionals can play in making patients aware of the symptoms and risk factors for diabetes, and in screening for hemoglobin A_{1C} (**Table 2**). A recent dental practice–based research study showed that dental offices were open to providing routine glucose testing for higher-risk patients,[36] becoming a part of what the American Diabetes Association recommends as "opportunistic screening" in a healthcare setting. The questions and observations that are a part of a routine dental visit give dental professionals an opportunity to target patients who carry a higher risk for diabetes mellitus.

Breast Cancer

Breast cancer, although not exclusively seen in women, is far more common in women than men. This disease is second only to lung cancer regarding the number of deaths in women with a female to male ratio of 100:1, and has the highest prevalence in women after age 70.[37] Treatment options today offer more targeted therapies, such as radiation, surgical removal, and chemotherapies, than the radical options of the past.

Dental professionals should be aware of the potential for bone metastasis in a patient with breast cancer. Bone metastases can include the mandible, making

Table 2
Symptoms and risks for type 2 diabetes

Symptoms	Risk Factors
Frequent urination	Obesity
Unusual thirst	Excessive abdominal fat
Extreme hunger	Family history
Unusual weight loss	Race and ethnicity (black, Hispanic, American
Extreme fatigue and irritability	Indian, and Asian American)
Frequent infections	Greater than age 45 y
Blurred vision	Continuous prediabetes blood sugar levels
Slow healing of cuts and bruises	History of gestational diabetes
Tingling or numbness in hands and feet	
Recurring skin, gum, or bladder infection	

oral radiographs, particularly panographic radiographs, an important diagnostic tool during survival follow-up. Breast cancer treatment may also include the use of intravenous bisphosphonates, which carries a risk of osteonecrosis of the jaw. This topic is discussed in greater depth elsewhere in this issue.

It is ideal for the patient to be cleared of any dental acute problems before beginning chemotherapy. Because of myelosuppression during treatment, the spread of a dental infection systemically can be life threatening. If dental treatment is needed during chemotherapy, it should be coordinated with the oncologist to ensure the patient has her highest blood cell count, which usually occurs just before the beginning of a new round of treatment. Specific guidelines for dental professionals regarding dental care for a patient during chemotherapy can be found in the Dental Oncology Program's guide.[38]

Sjögren Syndrome

Many autoimmune diseases primarily affect women. SS is such as example. This multisystem chronic inflammatory disease affects primarily the salivary and lacrimal glands, but includes extraglandular involvement. Lymphocytic infiltrates destroy the function of the patient's secretory glands. Dental professionals focus on the oral effects of this inflammatory process, but other exocrine glands found in the vagina, skin, respiratory, and gastrointestinal tract are also affected.[39] The female to male ratio of this disease is 9:1 and it is diagnosed primarily in women older than 50.[39,40] Any patient diagnosed with SS is at increased risk for non-Hodgkin lymphoma and should be seen annually for blood tests and a physician work-up.

Because of the low salivary flow, women with SS have been found to carry a significantly higher level of caries-causing bacteria compared with women with a normal salivary flow, even when they have good oral hygiene and no carious lesions.[41] In addition, Fontana and Zero[12] noted that a decreased salivary flow rate is a high risk for dental caries. Suggestions for addressing xerostomia and high caries risk are shown in **Box 2**. Patients with SS have varying degrees of salivary flow remaining, depending on the progression of their disease. Salivary stimulation of the remaining functioning glands can be accomplished mechanically of chemotherapeutically. Mechanical stimulation remains the first choice because it is the least invasive. Sugarless chewing gum is the easiest method, because the very act of chewing stimulates flow. However, if a patient cannot tolerate gum, one can consider sugarless lozenges as an alternative. It is helpful to have the patient consider this as prescription, because this is how most

---

Box 2
Treatment strategies for patients with SS

- Salivary stimulation by using sugarless gum or lozenges (suggest a prescription to use every 4 hours for 10 minutes at a time)
- Assess for adequate hydration
- Avoid cinnamon, strong mint, heavy lemon
- Suggest children's fluoridated toothpaste if there is oral sensitivity to regular paste
- Reduce or avoid liquids with alcohol or caffeine
- Try various salivary substitutes to find one that is comfortable
- Increased recall (three to four times a year)
- Additional fluoride, such as 1.1% sodium fluoride paste once or twice a day

Table 3 Ratio of women to men by age		
Age	Women	Men
55	100	100
65	116	100
85	250	100

Data from Administration on Aging. Available at: www.aoa.gov (2003 data); and Census 2000 Special Reports. Available at: www.census.gov/prod/2001pubs/czkbrol-9.pdf. Accessed February 15, 2013.

treatments are presented in today's society. Ask the patient to chew gum for approximately 10 minutes, every 4 hours during the daytime. This can help stimulate flow for comfort and keep thicker saliva from building up and blocking the duct openings.

Dentate patients with SS are at high risk for caries, and fluoride is a demonstrated effective treatment in adults.[42] A recent systematic review evaluating types of fluoride for adults found that the 1.1% sodium fluoride for home use and the 5% fluoride varnish applied professionally had some of the best evidence for their use in adults.[43] For root surface caries demineralization, even the 0.05% over-the-counter rinse could be effective if used for at least 1 minute twice a day.[43]

WOMEN AND LONG-TERM CARE

As women age, they often outlive their spouse and social support systems. As seen in **Table 3**, aging is definitely an issue dominated by women in persons older than age 75. When these women experience acute medical conditions, such as stroke or dementia, that cause significant disabilities requiring care, older women find they are at risk for long-term care, where women make-up most residents. Oral health care in long-term care facilities is woefully inadequate. As these women seek care in long-term care facilities, often their oral health may be neglected.

Daily oral care provides more than a method to decrease caries and periodontal disease, although those are primary positive results. A healthy mouth is important to quality of life and effects eating and social interacting, which can be significant sources of pleasure in a long-term setting where many other pleasurable activities are limited. Provision of regular oral hygiene care has actually been associated with reduced mortality from pneumonia in long-term care patients, which is the leading cause of death in that population.[44,45] It is known that oral plaque is a reservoir for the bacteria identified in aspiration pneumonia. Given the high number of medications taken and the reduced salivary flow that occurs, long-term care patients suffer with heavy plaque buildup. Daily oral hygiene care in a long-term care facility provides a dental and medical benefit when daily plaque and bacterial burden are removed.

SUMMARY

This article examines the sex and gender issues that affect oral and systemic health of women throughout their lifespan. Sex and gender remain important determinants of health. Women's health has identified that some diseases are more common in women, present differently in women, or require tailored treatment for women. This article identifies the effect of hormones on certain oral conditions and examines the role of certain chronic diseases on the oral health of women.

Because women comprise most of the aging population, there will be continued challenges to maintain good oral health throughout their lifetime. Oral healthcare clinicians are at the forefront in caring for patients and preventing and managing diseases. Future directions require additional research on evidence-based protocols and the implementation required to maintain good oral health for a lifetime. In addition, research on oral health literacy for men and women and for caregivers and health professionals is needed to better understand the relationships between oral health and systemic health.

REFERENCES

1. Koh HK, Oppenheimer SC, Massin-Short SB, et al. Translating research evidence into practice to reduce health disparities: a social determinants approach. Am J Public Health 2010;100(Suppl 1):S72–80.
2. Arias E. United States life tables, 2007. National vital statistics reports, vol. 59, No. 9. Hyattsville (MD): National Center for Health Statistics; 2011.
3. Wizemann TM, Pardue ML, editors. Exploring the biological contributions to human health: does sex matter? Washington, DC: Institute of Medicine; 2001.
4. Springer KW, Stellman JM, Jordan-Young RM. Beyond a catalogue of differences: a theoretical frame and good practice guidelines for researching sex/gender in human health. Soc Sci Med 2012;74(11):1817–24.
5. Arain FA, Kuniyoshi FH, Abdalrhim AD, et al. Sex/gender medicine. The biological basis for personalized care in cardiovascular medicine. Circ J 2009;73(10):1774–82.
6. Amos A, Greaves L, Nichter M, et al. Women and tobacco: a call for including gender in tobacco control research, policy and practice. Tob Control 2012; 21(2):236–43. http://dx.doi.org/10.1136/tobaccocontrol-2011-050280.
7. Doyal L, Naidoo S. Why dentists should take a greater interest in sex and gender. Br Dent J 2010;209:335–7.
8. Verdonk P, Benschop YW, de Haes HC, et al. From gender bias to gender awareness in medical education. Adv Health Sci Educ Theory Pract 2009;14(1):135–52.
9. US Public Health Service. Report of the Public Health Service Task Force on Women's Health Issues. Public Health Rep 1985;100:73–106.
10. Freund KM, Jacobs AK, Pechacek JA, et al. Disparities by race, ethnicity, and sex in treating acute coronary syndromes. J Womens Health (Larchmt) 2012;21(2): 126–32.
11. Niessen LC. Women's health. In: Patton LL, editor. The ADA practical guide to patients with medical conditions. 1st edition. Chicago: American Dental Association/John Wiley & Sons; 2012. p. 399–423.
12. Fontana M, Zero DT. Assessing patients' caries risk. J Am Dent Assoc 2006; 137(9):1231–9.
13. Leverett D. Appropriate uses of systemic fluoride: considerations for the 90s. J Public Health Dent 1991;51(1):42–7.
14. Martin JA, Hamilton BE, Ventura SJ, et al. Births: final data for 2009. Natl Vital Stat Rep 2011;60(91):1–104. Available at: http//www.cdc.gov/nchs/data/nvsr/nvsr60/nvsr60_01/pdf. Accessed October 14, 2012.
15. Offenbacher S, Katz V, Fertik G, et al. Periodontal infection as a possible risk factor for preterm low birth weight. J Periodontol 1996;67(Suppl 10):1103–13.
16. Michalowicz BS, DiAngelis AJ, Novak MJ, et al. Examining the safety of dental treatment in pregnant women. J Am Dent Assoc 2008;139(6):685–95.
17. Kent JA, Patel V, Varela NA. Gender disparities in health care. Mt Sinai J Med 2012;79:555–9.
18. Rathore SS, Chen J, Wang Y, et al. Sex difference in cardiac catheterization: the role of physician gender. JAMA 2001;286:2849–56.

19. Ayanian JZ, Epstein AM. Differences in the use of procedures between women and men hospitalized for coronary heart disease. N Engl J Med 1991;325:221–5.
20. Worrall-Carter L, Edward K, Page K. Women and cardiovascular disease: at a social disadvantage? Collegian 2012;19:33–7.
21. van der Meer MG, Cramer MJ, van der Graaf Y, et al. Gender difference in long-term prognosis among patients with cardiovascular disease. Eur J Prev Cardiol 2012;1(00):1–8.
22. Valentin A, Jordan B, Lang T, et al. Gender-related differences in intensive care: a multiple-center cohort study of therapeutic interventions and outcomes in critically ill patients. Crit Care Med 2003;31:1901–7.
23. Delta Dental Insurance. Available at: http://www.deltadentalins.com/oral_health/mensOralHealth.html. Accessed January 2, 2013.
24. Moore LC, Clark PC, Lee SY, et al. Smoking cessation in women at the time of an invasive cardiovascular procedure and 3 months later. J Cardiovasc Nurs 2012. [Epub ahead of print].
25. Charafeddine R, Van Oyen H, Demarest S. Trends in social inequalities in obesity: Belgium 1997-2004. Prev Med 2009;48:54–8.
26. Anand S, Islam S, Rosengren A, et al. Risk factors for myocardial infarction in women and men: insights from the INTERHEART study. Eur Heart J 2008;29(7):932–40.
27. Dantas AP, Fortes ZB, de Carvalho MH. Vascular disease in diabetic women: why do they miss the female protection? Exp Diabetes Res 2012;570–98.
28. Teng P, Yeh C, Lee M, et al. Change in depressive status and mortality in elderly persons: results of a national longitudinal study. Arch Gerontol Geriatr 2013;56(1):244–9.
29. Pennix BW, Guralnik JM, Mendes de Leon CF, et al. Cardiovascular event and mortality in newly and chronically depressed persons >70 year of age. Am J Cardiol 1998;81:988–94.
30. Erez HB, Weller A, Vaisman N, et al. The relationship of depression, anxiety and stress with low bone mineral density in post-menopausal women. Arch Osteoporos 2012. [Epub ahead of print].
31. Thibault JM, Steiner RW. Efficient identification of adults with depression and dementia. Am Fam Physician 2004;70(6):1101–10.
32. American Diabetes Association. Diabetes Statistics: data from the 2011 National Diabetes Fact Sheet (Released Jan 26, 2011). Available at: http://www.diabetes.org/diabetes-basics/diabetes-statistics/. Accessed October 22, 2012.
33. Centers for Disease Control and Prevention. Diabetes and women's health across the life stages: a public health perspective. 2001. Available at: http://www.cdc.gov/diabetes/pubs/pdf/womenshort.pdf. Accessed October 17, 2012.
34. Krämer HU, Rûter G, Schõttker B, et al. Gender differences in healthcare utilization of patients with diabetes. Am J Manag Care 2012;18(7):362–9.
35. Unden AL, Elofsson S, Andreasson A, et al. Gender differences in self-rated health, quality of life, quality of care and metabolic control in patients with diabetes. Gend Med 2008;5(2):162–80.
36. Barasch A, Safford MM, Qvist V, et al. Random blood glucose testing in dental practice. A community-based feasibility study from the Dental PBRN. J Am Dent Assoc 2012;143(3):262.
37. National Cancer Institute. Available at: http://seer.cancer.gov/statfacts/html/breast.html. Accessed January 2, 2013.
38. Rankin KV, Jones DL, Redding SW, editors. Oral health in cancer therapy. A guide for health care professionals. 3rd edition. 2008. Available at: http://doep.org/images/OHCT_III_FINAL.pdf. Accessed October 19, 2012.

39. Carr AJ, Ng W, Figueiredo F, et al. Sjogren's syndrome: an update for dental practitioners. Br Dent J 2012;213(7):353–7.
40. Garcia-Carrasco M, Cervera R, Rosas J, et al. Primary Sjogren's syndrome in the elderly: clinical and immunological characteristics. Lupus 1999;8(1):20–3.
41. Kolavic SA, Gibson G, Al-Hashimi I, et al. The level of cariogenic microorganisms in patients with Sjogren's syndrome. Spec Care Dentist 1997;17(2):65–9.
42. Griffin SO, Regnier E, Griffin PM, et al. Effectiveness of fluoride in preventing caries in adults. J Dent Res 2007;86(5):410–5.
43. Gibson G, Jurasic MM, Wehler CJ, et al. Supplemental fluoride use for moderate and high caries risk adults: a systematic review. J Public Health Dent 2011;71: 171–84.
44. Bassim CW, Gibson G, Ward T, et al. Modification of the risk of mortality from pneumonia with oral hygiene care. J Am Geriatr Soc 2008;56:1601–7.
45. Sjögren P, Nilsson E, Forsell M, et al. A systematic review of the preventive effect of oral hygiene on pneumonia and respiratory tract infection in elderly people in hospitals and nursing homes: effect estimates and methodological quality of randomized controlled trials. J Am Geriatr Soc 2008;56:2124–30.

Oral Health and Dental Care During Pregnancy

Barbara J. Steinberg, DDS[a,b,*], Irene V. Hilton, DDS, MPH[c,f], Hiroko Iada, DDS, MPH[d], Renee Samelson, MD, MPH[e]

KEYWORDS

- Pregnancy • Perinatal periodontal disease • Oral health • National consensus
- National guidelines

KEY POINTS

- A 2012 national experts' consensus statement concludes that dental care is safe and effective throughout all trimesters of pregnancy, and should not be withheld because of pregnancy.
- Research to date shows that routine preventive, diagnostic, and restorative dental treatment—including periodontal therapy—during pregnancy does not increase adverse pregnancy outcomes.
- The pregnant patient should be educated on the importance of oral health care for herself and her child and on expert recommendations for bolstering home oral hygiene care during pregnancy.
- Oral manifestations may be associated with pregnancy, including gingivitis, pregnancy epulis, and others.
- Research to date supports the safety of undertaking periodontal treatment during the perinatal period, with no associated adverse pregnancy outcomes. Whether perinatal periodontal treatment can reduce the risks for preterm birth or low birth weight has not been demonstrated thus far in US multicentered randomized controlled trials.

INTRODUCTION

Pregnancy is a unique period during a woman's life and is characterized by complex physiologic changes, which can adversely affect oral health.[1] Because oral health is an integral part of overall health, oral problems encountered in the pregnant patient must

[a] Drexel University College of Medicine, 2900 W, Queen Ln, Philadelphia, PA 19129, USA; [b] University of Pennsylvania School of Dental Medicine, 240 S, 40th Street, Philadelphia, PA 19104, USA; [c] San Francisco Department of Public Health, 25 Van Ness Avenue, San Francisco, CA 94102, USA; [d] University of North Carolina School of Dentistry, Manning Drive and Columbia Street, Chapel Hill, NC 27599, USA; [e] Department of Obstetrics and Gynecology, Albany Medical College, 16 New Scotland Avenue, Albany, NY 12208, USA; [f] University of California School of Medicine and School of Dentistry-San Francisco, 513 Parnassus Avenue, San Francisco, CA 94143
* Corresponding author. 7500 Bayshore Drive, Margate, NJ 08402.
E-mail address: bjsdds@aol.com

Dent Clin N Am 57 (2013) 195–210
http://dx.doi.org/10.1016/j.cden.2013.01.002
0011-8532/13/$ – see front matter © 2013 Elsevier Inc. All rights reserved.

dental.theclinics.com

be promptly and properly addressed.[1] Several national health organizations have issued statements in recent years calling for improved oral health care during pregnancy.[2]

Accumulated research shows that routine preventive, diagnostic, and restorative dental treatment—including periodontal therapy—during pregnancy does not increase adverse pregnancy outcomes.[3,4] The first national consensus statement issued in 2012 concluded such dental care is both safe and effective throughout pregnancy.[1] Nonetheless, many women currently do not seek or do not receive dental care during the perinatal period. Recent data suggest that about 50% of women do not have a dental visit during pregnancy, even when they perceive a dental need.[5,6] In addition, women with both private dental insurance and Medicaid coverage receive less dental care when they are pregnant than when they are not.[7,8] Factors for some women may include lack of insurance coverage or access, and it is possible that those with Medicaid coverage receive less dental care than those with other dental insurance plans. Research also suggests that misperceived barriers and inadequate knowledge about evidence-based perinatal dental care on the part of both patients and health care providers also play a role in underutilization.[9–12]

This article provides a summary of the most current evidence-based perinatal oral health guidelines, a review of common oral health manifestations during pregnancy, and insights into the safety and effectiveness of periodontal treatment on maternal and fetal outcomes.

PERINATAL ORAL HEALTH GUIDELINES

Over the last decade, several state organizations have issued evidence-based guidelines on perinatal oral health, including California, New York, South Carolina, and Washington.[13–16] The American Academy of Pediatric Dentistry also issued guidelines, highlighting the important influence of maternal oral health care and knowledge on their children's oral health.[17] These guidelines and a review of the recent medical literature culminated in the first national guidelines issued in 2012: *Oral Health Care During Pregnancy: A National Consensus Statement of an Expert Workgroup Meeting.*[1] This workgroup and meeting were sponsored by the Health Resources and Services Administration's Maternal and Child Health Bureau in collaboration with the American College of Obstetricians and Gynecologists and the American Dental Association. Key concepts from the 2012 consensus statement are reviewed here.

When to Consult with Prenatal Care Health Professionals

In general, the national consensus states that dental care can be safely delivered during all trimesters of pregnancy.[1] It is important, however, to consult with a patient's prenatal care provider when considering any of the following[1]:

- Comorbid conditions that could affect management of the patient's oral problems, such as diabetes, hypertension, pulmonary or cardiac disease, and bleeding disorders
- The use of intravenous sedation or general anesthesia
- The use of nitrous oxide as an adjunct to local anesthetics

Safety of Dental Treatment During Pregnancy

Pregnant women deserve the same level of care as any other dental patient, and clinicians now have an evidence base that shows appropriate dental care as being both necessary and safe during the perinatal period.[1,13] There have been three published US randomized clinical trials in which standard dental treatment was provided to pregnant women. Overall, these studies confirmed the safety of this treatment to the pregnant woman and the fetus. Among women who know they are pregnant, the risk of miscarriage before 20 weeks of pregnancy is between 15% and 20%, and most miscarriages are not preventable.[18] By definition, the risk of teratogenicity (the ability to cause birth defects), whether from imaging procedures, medications, or other medical treatments, must take place prior to 12 weeks gestation. There is little evidence that the medications used in standard dental practice have a teratogenic effect. Necessary dental imaging studies with appropriate maternal body shielding have not been associated with adverse pregnancy outcomes.

The following sections review the evidence-based consensus on dental-related treatments.

Medications and anesthesia

There is considerable confusion among dental health care providers about medication safety during pregnancy. The national consensus panel released evidence-based guidelines related to pharmaceutical agents, including analgesics, antibiotics, anesthetics, and antimicrobials (**Table 1**).

Few clinical drug trials have included pregnant women; therefore, successful long-term clinical use without known adverse effects is the best available evidence supporting the safety of a given drug.[13]

Older, reliable anesthetics and medications that have a solid track record of low-incidence adverse effects should always be the first choice.[13,14] Some examples include local anesthetics such as lidocaine 2% with 1:100,000 epinephrine and mepivacaine 3%; antibiotics such as penicillin, amoxicillin, and clindamycin; antifungals such as nystatin; and short-term use of analgesics such as acetaminophen with codeine.[13] Providers should also be familiar with medications that are contraindicated in pregnancy, and all guidelines mentioned earlier include these agents.[13–17]

A dental provider must always ask if the benefit to the mother and fetus of taking a medication, whether to control infection, pain, or other disease processes, is greater than the potential downside of not using the medication to manage or treat the underlying problem. It is judicious to contact the patient's primary care provider or obstetrician/gynecologist if there are questions or concerns.

Radiographs

The 2012 consensus statement and other guidelines advise that radiographic imaging is not contraindicated during pregnancy.[1] As for any patient, the standard of care is to take the minimum number of images required for a comprehensive examination, diagnosis, and treatment plan. As with all patients, a thyroid collar and abdominal apron should be used.[19]

Sedation and anesthesia

The use of nitrous oxide should be limited to situations whereby topical and local anesthetics are inadequate and care is essential.[1] As mentioned earlier, the patient's prenatal care provider should always be consulted when considering the use of nitrous oxide, intravenous sedation, or general anesthesia.[1]

Extractions, Restorations, Root Canals, and Other Dental Treatments

Data from the Obstetrics and Periodontal Therapy Trial showed that women who receive fillings or who undergo extractions or root canal treatment during the second trimester of pregnancy do not experience higher rates of adverse birth outcomes compared with women who do not undergo these dental treatments.[3] Oral health professionals should recommend prompt treatment when needed, and collaborate

Table 1
Pharmacologic considerations for pregnant women

Pharmaceutical Agent	Indications, Contraindications, and Special Considerations
Analgesics	
Acetaminophen Acetaminophen with codeine, hydrocodone, or oxycodone Codeine Meperidine Morphine	May be used during pregnancy
Aspirin Ibuprofen Naproxen	May be used in short duration during pregnancy; 48–72 h. Avoid in first and third trimesters
Antibiotics	
Amoxicillin Cephalosporins Clindamycin Metronidazole Penicillin	May be used during pregnancy
Ciprofloxacin Clarithromycin Levofloxacin Moxifloxacin	Avoid during pregnancy
Tetracycline	Never use during pregnancy
Anesthetics	Consult with a prenatal care health professional before using intravenous sedation or general anesthesia
Local anesthetics with epinephrine (eg, bupivacaine, lidocaine, mepivacaine)	May be used during pregnancy
Nitrous oxide (30%)	May be used during pregnancy when topical or local anesthetics are inadequate. Pregnant women require lower levels of nitrous oxide to achieve sedation; consult with prenatal care health professional
Over-the-counter antimicrobials	Use alcohol-free products during pregnancy
Cetylpyridinium chloride mouth rinse Chlorhexidine mouth rinse Xylitol	May be used during pregnancy

The pharmacologic agents listed are to be used only for indicated medical conditions and with appropriate supervision.

Reprinted from Oral Health During Pregnancy Expert Workgroup. Oral health during pregnancy: a national consensus statement—summary of an expert workgroup meeting. Washington, DC: National Maternal and Child Oral Health Resource Center; 2012.

with the patient to determine appropriate treatments and restorative materials because of the risks associated with untreated caries in pregnant women.[13] For amalgam, there is no evidence of any harmful effects from both population-based studies and reviews, and there should be no additional risk if standard safe amalgam practices, including rubber-dam placement and use of high-volume suction, are used.[13,20,21] For composite resins, the current evidence base shows that short-term exposure associated with placement does not pose any health risk. However, data are lacking on the effects of long-term exposure.[13] With any material, best practices should be used to minimize risk, such as rubber-dam placement and immediate rinsing of cured surfaces to remove the unpolymerized layer.[22]

With regard to periodontal disease, meta-analyses of clinical trials have shown that women who receive anesthesia and scaling and root planing (SRP) during the second trimester do not experience higher rates of adverse birth outcomes in comparison with women who do not undergo these treatments.[23–26] Additional information about periodontal disease during pregnancy is included later in this article.

Advising and Educating Patients During Pregnancy

Educating women about oral health care

Pregnancy provides a unique opportunity to deliver oral health preventive information and services that benefit 2 individuals at the same time: the mother and her child. The basis for developing the appropriate preventive approach is risk assessment, which will identify the lifestyle and behavior changes a woman can make to lower her risk for dental disease. Many of these habits and decisions will also affect her child's oral health.

Educating women about how their own oral health can affect their child's is a powerful tool.[1] A survey of pregnant Minnesota women with public and private insurance showed a preference for infant-specific educational information over education on topics that concerned both mother and infant.[8] In addition, 68% of the women preferred receiving oral health information by mail, compared with 34.4% who favored face-to-face delivery. How information is presented in person is critical. Behavioral approaches that determine readiness for change are more appropriate than simply telling a patient what to do.[27] When selecting health education materials for pregnant women, characteristics of the dental practice and the community it serves are important. Having materials that are appropriate to the literacy level, language, and culture of the patient is critical to reinforcing the verbal message.

Recommended oral hygiene during pregnancy

According to the National Consensus, pregnant women should be advised to continue with routine dental visits every 6 months and to schedule a dental appointment as soon as possible if oral health problems or concerns arise.

Pregnant women should also be advised to adhere to the following oral hygiene regimen at home[1]:

- Brush teeth with fluoridated toothpaste twice daily, and clean between teeth daily with floss or an interdental cleaner.
- Rinse daily with an over-the-counter fluoridated, alcohol-free mouth rinse. After eating, chew xylitol-containing gum or use other products, such as mints, with xylitol to help reduce bacteria that can cause decay.
- After vomiting, rinse the mouth with 1 teaspoon of baking soda dissolved in a cup of water to stop acid from attacking teeth.
- Eat healthy foods and minimize sugar consumption.

In certain instances, chlorhexidine antimicrobial rinse (alcohol-free formulation) may be indicated for optimal gingival health.[13]

Patient comfort during pregnancy

With very simple modifications, dental treatment can be comfortable for the patient throughout pregnancy. The following steps can help[1]:

- Treatment at any time during the pregnancy, including the first trimester, can be safe and effective. However, the early second trimester (at 14–20 weeks) is traditionally considered more comfortable, because nausea and postural issues are often less of a problem.

- Instruct your scheduling person to query "What time of day do you feel best coming in for your appointment?"
- Position pregnant patients for comfort. Postural hypotensive syndrome is a clinical concern and occurs in 15% to 20% of term pregnant women when supine.[13] To decrease the risk for hypotension, place a small pillow under the patient's right hip and ensure her head is raised above her feet when reclining. If a patient feels dizzy or faint or reports chills, position her on her left side to relieve pressure and restore circulation. These symptoms are commonly caused by the weight of the pregnant uterus impinging on the inferior vena cava, thus impacting returning venous circulation.
- For women in later stages of pregnancy who must undergo longer procedures, be mindful of the need for frequent postural changes or a restroom break during treatment.

COMMON ORAL HEALTH MANIFESTATIONS DURING PREGNANCY
Pregnancy Gingivitis

Gingivitis is one of the most common findings during pregnancy, affecting 60% to 75% of all pregnant women.[13,28] It is characterized by erythema of the gingiva, edema, hyperplasia, and increased bleeding (**Fig. 1**).[29–31] Gingival inflammatory changes are generally observed in the second or third month of pregnancy, persist or increase during the second trimester, and then decrease in the last month of pregnancy, eventually regressing after parturition.[30,31] Histologically there are no differences between pregnancy gingivitis and other forms, but pregnancy gingivitis is characterized by an exaggerated response to local irritants, including bacterial plaque and calculus.

The underlying mechanism for this enhanced inflammatory response during pregnancy is elevated levels of progesterone and estrogen.[32–34] The severity of the response is directly attributed to the levels of these hormones. Sex hormones also

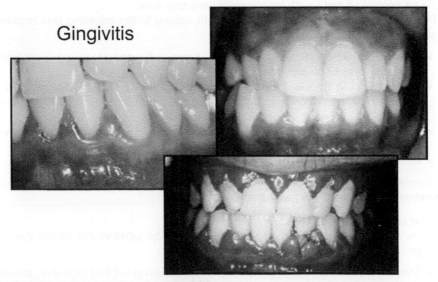

Gingivitis

Fig. 1. Mild and severe pregnancy gingivitis.

have an effect on the immune system. Sex hormones depress neutrophil chemotaxis and phagocytosis, as well as T-cell and antibody responses.[32–34] Specific estrogen receptors have been identified in gingival tissues.[35] Estrogen can increase cellular proliferation of gingival blood vessels, decreased gingival keratinization, and increased epithelial glycogen. These changes diminish the epithelial barrier function of the gingiva.[29,30,36]

Progesterone increases vascular membrane permeability, edema of the gingival tissues, gingival bleeding, and increased gingival crevicular fluid flow.[29,30,32,37] Progesterone also reduces the fibroblast proliferation rate and alters the rate and pattern of collagen production, reducing the ability of the gingiva to repair.[35] The breakdown of folate, a requirement for maintaining healthy oral mucosa, is increased in the presence of higher levels of sex hormones.[38] The subsequent relative folate deficiency increases the inflammatory destruction of the oral tissue by inhibiting its repair.

Sex hormones can also affect gingival health during pregnancy by allowing an increase in the anaerobic-to-aerobic subgingival plaque ratio, leading to a higher concentration of periodontopathic bacteria.[39] A 55-fold increase in the level of *Prevotella intermedia* has been shown in pregnant women in comparison with nonpregnant women.[40] *P intermedia* is able to substitute progesterone and estrogen for vitamin K, an essential growth factor.[41]

To summarize, the increased levels of sex hormones found in pregnancy help depress the immune response, compromise the local defense mechanism necessary for good oral health, and reduce the natural protection of the gingival environment. These changes, combined with a microbial shift favoring an anaerobic flora dominated by *P intermedia*, are partly responsible for the exaggerated response to bacterial plaque in pregnancy.[38–40] Generalized supragingival and/or subgingival periodontal therapies should be initiated in women with gingivitis to eliminate plaque buildup, as should intensive education on oral hygiene.[1] Moreover, periodontal therapy can be effective in reducing signs of periodontal disease and the level of periodontal pathogens.[1] Necessary periodontal care is important and should be undertaken, not postponed, during pregnancy.[1]

Pregnancy Tumor (Epulis Gravidarum)

Pregnancy can also cause single tumor-like growths of gingival enlargement referred to as pregnancy tumor, epulis gravidarum, or pregnancy granuloma. The histologic appearance is a pyogenic granuloma observed in 0.2% to 9.6% of pregnant patients, usually during the second or third trimester.[30,42] This lesion occurs most frequently in an area of inflammatory gingivitis or other areas of recurrent irritation, or as a result of trauma.[13,43] It often grows rapidly, although it seldom becomes larger than 2 cm in diameter. Poor oral hygiene is variably present, and often there are deposits of plaque and calculus on the teeth adjacent to the lesion.[13,28] The gingiva enlarges in a nodular fashion to give rise to the clinical mass (**Fig. 2**). The fully developed pregnancy epulis is a sessile or pedunculated lesion that is usually painless. The color varies from purplish red to deep blue, depending on the vascularity of the lesion and the degree of venous stasis. The surface of the lesion may be ulcerated and covered by yellowish exudate, and gentle manipulation of the mass easily induces hemorrhage. Bone destruction is rarely observed around pregnancy granulomas.[28]

SRP and intensive instruction on oral hygiene can, and should, be initiated before delivery to reduce plaque retention.[13,28,44] In some situations the lesion may need to be excised during pregnancy, such as when it causes discomfort for the patient, disturbs the alignment of the teeth, or bleeds easily on mastication.[13,28] The patient should be advised, however, that a pregnancy granuloma excised before term may

Pregnancy granuloma

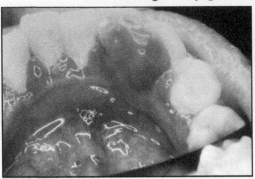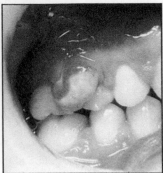

Fig. 2. Pregnancy tumor (epulis gravidarum).

recur.[13,28,45] In general, the pregnancy granuloma will regress postpartum; however, surgical excision may be required for complete resolution.[28]

Caries

The relationship between dental caries and pregnancy is not well defined. Changes in salivary composition in late pregnancy and during lactation may temporarily predispose to erosion as well as dental caries.[13,46] There are no convincing data, however, to show that the incidence of dental caries increases during pregnancy or in the immediate postpartum period, although existing untreated caries will likely progress.

Pregnancy may cause food cravings, and if these are for cariogenic foods, the pregnant woman may increase her risk for caries at this time. All pregnant patients, therefore, should be advised to bolster their daily oral hygiene routine.[1] For recommendations per the National Consensus, see the earlier section on recommended oral hygiene during pregnancy.

Xerostomia

Some pregnant women may experience temporary dryness of the mouth, for which hormonal alterations associated with pregnancy are a possible explanation.[28,47,48] More frequent consumption of water and sugarless candy or gum may help alleviate this problem. More frequent fluoride exposure (toothpaste, mouth rinse) is also recommended for women who experience xerostomia, to help remineralize teeth and reduce the risk for caries.[13,47]

Perimylolysis

Although nausea and vomiting are predominantly associated with early pregnancy, some women continue to experience this past the first trimester. Hyperemesis gravidarum, a severe form of nausea and vomiting that occurs in 0.3% to 2% of pregnant women, can lead to loss of surface enamel (perimylolysis) primarily through acid-induced erosion.[13,49,50]

Pregnant patients should be queried about nausea and vomiting during their dental visits. Those who experience vomiting should be instructed to rinse the mouth immediately afterward with a teaspoon of baking soda dissolved in a cup of water, which can prevent acid from attacking teeth.[1] These patients should also be advised to avoid brushing teeth immediately after vomiting. More frequent fluoride exposure to remineralize teeth is also recommended for women who experience repeated nausea and vomiting during pregnancy.

Tooth Mobility

Generalized tooth mobility in the pregnant patient is probably related to the degree of gingival diseases that disturb the attachment apparatus and to mineral changes in the lamina dura.[13,28,51] Longitudinal studies demonstrate that as gingival inflammation increases, so do probing depths attributable to the swelling of the gingiva.[13,52] Although most research concludes that generally no permanent loss of clinical attachment occurs during pregnancy,[13,53,54] in some individuals the progression of periodontitis occurs, and may be permanent.[13,55]

PERINATAL PERIODONTAL HEALTH AND OBSTETRIC OUTCOMES
The Association Between Maternal Periodontal Disease and Adverse Pregnancy Outcomes

Accumulated scientific evidence to date on the association between maternal periodontal disease and risk of preterm birth (PTB) and low birth weight (LBW) is mixed, but generally points to a positive association.[13,56–59] In general, studies performed in economically disadvantaged populations show these positive associations.[58] The first report suggesting that maternal periodontal infection may be a possible risk factor for preterm LBW was published in 1996.[60] The etiology of these adverse birth outcomes continues to be debated, but it has been suggested that bacterial infection and/or inflammation could be causative factors.[61,62]

Periodontal disease is a chronic infection caused by anaerobic gram-negative bacteria of the plaque biofilm.[63] As biofilm becomes mature and more pathogenic, oral bacteria can be disseminated systemically and colonize the maternal-fetal-placental complex, causing inflammatory responses.[56,60,63] Alternatively, periodontal disease can cause abnormal immunologic changes systemically, which lead to pregnancy complications.[56] These biological pathways explain how periodontal disease may potentiate as a maternal and/or fetal response, resulting in adverse pregnancy outcomes.[56,60] In 2011, Han and colleagues[64] reported the first human evidence of an oral pathogen that originated in the mother's subgingival plaque, *Fusobacterium nucleatum*, having translocated to her placenta and fetus, potentially causing the acute inflammation that led to term stillbirth.

One of the obstacles to clarity on this issue has been the variability in how both periodontal disease and adverse obstetric outcomes have been defined in the epidemiologic studies thus far. Commonly accepted clinical measures of periodontal disease are clinical attachment loss and probing depth, although there is no universally accepted standard in the case definition of periodontal disease.[58,65] Furthermore, because chronic periodontitis, the most common form of the disease especially in its advanced stage, is typical among older adults, the prevalence of periodontal disease among younger pregnant women may be directly affected by the case definition.[65]

There is also variability in the definition of adverse pregnancy outcomes. Many studies used PTB and/or LBW as the outcome measure. PTB is childbirth occurring at less than 37 weeks or 259 days of gestation.[66] LBW is considered less than 2500 g or 5.5 pounds at birth. Although there is a relationship between PTB and LBW, each may have distinct causes.[62] Birth weight is determined by 2 processes: duration of gestation and rate of fetal growth.[62] Thus, newborns may have LBW because they are born too early or are small for gestational age (SGA), a proxy for intrauterine growth restriction.[62] Some SGA newborns are merely constitutionally small rather than nutritionally growth restricted. Conversely, some intrauterine growth–restricted newborns who would otherwise be constitutionally large do not meet the standard criteria for SGA.[62] Moreover, newborns may be growth restricted or preterm without having LBW.[62] While the use of more precise case definitions of adverse pregnancy outcomes might be considered ideal, a valid estimation of gestational age may be difficult in populations with late or infrequent access to prenatal care, uncertainty about the date of the last menstrual period, and unavailability of early ultrasound examination.[62]

Another methodological issue that makes the interpretation of the current body of research challenging is that periodontal disease and adverse birth outcomes share several common risk factors, including smoking, stress, socioeconomic disadvantages, older age, chronic diseases such as diabetes, and genetic susceptibility.[62,65] Thus, questions remain about whether the observed associations represent a causal relationship or are due to the confounding effects of other variables.[58] Increases in maternal age, rates of multiple births, use of early cesarean sections, and use of assisted reproductive technologies in recent years have also modified the demographics and outcomes of pregnancy.[62,67] There is a clear need for methodologically rigorous studies that use consistent and valid case definitions and control for key confounders.

Randomized controlled trials in the United States have demonstrated that routine dental treatment during pregnancy, including periodontal therapy, does not increase the incidence of adverse pregnancy outcomes.[3,60] The 2012 national consensus guidelines emphasize the importance of oral health care during pregnancy and of interprofessional collaboration to improve health care access and overall wellbeing of women during the perinatal period. In addition, the national consensus statement recognizes the importance of maternal oral health care and education on the oral health of their children.[1]

However, whether periodontal therapy is effective in reducing the risk for adverse pregnancy outcomes is still under investigation. Clinical intervention trials conducted during the past decade have produced conflicting results on these outcomes.[24–26,68–75] A meta-analysis published in 2012 showed a pooled risk ratio (RR) of 0.81 (95% confidence interval [CI] 0.64–1.02) for the effect of SRP during pregnancy on the rate of PTB (<37 weeks' gestation) using the data from 11 randomized controlled trials (N = 2875) with fair to good quality.[75] Pooled RR was 0.72 (95% CI 0.48–1.07) for the rate of LBW (N = 2076; data from 8 studies), indicating a statistically insignificant protective effect of periodontal treatment on LBW.[75]

In the 3 multicenter randomized controlled trials conducted to date in the United States, periodontal treatment during pregnancy did not decrease the rate of PTB (<35 or 37 weeks) when compared with women who were treated postpartum (Table 2). Of the 3 robust randomized controlled trials, the Obstetrics and Periodontal Therapy (OPT) study[68] and the Maternal Oral Therapy to Reduce Obstetric Risk (MOTOR) study[69] used less than 37 weeks' gestation as the end point, whereas the Periodontal Infections and Prematurity Study (PIPS)[72] used less than 35 weeks' gestation. The PIPS trial was terminated owing to loss of funding and inability to recruit the intended number of study participants, so the results are less reliable than those of the other 2 studies.[76] Furthermore, giving unnecessary weight to a trend in increasing indicated preterm delivery at less than 32 weeks in women randomized to the treatment arm in this study must be interpreted with caution.[76] A secondary analysis in the PIPS study suggested a possible weak association between scaling and root planing and miscarriage.[76] An Australian single-center randomized controlled trial also showed no difference in PTB outcomes (<37 weeks) for women treated with periodontal

Table 2
Summary of high-quality randomized controlled trials investigating effect of perinatal periodontal treatment on pregnancy outcomes

Study	Sample Size (N)	Mean Age (y)	Gestational Age at Enrollment	Definition of Periodontal Disease	Primary Pregnancy Outcomes	Interventions	HR/OR/RR (95% CI)
Michalowicz et al,[68] 2006 The Obstetrics and Periodontal Therapy (OPT) Study	823 I = 413 C = 410 Multicenter (MN, KY, NY)	I = 26.1 ± 5.6 C = 25.9 ± 5.5	<16 wk and 6 d	≥4 mm PD on ≥4 teeth CAL ≥2 mm BOP at 35% sites	GA at end of pregnancy (birth <37 and <35 wk GA)	SRP Up to 4 visits allowed, before 21 wk GA	HR 0.93 (0.63–1.37)
Offenbacher et al,[69] 2009 The Maternal Oral Therapy to reduce Obstetric Risk (MOTOR) Study	1806 I = 903 C = 903 Multicenter (NC, AL, TX)	I = 25.3 ± 5.5 C = 25.4 ± 5.5	<23 and 6/7 wk	CAL ≥3 mm at ≥3 sites	Birth <37 wk GA	SRP Up to 4 sessions, early in second trimester	OR 1.219 (0.0893–1.664)
Newnham et al,[70] 2009 The Smile Study	1087 I = 546 C = 541 Single-center (Australia)	I = 30.5 ± 5.5 C = 30.5 ± 5.5	12–20 wk	PD ≥4 mm at ≥12 sites	Birth <37 wk GA	SRP 3 sessions weekly commencing at 21 wk of GA (Additional 3 sessions offered if initial series treatment was not successful)	OR 1.05 (0.7–1.58)
Macones et al,[72] 2010 The Periodontal Infections and Prematurity Study (PIPS)	756 I = 376 C = 380 Multicenter within PA	I = 24.1 ± 5.2 C = 24.4 ± 5.7	6–20 wk	CAL ≥3 mm on ≥3 teeth	Birth <35 wk GA	SRP	RR 1.19 (0.62–2.28)

Abbreviations: AL, Alabama; BOP, bleeding on probing; C, control group; CAL, clinical attachment level; CI, confidence interval; GA, gestational age; HR, hazard ratio; I, intervention group; KY, Kentucky; MN, Minnesota; NC, North Carolina; NY, New York; OR, odds ratio; PA, Pennsylvania; PD, probe depth; RR, relative risk; SRP, scaling and root planing; TX, Texas.

therapy during pregnancy in a comparison with women treated postpartum (odds ratio 1.05, 95% CI 0.7–1.58).[70]

In most of these perinatal intervention studies, SRP was the periodontal treatment provided.[56] It has been suggested that a single treatment of SRP during the second trimester or mechanical debridement alone may not be sufficient to effectively treat advanced stages of periodontal disease.[56,74]

The 2009 Institute of Medicine report on comparative effectiveness research (CER) recommends studies that compare the effectiveness of the various delivery models, the clinical effectiveness and cost-effectiveness of surgical care, and a medical model of prevention and care in managing periodontal disease to increase tooth longevity and reduce systemic secondary effects in other organ systems.[77] Such studies would generate evidence to assist clinicians, patients, and policy makers in making informed decisions that improve perinatal health and oral health care and its outcomes at both the individual and population levels.[77] There is an urgent need of such research and effective strategies for disseminating and adopting CER findings in obstetric and dental practice.

SUMMARY AND FUTURE DIRECTIONS

The first national consensus statement issued in 2012 concluded that dental care is both safe and effective throughout pregnancy.[1] Oral health care providers must be judicious in educating the pregnant patient on the importance of oral health, for herself and her child. Patients should also be advised of common oral manifestations and of guidelines for bolstering their usual daily oral hygiene care. As for periodontal disease, research to date shows that conventional treatment does not adversely affect pregnancy outcomes, and guidelines recommend undertaking such treatment as needed. Whether such perinatal therapy can reduce a woman's risk of LBW or PTB is still inconclusive, and more well-designed research is needed. In conclusion, it is well-documented in the medical literature that maintaining good oral health during pregnancy can be critical to the overall health of both pregnant women and their infants.[13]

REFERENCES

1. Oral Health Care During Pregnancy Expert Workgroup. Oral health care during pregnancy: a national consensus statement—summary of an expert workgroup meeting. Washington, DC: National Maternal and Child Oral Health Resource Center; 2012.
2. Buerlein J, Peabody H, Santoro K. NIHCM Foundation. Improving access to perinatal oral health care: strategies & considerations for health plans: issue brief July 2010. National Institute for Health Care Management. Available at: http://nihcm. org/pdf/NIHCM-OralHealth-Final.pdf. Accessed December 10, 2012.
3. Michalowicz BS, DiAngelis AJ, Novak MJ, et al. Examining the safety of dental treatment in pregnant women. J Am Dent Assoc 2008;139:685–95.
4. Association of State and Territorial Dental Directors. Perinatal oral health policy statement. Adopted July 26, 2012. Available at: www.astdd.org/docs/Perinatal_ Oral_Health_Policy_Statement_July_26_2012.pdf. Accessed December 10, 2012.
5. Iida H, Kumar JV, Radigan AM. Oral health during perinatal period in New York State. Evaluation of 2005 pregnancy risk assessment monitoring system data. N Y State Dent J 2009;75:43–7.
6. Hwang SS, Smith VC, McCormick MC, et al. Racial/ethnic disparities in maternal oral health experiences in 10 states, pregnancy risk assessment monitoring system, 2004-2006. Matern Child Health J 2011;15:722–9.

7. Jiang P, Bargman EP, Garrett NA, et al. A comparison of dental service use among commercially insured women in Minnesota before, during and after pregnancy. J Am Dent Assoc 2008;139:1173–80.
8. Thoele MJ, Asche SE, Rindal DB, et al. Oral health program preferences among pregnant women in a managed care organization. J Public Health Dent 2008;68: 174–7.
9. Al Habashneh R, Guthmiller JM, Levy S, et al. Factors related to utilization of dental services during pregnancy. J Clin Periodontol 2005;32:815–21.
10. Strafford KE, Shellhaas C, Hade EM. Provider and patient perceptions about dental care during pregnancy. J Matern Fetal Med 2008;21:63–71.
11. Huebner CE, Milgrom P, Conrad D, et al. Providing dental care to pregnant patients: a survey or Oregon general dentists. J Am Dent Assoc 2009;140:211–22.
12. Da Costa EP, Lee JY, Rozier RG, et al. Dental care for pregnant women: an assessment of North Carolina general dentists. J Am Dent Assoc 2010;141:986–94.
13. California Dental Association Foundation. Oral health during pregnancy and early childhood. Evidence-based guidelines for health professionals, 2010. Available at: www.cdafoundation.org/Portals/0/pdfs/poh_guidelines.pdf. Accessed December 10, 2012.
14. New York State Department of Health. Oral health care during pregnancy and early childhood. Practice guidelines, 2006. Available at: www.health.ny.gov/publications/0824.pdf. Accessed December 10, 2012.
15. South Carolina Oral Health Advisory Council and Coalition. Oral health care for pregnant women, 2009. Available at: www.scdhec.gov/administration/library/CR-009437.pdf. Accessed December 10, 2012.
16. Northwest Center to Reduce Oral Health Disparities. Guidelines for oral health care in pregnancy, 2009. Available at: http://depts.washington.edu/nacrohd/sites/default/files/oral_health_pregnancy_0.pdf. Accessed December 10, 2012.
17. American Academy of Pediatric Dentistry Council on Clinical Affairs. Guidelines on perinatal oral health care, 2011. Available at: www.aapd.org/media/Policies_Guidelines/G_PerinatalOralHealthCare.pdf. Accessed December 10, 2012.
18. National Institutes of Health. MedlinePlus: miscarriage. Last updated November 2010. Available at: www.nlm.nih.gov/medlineplus/ency/article/001488.htm. Accessed December 10, 2012.
19. American Dental Association Council on Scientific Affairs. The use of dental radiographs: update and recommendations. J Am Dent Assoc 2006;137:1304–12.
20. US Food and Drug Administration. Dental amalgam. Last updated August 2009. Available at: www.fda.gov/MedicalDevices/ProductsandMedicalProcedures/DentalProducts/DentalAmalgam/ucm171094.htm. Accessed December 10, 2012.
21. Life Sciences Research Organization Inc. Review and analysis of the literature on the health effects of dental amalgam. Available at: www.lsro.org/presentation_files/amalgam/amalgam_execsum.pdf. Accessed December 10, 2012.
22. Fleisch AF, Sheffield PE, Chinn C, et al. Bisphenol A and related compounds in dental materials. Pediatrics 2010;126:760–8.
23. Baccaglini LA. Meta-analysis of randomized controlled trials shows no evidence that periodontal treatment during pregnancy prevents adverse pregnancy outcomes. J Am Dent Assoc 2011;142:1192–3.
24. Polyzos NP, Polyzos IP, Zavos A, et al. Obstetric outcomes after treatment of periodontal disease during pregnancy: systematic review and meta-analysis. BMJ 2010;341:c7017.
25. Chambrone L, Pannuti CM, Guglielmetti MR, et al. Evidence grade associating periodontitis with preterm birth and/or low birth weight. II: a systematic review

or randomized trials evaluating the effects of periodontal treatment. J Clin Perio-dontol 2011;38:902–14.

26. Uppal A, Uppal S, Pinto A, et al. The effectiveness of periodontal disease treatment during pregnancy in reducing the risk of experiencing preterm birth and low birth weight: a meta-analysis. J Am Dent Assoc 2010;141:1423–34.

27. Hilton I. Application of the perinatal oral health guidelines in clinical practice. J Calif Dent Assoc 2010;38:673–9.

28. Niessen LC. Women's health. In: Patton LL, editor. The ADA practical guide to patients with medical conditions. Ames (IA): American Dental Association and Wiley-Blackwell; 2012. p. 399–417.

29. Sooriyamoorthy M, Gower D. Hormonal influences on gingival tissues: relationship to periodontal disease. J Clin Periodontol 1989;16:201–8.

30. Amar S, Chung K. Influence of hormonal variation on the periodontium in women. Periodontol 2000 1994;6:78–87.

31. Ferris G. Alteration in female sex hormones: their effect on oral tissues and dental treatment. Compend Contin Educ Dent 1993;14:1558–70.

32. Zachariasen R. The effect of elevated ovarian hormones on periodontal health: oral contraceptives and pregnancy. Women Health 1993;14:1558–70.

33. Raber-Durlacher J, Zeijlemaker W, Meinesz A, et al. CD4 to CD8 ratio and in vitro lymphoproliferative responses during experimental gingivitis in pregnancy and post-partum. J Periodontol 1991;62:663–7.

34. Raber-Durlacher J, Leene W, Palmer-Bouva C, et al. Experimental gingivitis during pregnancy and post-partum: immunohistochemical aspects. J Periodontol 1993; 64:211–8.

35. Vittek J, Hernandez M, Wenk E, et al. Specific estrogen receptors in human gingiva. J Clin Endocrinol Metab 1982;54:608–12.

36. Mariotti A. Sex steroid hormones and cell dynamics in the periodontium. Crit Rev Oral Biol Med 1994;5:27–53.

37. O'Neil T. Plasma female sex-hormone levels and gingivitis in pregnancy. J Periodontol 1979;50:270–82.

38. Thomson M, Pack A. Effects of extended systemic and topical folate supplementation on gingivitis in pregnancy. J Clin Periodontol 1982;9:275–80.

39. Kornman K, Loesche W. The subgingival microflora during pregnancy. J Periodont Res 1980;15:111–22.

40. Jensen J, Liljemark W, Bloomquist C. The effect of female sex hormones on subgingival plaque. J Periodontol 1981;52:599–602.

41. Kornman K, Loesche W. Effects of estradiol and progesterone on *Bacteroides melaninogenicus*. Infect Immun 1982;35:256–63.

42. Arafat A. The prevalence of pyogenic granuloma in pregnant women. J Baltimore Coll Dent Surg 1974;29:64–70.

43. Demir Y, Demir S, Aktepe F. Cutaneous lobular capillary hemangioma induced by pregnancy. J Cutan Pathol 2004;31:77–80.

44. Steinberg B. Women's oral health issues. J Calif Dent Assoc 2000;28:663–7.

45. Rose LF. Sex hormonal imbalances, oral manifestations and dental treatment. In: Genco RJ, Goldman HM, Cohen DW, editors. Contemporary periodontics. St Louis (MO): Mosby Publishing Co; 1990. p. 221–7.

46. Laine MA. Effect of pregnancy on periodontal and dental health. Acta Odontol Scand 2002;260:257–64.

47. Steinberg BJ, Minsk L, Gluch JI, et al. Women's oral health issues. In: Clouse AL, Sherif K, editors. Women's health in clinical practice: a handbook for primary care. Totowa (NJ): Human Press Inc; 2008. p. 273–93.

48. El-Ashiry GM, El-Kafrawy AH, Nasr MF, et al. Comparative study of the influence of pregnancy and oral contraceptives on the gingivae. Oral Surg Oral Med Oral Pathol 1970;30:472–5.
49. Ismail SK, Kenney L. Review of hyperemesis gravidarum. Best Pract Res Clin Gastroenterol 2007;21:755–69.
50. Pirie M, Cooke I, Linden G, et al. Dental manifestations of pregnancy. Obstetrician Gynaecologist 2007;9(1):21–6.
51. Rateitschak KG. Tooth mobility changes in pregnancy. J Periodont Res 1967;2: 199–206.
52. Gürsoy M, Pajukanta R, Sorsa T, et al. Clinical changes in periodontium during pregnancy and postpartum. J Clin Periodontol 2008;35:576–83.
53. Tilakaratne A, Soory M, Ranasinghe AW, et al. Periodontal disease status during pregnancy and 3 months postpartum in a rural population of Sri-Lankan women. J Clin Periodontol 2000;27:787–92.
54. Silness J, Löe H. Periodontal disease in pregnancy. II. Correlation between oral hygiene and oral condition. Acta Odontol Scand 1964;22:121–35.
55. Moss KL, Beck JD, Offenbacher S. Clinical risk factors associated with incidence and progression of periodontal conditions in pregnant women. J Clin Periodontol 2005;32:492–8.
56. Han YW. Oral health and adverse pregnancy outcomes–What's next? J Dent Res 2011;90:289–93.
57. Offenbacher S, Boggess KA, Murtha AP, et al. Progressive periodontal disease and risk of very preterm delivery. Obstet Gynecol 2006;107:29–36.
58. Xiong X, Buekens P, Fraser WD, et al. Periodontal disease and adverse pregnancy outcomes: a systematic review. BJOG 2006;113:135–43.
59. Srinivas SK, Sammel MD, Stamilio DM, et al. Periodontal disease and adverse pregnancy outcomes: is there an association? Am J Obstet Gynecol 2009;200: 497.e1–8.
60. Offenbacher S, Katz V, Fertik G, et al. Periodontal infection as a possible risk factor for preterm low birth weight. J Periodontol 1996;67:1103–13.
61. Gibbs RS. The relationship between infections and adverse pregnancy outcomes: an overview. Ann Periodontol 2001;6:153–63.
62. Kramer MS. The epidemiology of adverse pregnancy outcomes: an overview. J Nutr 2003;133(Suppl):1592S–6S.
63. Bobetsis YA, Barros SP, Offenbacher S. Exploring the relationship between periodontal disease and pregnancy complications. J Am Dent Assoc 2006; 137(Suppl):7S–13S.
64. Han YW, Fardini Y, Chen C, et al. Term stillbirth caused by oral *Fusobacterium nucleatum*. Obstet Gynecol 2010;115:442–5.
65. Burt BA, Eklund SA. Dentistry: dental practice, and the community. 6th edition. St Louis (MO): Elsevier Saunders; 2005.
66. Back S, Wojdyla D, Say L, et al. The worldwide incidence of preterm birth: a systematic review of maternal mortality and morbidity. Bull World Health Organ 2010;88:31–8.
67. Blondel B, Kogan MD, Alexander GR, et al. The impact of the increasing number of multiple births on the rates of preterm birth and low birthweight: an international study. Am J Public Health 2002;92:1323–30.
68. Michalowicz BS, Hodges JS, Diangelis AJ, et al. Treatment of periodontal disease and the risk of preterm birth. N Engl J Med 2006;355:1885–94.
69. Offenbacher S, Beck JD, Jared HL, et al. Effects of periodontal therapy on rate of preterm delivery: a randomized controlled trial. Obstet Gynecol 2009;114:551–9.

70. Newnham JP, Newnham IA, Ball CM, et al. Treatment of periodontal disease during pregnancy: a randomized controlled trial. Obstet Gynecol 2009;114: 1239–48.
71. Michalowicz BS, Hodges JS, Novak MJ, et al. Changes in periodontitis during pregnancy and the risk of pre-term birth and low birthweight. J Clin Periodontol 2009;36:308–14.
72. Macones GA, Parry S, Nelson DB, et al. Treatment of localized periodontal disease in pregnancy does not reduce the occurrence of preterm birth: results from the Periodontal Infections and Prematurity Study (PIPS). Am J Obstet Gynecol 2010;202:147.e1–8.
73. Jeffcoat M, Parry S, Sammel M, et al. Periodontal infection and preterm birth: successful periodontal therapy reduces the risk of preterm birth. BJOG 2011; 118:250–6.
74. Xiong X, Buekens P, Goldenberg RL, et al. Optimal timing of periodontal disease treatment for prevention of adverse pregnancy outcomes: before or during pregnancy? Am J Obstet Gynecol 2011;205:111.e1–6.
75. Kim AJ, Lo AJ, Pullin DA, et al. Scaling and root planing treatment for periodontitis to reduce preterm birth and low birth weight: a systematic review and meta-analysis of randomized controlled trials. J Periodontol 2012;83:1508–19.
76. Boggess KA. Treatment of localized periodontal disease in pregnancy does not reduce the occurrence of preterm birth: results from the Periodontal Infections and Prematurity Study (PIPS). Am J Obstet Gynecol 2010;202:101–2.
77. Institute of Medicine. Initial national priorities for comparative effectiveness research. Washington, DC: The National Academies Press; 2009.

Dietary Behaviors and Oral-Systemic Health in Women

Juhee Kim, MS, ScD[a],*, Rita DiGioacchino DeBate, PhD, MPH, FAED[b],
Ellen Daley, PhD, MPH[b]

KEYWORDS

• Food habits • Dental care • Public health practice • Diet • Eating disorders

KEY POINTS

• Specific dietary behaviors and food consumption significantly affect oral health.
• Compared with men, women tend to report more weight-related unhealthy eating behaviors, including those of eating disorders.
• Certain food consumption and dietary behaviors are known risk factors for both obesity and dental disease.
• Oral health care providers (OHPs) must have an active role in early diagnosis, oral treatment, and referral of patients with unhealthy dietary behaviors because they are often the first health providers to observe overt health effects.
• The impact of OHPs is enhanced with their taking an active role combating a broad spectrum of weight-related disorders and oral diseases by providing preventive strategies at the personal and community levels.

INTRODUCTION

The impact of specific dietary behaviors and food consumption is evident and of increasing importance in obesogenic and cariogenic food arenas. Generally, studies conclude that women and men have different dietary behaviors. Understanding the influences of dietary behaviors on oral health from the perspective of gender disparities is limited, however, calling for review to shed some light on these complex interactions. This article provides the intersections of dietary factors and oral-systemic health that are at greater risk for women than men. Additionally covered are US government initiatives and leadership structures that are set to address oral health disparities. Lastly, current efforts on dental office–based and community-based interventions that designed to directly or indirectly influence dietary oral-systemic health are discussed.

[a] Department of Public Health, Center for Health Disparities, Brody School of Medicine, East Carolina University, 1800 West 5th Street, Medical Pavilion Suite 9, Greenville, NC 27834, USA; [b] Department of Community and Family Health, Center for Transdisciplinary Research in Women's Health, College of Public Health, University of South Florida, 13201 Bruce B. Downs Boulevard, MDC 56, Tampa, FL 33612, USA
* Corresponding author.
E-mail address: kimju@ecu.edu

Dent Clin N Am 57 (2013) 211–231
http://dx.doi.org/10.1016/j.cden.2013.01.004
0011-8532/13/$ – see front matter © 2013 Elsevier Inc. All rights reserved.

WEIGHT-PREOCCUPIED SOCIETY AND OBESITY

According to the World Health Organization, overweight (body mass index [BMI] $\geq$25) and obesity (BMI $\geq$30) compose the 5th leading risk for deaths globally.[1] In the United States, approximately 2 in 3 adults and 1 in 3 children are reported to be overweight or obese.[2,3] The percentage of obese adults increases with age, especially among women. Although an estimated 32% of women between 20 and 39 years of age are obese, the percentage climbs to 36% between ages 40 and 59 and tops 42% for women ages 60 and older.[3] The rate of obesity, however, is similar between girls (15%) and boys (18.6%).[3] Moreover, 2.8% of men and 6.9% of women are reported to be morbidly obese; significant differences also exist by ethnicity, with lower rates of obesity among white adults than black or Hispanic adults.[4] In the United States, approximately 60% of non-Hispanic black women 20 years of age and older are obese compared with slightly more than 40% of Hispanic women and approximately 35% of non-Hispanic white women.[5] Models predict that by the year 2015, three-quarters of adults in the United States will be overweight and 40% obese.[6]

Girls and young women face different developmental stages and challenges in childhood, adolescence, and pregnancy. Weight concerns and dieting behaviors are more common among women than men. Among social factors, social pressure for thinness has been widely accepted as an explanatory factor that contributes to gender disparities in distorted body image, weight preoccupation,[6] and, in consequence, dieting and eating disorders.[7–9] Compared with men, women tend to report more unhealthy eating behaviors, such as dieting and eating disorders.[10–12] The general consensus is that weight concern is a powerful medium that distorts body image, which, in turn, contributes to distorted eating behaviors, particularly more for women than men. These unhealthy eating behaviors make individuals susceptible to health risks. Less attention is given, however, to whether dieting or eating disorders are directly related to oral health.

CARIOGENIC FOOD CONSUMPTION AND DIETARY BEHAVIORS

Certain food consumption and dietary behaviors are known risk factors for both obesity and dental caries. During the past 3 decades, Americans have dramatically increased their consumption of sugar-sweetened beverages (SSBs), including soda, fruit drinks and punches, and sport drinks.[13,14] Since the 1970s, soda consumption has approximately tripled. Concurrently, the rates of weight gain, obesity, type 2 diabetes mellitus, and cardiovascular disease (CVD) have risen.[15,16] SSBs are the largest source of refined sugar consumed in the United States. In 2004, adolescents consumed an average of 300 calories per day from SSBs, accounting for 13% of their daily caloric intake.[14] The high consumption of SSBs is a significant determinant of dental caries, obesity, bone mineral density (BMD), anxiety, and poor sleep.[17–20]

High consumption of SSBs, when combined with gingival plaque deposits, is a significant risk factor for dental caries among low-income youth and adults. A longitudinal cohort study from birth to preschool age by Marshall and colleagues[21] confirmed that regular soda consumption, including 100% fruit juice or powdered beverages, was the strongest risk factor for dental caries among dietary factors. The increased consumption of SSBs with a concurrent reduced intake of milk during the teenage years may increase the risk of osteoporosis in older women.[17,21]

Recent focus has extended to other deleterious dietary behaviors, including snacking on chips and sugar-dense foods as well as the frequency of processed starch consumption.[22–24] Dietary habits, such as skipping breakfast and eating inadequate fruits or vegetables, were also associated with dental caries in children.[25]

Furthermore, inappropriate feeding practices, such as at-will feeding and bedtime bottle feeding, contribute significantly to the development of dental caries.[26–28] In summary, poor dietary choices, such as these, combined with SSB consumption are common indicators of obesity and dental caries, making consideration of food environment and choice in relation to oral health essential.

ORAL-SYSTEMIC DIETARY CONNECTIONS

Although oral-systemic connections have been documented since the seventeenth century, only recently have medicine and dentistry become confluent with respect to the overall health and well-being of the patient population.[29] Several reviews have outlined the many oral-systemic connections that have been studied or theorized.[29–40] Several mechanisms have linked how oral-systemic connections are made throughout the body, including oral manifestations of systemic diseases, oral causes of systemic diseases, and, in some cases, simply correlations between oral health and systemic health issues. As an example, severe generalized periodontitis may negatively affect the control of underlying systemic diseases.[41–43]

A growing body of research points to the relationship between oral health and systemic diseases, such as heart diseases, diabetes, and poor pregnancy outcomes.[44–49] Oral health has been declared as 1 of the 12 Leading Health Indicators in *Healthy People 2010*.[50] The oral-systemic women's health issues that have dietary connections are discussed.

Diabetes

In the United States, approximately 25.8 million people have diabetes and approximately 35% of adults, ages 20 and older, are considered prediabetic, with conditions that are exacerbated by being overweight or obese.[51] Similarly, hyperinsulinemia and the insulin-resistant state are related to increased weight,[52] which, in combination, contribute to diabetes and kidney disease–related deaths.[53] As the 7th leading cause of death in the United States, the lifetime risk of developing diabetes for an individual born in 2000 is 33% for men and 39% for women.[54] Although the all-cause mortality rate among diabetic men has decreased over the past 4 decades, the rates of all-cause mortality among diabetic women have shown no reduction.[54]

A bidirectional relationship exists between periodontitis and diabetes. Diabetes has an adverse effect on periodontal health,[55] and periodontal disease is a widely accepted complication associated with type 2 diabetes mellitus.[56,57] Periodontal disease may contribute to systemic inflammation that generates inflammatory cytokines, which can lead to worsening insulin resistance and type 2 diabetes mellitus.[58] At the same time, diabetes can have adverse effects of the periodontium, including decreased collagen turnover, impaired neutrophil function, and periodontal destruction.[59] In a study among Pima Indians with and without type 2 diabetes mellitus, diabetes increased the risk of developing periodontitis 3-fold.[60] Moreover, studies have shown that diabetes increases the risk of alveolar bone and attachment loss.[43,61] There is strong evidence to suggest that the incidence and severity of periodontitis are influenced by the presence of type 2 diabetes mellitus and, among individuals with type 2 diabetes mellitus, that the incidence and prevalence of periodontitis are affected by patient control.[61–66] Diabetes patients, especially those with poorly controlled diabetes mellitus or hyperglycemia, are more susceptible to loss of periodontal attachment.[61,67,68]

Diabetes is a risk factor for other oral pathologies as well. Diabetes is associated with increased risk of gingivitis; candidiasis; oral lichen planus; premalignant lesions, like leukoplakia; and oral malignancies.[58,69] Oral symptoms commonly associated with type 2 diabetes mellitus include dry mouth, gingival bleeding and swelling, and advanced pocket formation.[70] Diabetes-associated xerostomia may make oral tissue more susceptible to damage by trauma and opportunistic infections, such as candidiasis. It can also lead to accumulation of bacterial plaque and food debris, which are associated with increased risk for dental caries and periodontitis.[71] Prolonged xerostomia increases the risk of local accumulation of plaque and debris, which can increase the risk of opportunistic infections, altered taste, oral malodor, and oral mucosal soreness.[72]

Additionally, glycemic control and disease duration seem to have different effects on oral health. Poor control and duration of diabetes are both associated with more severe periodontal disease[58] and individuals with poor glycemic control have higher prevalence and severity of gingival inflammation and periodontal destruction.[73–75] Xerostomia and parotid gland enlargement may also be related to the degree of glycemic control.[76–78] Similarly, poorly controlled diabetes mellitus may increase the risk of developing superficial and systemic fungal infections[79–81]; the clinical course of oral candidosis may be more severe among patients with type 2 diabetes mellitus than in healthy patients and exacerbated most among type 2 diabetes mellitus patients with poor glycemic control.[72,81] It is unclear whether improved oral hygiene improves glycemic control.[36] Evidence suggests that improvements in oral hygiene among diabetics can improve diabetes control and may reduce Hemoglobin A1c.[82]

Cardiovascular Disease

Women represent an increasingly larger proportion of patients with coronary artery disease due to their living longer than their male counterparts. The incidence of heart disease throughout their life span poses an increased financial burden on the health care system.[83] Oral health has been associated with CVD since as early as 1989, when Mattila and colleagues[84] reported an association between poor dental health and acute myocardial infarction. Periodontal disease specifically has been linked to CVD since 1996, when the newly formed area of periodontal medicine paved the way for looking at oral-systemic links, such as CVD.[85] Since that time, there have been several research studies connecting CVD and periodontitis.[84,86–91] This literature has grown to the extent that 6 meta-analyses have been conducted, all showing that patients with periodontitis are at increased risk for developing CVD.[32,88,92–96] Furthermore, a systematic review demonstrated that periodontitis is associated with systemic concentrations that are linked to atherosclerosis—raised concentrations of C-reactive protein, fibrinogen, and cytokines.[97]

Although these connections have been made extensively, some studies have found mixed results, particularly in connections to coronary heart disease.[98–100] Although many studies demonstrate increased risk of CVD with periodontitis, epidemiologic studies cannot establish causality, and the question of the mechanism is being investigated. Four potential mechanisms that foster this oral-systemic connection have also been posited: common susceptibility to infections (causing both periodontitis and atherosclerosis), systemic inflammation, infection from periodontitis entering the blood, and immune response to periodontitis, causing inflammation.[32,101]

Excess weight is associated with an increased risk of CVD and a woman's risk of coronary heart disease is graded: as more excess weight is accumulated, the risk of coronary heart disease increases.[80] In a large prospective cohort study conducted among women in the United States, researchers found that after controlling for obesity, even mild-to-moderate weight gain increased a middle-aged woman's risk of coronary disease.[102]

Reproductive Complication

Pregnancy has been linked to some of the most significant hormonal-oral changes.[40] Oral manifestations include increased caries,[103] acid erosion,[39] and increased salivation[104] from vomiting as well as xerostomia,[39] increased tooth mobility,[39] and tooth loss.[105–107] Research has suggested several potential risk factors that periodontal disease may carry for adverse pregnancy outcomes. Correlations were established between periodontitis and preterm low-birth-weight infants,[85,108] and a direct relationship between the severity of periodontitis and the risk of preterm birth was established.[109–124] These connections have been researched extensively enough for the conduct of 4 meta-analyses, 3 that concluded a positive association between pregnant women with periodontal disease and risk of preterm birth[125–127] and 1 that demonstrated indications of this association but with a lack of conclusive evidence.[128]

A systematic review of 25 studies reported that 18 of the reviewed studies demonstrated an association between periodontal treatment and a reduction in preterm birth and preterm low-birth-weight babies.[127] In 2009, a meta-analysis conducted by Polyzos and colleagues[129] demonstrated a significantly lower rate of preterm birth but only a borderline significantly lower rate of low-birth-weight infants when pregnant women were treated for periodontal disease with scaling and root planning. (For a review of this topic, see the article by Steinberg and colleagues elsewhere in this issue.) Given the varied results, more research is needed to understand how periodontal treatment may have an impact on adverse birth outcomes.[130–135]

Excess weight also puts women at risk for experiencing an array of pregnancy-related complications, mainly due to elevated rates of chronic hypertension and diabetes prior to conception.[136] Compared with women with normal BMI, obese pregnant women are more likely to develop gestational diabetes mellitus[137–141] and pregnancy-induced hypertension.[138,139,141,142] While giving birth, they face increased rates of labor induction, delivery by cesarian section,[137,140] and wound infection.[139,142,143]

Osteoarthritis

Osteoporosis has been associated with increased rates of bone loss,[39,144,145] accelerated alveolar bone resorption,[39,146,147] and periodontitis.[133,134,148] Overweight women are at greater risk of developing osteoarthritis[149] and tend to suffer more from its effects than similarly overweight or obese men.[149] The prevalence of osteoarthritis increases with additional severity of overweight and obesity.[80] Additionally, some medications used to treat osteoporosis may cause osteonecrosis of the teeth.[150] Osteoporosis is not believed to cause periodontitis but may increase the severity of already existing periodontitis[39,148,151]; this relationship, however, remains unclear.[35,38,39]

Other osteopathic conditions, such as osteoporosis and osteopenia, are common among competitive female athletes and those with some types of disordered eating. Disordered eating is associated with menstrual irregularity and menstrual irregularity is correlated with low BMD.[152,153] A study among young competitive female distance runners found that disordered eating was associated with low BMD even in the absence of menstrual irregularity.[152] Anorexia nervosa (AN) that begins during the teenage years can also cause deficiencies in bone mass accrual and short stature[152] as well as increase the likelihood of being osteopenic, even after years of weight and menstrual recovery.[152–154]

Grocholewicz and Bohatyrewicz[155] reported a negative correlation between lumbar BMD and periodontal disease as well as between the radius BMD and papillary bleeding index.

EATING DISORDERS AND DISORDERED EATING

Girls and women are disproportionately affected by eating disorders and disordered eating. Studies have consistently reported higher rates of AN, bulimia nervosa (BN), and binge-eating behaviors among girls and women,[156–160] with the lifetime prevalence of AN and BN 1.75 to 3 times higher among women.[161] It is suggested that dieting may be a precursor to disordered eating behaviors.[162–167] Moreover, mounting evidence suggests that obesity, disordered eating behaviors, and eating disorders are interrelated, often occurring in the same individuals.[163]

Although eating disorders are defined as psychiatric diagnoses, they are associated with nutritional, medical, and dental problems. AN is often practiced by severe food restriction or starving oneself, thus leading to underweight status. BN is characterized by binge eating and inappropriate compensatory behaviors, such as vomiting, laxative use, and excessive exercise, in order to control body weight.[12] Eating disorders are associated with psychological disorders and systemic diseases, including oral health.[168,169] AN and BN have both been associated with increased oral health problems, and some cases are linked to dental caries and periodontal diseases.[170,171] Compared with AN patients, BN patients reported worse oral health status, especially dental erosion, dry or cracked lips, and burning tongue syndrome.[172]

Disordered eating includes a broad range of behaviors that elude clear definitional boundaries. In practice, disordered eating is often used to describe a wide array of irregular eating behaviors that do not collectively meet the clinical criteria for diagnosis as eating disorders. Unhealthy eating behaviors may include excessive dieting, fasting, extreme body dissatisfaction, binge eating, compulsive exercising, and purging.[173,174] Boutelle and colleagues[175] found that overweight adolescents were more likely than peers with healthy weights to partake in unhealthy weight control measures, such as using laxatives or diet pills or vomiting. Similarly, obese children are 3 times more likely than healthy controls to develop BN.[176] In a longitudinal study of adolescents, researchers found that those who used unhealthful weight control behaviors at baseline (including using diet pills, food substitutes, cigarettes, diet pills, vomiting, or laxatives to control weight) increased their BMI more than those who did not engage in any weight control behaviors. Five years later, these youth were also at increased risk for binge eating with loss of control and extreme weight control behaviors.[177]

Even though oral health problems are secondary conditions in eating disorder patients, the true problems of dental diseases are often not recognized or are hidden by patients, remaining undetected by dental professionals.[178–180] Oral health education and training in the association between eating disorders and oral health is a great necessity because dental care professionals can play an important role in early detection and diagnosis of eating disorders, thus promoting oral health.

PREVENTIVE PUBLIC HEALTH ACTIVITIES
Government Initiatives

In 2000, the surgeon general's first report on oral health, *Oral Health in America,*[181] addressed the need of public health efforts to improve oral health disparities in the United States. By building on the recommendations of the surgeon general's report, *Healthy People 2010* and *Healthy People 2020* provided the specific goals and objectives to work with national and state public health agencies.[182,183] For the first time, in *Healthy People 2020*, the US Department of Health and Human Services included "oral health" as 1 of the 12 Leading Health Indicators and introduced the importance of oral-systemic diseases. To prevent oral-systemic diseases, *Healthy People 2020* recommends increasing regular dental care visits, which is 1 of the 17 oral health objectives: "Persons aged 2 years and older who used the oral health care system in the past 12 months."[182]

Among the objectives, increasing the proportion of site-specific access to preventive care with an oral health component was clearly stated along with increasing the proportion of the population who use the oral health care system and preventive dental service. The access to site-specific public health channels such as schools, local health departments, and Federally Qualified Health Centers, was listed as a separate objective for preventive oral health services where comprehensive oral-systemic health screening and interventions can be incorporated (**Box 1**). In particular, increasing access to preventive dental care service for low-income children and adolescents was a separate objective, reflecting the need to address disparities of populations at risk. Given the problems of reproductive complications and their health implications to children, women in poverty may be a special population in need as well.

The *Oral Health Initiative 2010* was announced to support and enhance current public health efforts to improve the oral health of the public.[183] The key message is, "oral health is integral to overall health," and a systems approach is proposed that focuses on 4 areas: (1) emphasize oral health promotion/disease prevention, (2) increase access to care, (3) enhance oral health workforce, and (4) eliminate oral health disparities. Among the 9 new initiatives, there were no initiatives that can be directly connected to oral-systemic diseases or dietary factors; in fact, none of the initiatives used the words oral-systemic disease (**Box 2**). It is encouraging, however, to have "oral health as part of women's health across the lifespan" as one of the initiatives. The last initiative in **Box 2** presents a developmental perspective on women's oral health issues from infancy to the postmenopausal period to medical and dental care services.

Community Interventions on SSB Consumption

Community-based nutrition interventions aimed at curve obesity epidemics have been tested and placed at different levels. Among those recent efforts, there is no question that community interventions focused on SSBs may present a valuable opportunity in preventive oral health interventions. The recent increases in soft drink consumption among children and youth not only reflect the recent advertisement and business advances by manufacturers of these beverages but also the widespread availability within communities, including school settings.[184,185]

Box 1
Oral health objectives on "Access to Preventive Services" and "Oral Health Interventions" in *Healthy People 2020*

OH–7: Increase the proportion of children, adolescents, and adults who used the oral health care system in the past 12 months.

OH–8: Increase the proportion of low-income children and adolescents who received any preventive dental service during the past year.

OH–9: Increase the proportion of school-based health centers with an oral health component.

OH–10: Increase the proportion of local health departments and Federally Qualified Health Centers that have an oral health component.

OH–11: Increase the proportion of patients who receive oral health services at Federally Qualified Health Centers each year.

OH–14: (Developmental) Increase the proportion of adults who receive preventive interventions in dental offices.

Abbreviation: OH, Oral health.

Box 2
Oral Health Initiative 2010 **(leading agency)**

- Head Start Dental Home Initiative (Administration for Children and Families)
- National Oral Health Surveillance Plan (Centers For Disease Control and Prevention and National Institutes of Health)
- Review of Innovative State Medicaid dental Programs (Centers for Medicare and Medicaid Services)
- National Study on Oral Health Access to Services (Centers for Medicare and Medicaid Services)
- Early Childhood Caries Initiative (Indian Health Service)
- Clinical and Translational Science Program (National Institutes of Health)
- A Cultural Competency E-learning Continuing Education Program for Oral Health Professionals (Office of Minority Health)
- Oral Health as Part of Women's Health Across the Lifespan (The Office on Women's Health)

SSBs represent the most frequent purchase among youth. The recommendation that reducing these added dietary sugars might be feasible by reducing the availability of vending machines in school settings.[186,187] Cullen[188] conducted a school interventional study to investigate whether school food environment changes influenced soda purchases in a middle school in Texas. She found that healthier alternatives, such as increasing access to bottled water and whole fruit juices, can be made available to youth with favorable uptake. This study demonstrated that vending machine changes (including soda machines) can be implemented in school setting. In efforts to curb high rates of SSB consumption, researchers suggest reducing soda bottle sizes and adding more water bottles as an alternative.

Banning all SSBs in schools was recommended by the Institute of Medicine in 2007 to establish healthy school environments.[186] Many state school beverage policies, however, focused only on soda bans yet allowed other sweetened beverages, such as sports drinks and fruit juices.[189] Tabera[190] conducted an evaluation study on children's access to, purchase of, and consumption of SSBs. They found that policies banning all SSBs may reduce access and purchase of SSBs but not consumption. Also, they reported that there were no differences detected between states having only a soda ban and those with no policy. The results indicated no positive effect of school beverage policies on children's SSB consumption. Thus, more a comprehensive approach is desired in the development of school-based beverage policy interventions.

As an example of community-wide intervention on SSB consumption, New York City became the first major metropolitan city to enact a ban on the size of soda cans and bottles. The intent of such a ban is to reduce excess caloric intake by the city's residents in hopes to help curb the increasing obesity epidemic and improve overall community health. This ban essentially limits soda larger than 16 ounces in size to be sold at restaurants, fast food chains, theaters, delis, and office cafeterias. This revolutionary city-wide stipulation is the first of its kind in the United States, although the city of New York has passed previous bans on smoking in bar settings, removed whole milk selections from city schools and trans fat additives in food, and required calorie labeling in restaurants.[191]

Although community-based food ban policies are in their infancy, their basis is justifiable to improving the community health of residents of all.[192] Currently, community-level efforts are discussed only regarding obesity prevention and do not include the angle of oral health. There is well-established evidence that high SSB consumption poses serious potential harm to oral health. Therefore, community-based interventions aimed at targeting dietary behaviors at various levels (schools, restaurants, and so forth) may provide the optimal opportunity in regards to oral-systemic diseases prevention.

FROM RESEARCH TO PRACTICE
Diabetes

Greenberg and colleagues[193] conducted a national random sample of general dentists in the United States in order to assess attitudes, willingness, and perceived barriers regarding chairside medical screening in the dental office. The majority of dentists believed it was important to screen for hypertension (85.8%), CVD (76.8%), type 2 diabetes mellitus (76.6%), hepatitis (71.5%), and HIV (68.8%). Likewise, the majority of dentists were willing to refer patients for consultation with physicians (96.4%), collect oral fluids for salivary diagnostics (87.7%), and conduct medical screenings that yield immediate results (83.4%).

In a cross-sectional survey of 265 randomly selected dentists in 3 states, researchers found 61% believed that addressing diabetes was an important responsibility. Athough the vast majority (86%) of dentists advised patients with diabetes about the risk of periodontal disease, only 47% reported that they knew how to assess for diabetes, 42% felt well prepared to intervene with patients with diabetes, and 18% provided diabetic-related services.[194]

Eating Disorders

OHPs (ie, dentists and dental hygienists) have a role in prevention, early diagnosis and oral treatment, and referral of patients who engage in unhealthy weight control behaviors[195,196] because they are often the first health professionals to observe overt health effects.[196,197] Oral health issues resulting from unhealthy weight control behaviors present themselves as signs of malnutrition,[168,198–207] dehydration,[204,207–209] and vomiting.[168,198–200,203,206,208,210]

Failure of OHPs to identify oral signs and oral health issues may lead to irreversible damage to the oral cavity and progression to weight-related disorders and associated systemic health problems.[195,211–213] OHPs must learn to provide screening, baseline education, and referrals as part of comprehensive patient care[213,214] (see American Dietetic Association for specific guidelines[195]). Despite the growing evidence of the role of nutrition in oral-systemic health issues, nutrition education in dental education has faced challenges.[215] Although the fundamentals of macronutrients and micronutrients in human metabolism and oral health are taught in biochemistry and pathology courses, translation of nutrition and diet into patient care practice is limited.[195] In addition, limited patient contact time and lack of strong evidence-based practice outcomes have contributed to inconsistent integration of health behavior management into oral health practice.[215]

The following components, based on the information–motivation–behavioral skills model, health belief model, and brief motivational interviewing,[216] are part of a training program to increase the capacity of OHPs to practice early identification of disordered eating behaviors among their patients:

- Didactic component: eating disorders and oral findings—describes the main types of eating disorders and associated disordered eating behaviors, characteristics, and health issues. In addition, this component displays the oral findings of disordered eating behaviors and information for differential diagnosis.

- Behavioral skills component: EAT (Evaluate, Assess, Treat) framework and skills—based on the Brief Motivational Interviewing,[200] the EAT framework and skills component is the critical skill–based portion of the intervention. The EAT framework is divided into 3 steps that include (1) evaluating patients presenting signs of disordered eating behaviors and perform differential diagnosis, (2) assessing patient readiness for addressing disordered eating behaviors, and (3) patient-specific treatment strategies based on a patient's stage of readiness.
- Practice component: EAT case studies—4 interactive case studies provide an opportunity for learners to practice secondary prevention behaviors with 4 different patients (varying in age and gender) at different stages of readiness to address the underlying cause of the various oral health issues identified. The video case studies provide an opportunity for learners to practice secondary prevention behavioral skills, leading to increased self-efficacy.
- Resource and referral components: provide OHPs with the resources necessary for supporting secondary prevention behaviors, including (1) printer-friendly education materials for patients, parents, and dental office staff; (2) printer-friendly patient-specific treatment plan templates available for OHPs; and (3) a Web link to nutrition and disordered eating treatment networks.

A prospective group randomized controlled trial involving 27 dental and dental hygiene classes from 12 accredited oral health education programs in the United States was implemented to assess the efficacy of the Web-based training program on attitudes, knowledge, self-efficacy, and skills related to the secondary prevention of disordered eating behaviors. Mixed-model analysis of covariance indicated large improvements among students in the intervention group on all 6 outcomes of interest.

Obesity

It is imperative that dentists along with other health professional take a leadership role for nutrition/healthy lifestyle counseling of their patients, especially in those with high risks for dental caries. Dovey[217] recommends that dental clinics serve as an important source of health promotion and diseases prevention, suggesting that dentists could screen for obesity, thus offering better integration of children's dental services and other child health care services.

Incorporating nutrition/healthy lifestyle counseling into pediatric dental practices is reviewed and recommended by Vann and colleagues.[218] After height and weight are recorded, health care providers can easily calculate BMI and establish conversations about nutrition and healthy lifestyle with parents. Vann and colleagues[218] also suggested that by embracing an awareness of the childhood obesity epidemic, pediatric dental providers can serve as community model for healthy lifestyle practices by sponsoring and promoting both office-based and community-based lifestyle programs.

FUTURE/IMPLICATIONS FOR DIETARY ORAL-SYSTEMIC RESEARCH AND PRACTICE

Women are disproportionately affected by diet-related oral and systemic health issues. Growing evidence shows that many of the same factors contribute to both oral health and obesity. Dental practitioners are in a pivotal position to provide guidance for the prevention and reduction of both. The American Academy of Pediatric Dentistry policy on nutrition points out that discussions relative to diet and dental caries should be the essential components of oral health anticipatory guidance for children and that dietary discussions are central in providing counseling for caregivers of children with increased caries risk.[219] An American Dietetic Association 2007 position report states, "oral health and nutrition have a synergistic bidirectional relationship."[195] The American Academy of Pediatric Dentistry revised a policy on dental homes in 2004 that is similar to the medical homes proposed by the American Academy of Pediatrics: dental homes offer patient-centered comprehensive, continuous, coordinated, and prevention-based care.[220,221] There is a clear consensus across the multiple health care professions that the integration of oral health with nutritional and medical services, education, and research is necessary. Literature on implementation and evaluation of this new model of care, however, is scarce.

The oral health community continues to recognize the importance of looking at the ways to understand and improve oral health disparities and associated social environmental conditions. Oral health professionals and government agencies need to expand their efforts synergistically in office settings and education institutions. Public health interventions targeting obesity prevention can be strategically incorporated with oral health interventions in a congruent way. How and whether these scientific findings would be translated in the development of programs and policies for dental office and oral health programs remain to be determined.

By acknowledging the infancy stage of oral-systemic disease research and practice, this article attempts to emphasize the importance of a gendered perspective on diet-related oral health issues. There is scarce information, however, in the literature for women-centered research and practices that would be responsive to the increased diseases and illness associated with diet. Failure to identify and address the need of women, however, would deepen the current health disparities being addressed. Strategies across oral health and all disciplines will provide for a more comprehensive integrative approach to better the health and well-being of the patient population.

REFERENCES

1. World Health Organization. Obesity and overweight. Fact sheet N311. Geneva (Switzerland): World Health Organization; 2011.
2. Flegal KM, Carroll MD, Ogden CL, et al. Prevalence and trends in obesity among US adults, 1999-2000. JAMA 2002;288:1723-7.
3. Ogden CL, Carroll MD, Kit BK, et al. Prevalence of obesity in the United States, 2009-2010. NCHS Data Brief 2012;(82):1-8.
4. Ogden CL, Carroll MD, Curtin LR, et al. Prevalence of overweight and obesity in the United States, 1999-2004. JAMA 2006;295:1549-55.
5. Centers for Disease Control and Prevention. QuickStats: prevalence of obesity among adults aged 20 years by race/ethnicity and sex - National Health and Nutrition Examination Survey, United States, 2009-2010. MMWR Morb Mortal Wkly Rep 2012;61:130.
6. McCabe MP, Ricciardelli LA. A prospective study of pressures from parents, peers, and the media on extreme weight change behaviors among adolescent boys and girls. Behav Res Ther 2005;43(5):653-68.
7. McCabe MP, Ricciardelli LA. Parent, peer, and media influences on body image and strategies to both increase and decrease body size among adolescent boys and girls. Adolescence 2001;36(142):225-40.
8. Anderson CB, Bulik CM. Gender differences in compensatory behaviors, weight and shape salience, and drive for thinness. Eat Behav 2004;5(1):1-11.
9. Ricciardelli LA, McCabe MP. Dietary restraint and negative affect as mediators of body dissatisfaction and bulimic behavior in adolescent girls and boys. Behav Res Ther 2001;39(11):1317-28.
10. Neumark-Sztainer D, Sherwood NE, French SA, et al. Weight control behaviors among adult men and women: cause for concern? Obes Res 1999;7(2):179-88.

11. Wardle J, Haase AM, Steptoe A, et al. Gender differences in food choice: the contribution of health beliefs and dieting. Ann Behav Med 2004;27(2):107–16.

12. American Psychiatric Association. Diagnostic and statistical manual of mental disorders. Washington, DC: American Psychiatric Association; 2000.

13. French SA, Lin B, Guthrie JF. National trends in soft drink consumption among children and adolescents age 6 to 17 years: Prevalence, amounts, and sources, 1977/1978 to 1994/1998. J Am Diet Assoc 2003;103(10):1326–31.

14. Wang YC, Bleich SN, Gortmaker SL. Increasing caloric contribution from sugar-sweetened beverages and 100% fruit juices among US children and adolescents, 1988-2004. Pediatrics 2008;121(6):e1604–14.

15. Position of the American Dietetic Association: nutrition intervention in the treatment of Anorexia Nervosa, Bulimia Nervosa, and other eating disorders. J Am Diet Assoc 2006;106(12):2073–82.

16. Hu FB, Malik VS. Sugar-sweetened beverages and risk of obesity and type 2 diabetes: epidemiologic evidence. Physiol Behav 2010;100(1):47–54.

17. Marshall TA, Eichenberger Gilmore JM, Broffitt B, et al. Diet quality in young children is influenced by beverage consumption. J Am Coll Nutr 2005;24(1): 65–75.

18. Whiting SJ, Healey A, Psiuk S, et al. Relationship between carbonated and other low nutrient dense beverages and bone mineral content of adolescents. Nutr Res 2001;21(8):1107–15.

19. Pollak CP, Bright D. Caffeine consumption and weekly sleep patterns in US seventh-, eighth-, and ninth-graders. Pediatrics 2003;111(1):42–6.

20. Tahmassebi JF, Duggal MS, Malik-Kotru G, et al. Soft drinks and dental health: A review of the current literature. J Dent 2006;34(1):2–11.

21. Marshall TA, Levy SM, Broffitt B, et al. Dental caries and beverage consumption in young children. Pediatrics 2003;112(3):184–91.

22. Burt BA, Ismail AI. Diet, nutrition, and food cariogenicity. J Dent Res 1986; 65(Special Issue):1475–84.

23. Johansson I, Holgerson PL, Kressin NR, et al. Snacking habits and caries in young children. Caries Res 2010;44(5):421–30.

24. Chankanka O, Marshall TA, Levy SM, et al. Mixed dentition cavitated caries incidence and dietary intake frequencies. Pediatr Dent 2011;33(3):233–40.

25. Dye BA. The relationship between healthful eating practices and dental caries in children aged 2–5 years in the United States, 1988–1994. J Am Dent Assoc 2004;135(1):55.

26. Ismail AI. Prevention of early childhood caries. Community Dent Oral Epidemiol 1998;26(Suppl 1):49–61.

27. Alm AA. Body adiposity status in teenagers and snacking habits in early childhood in relation to approximal caries at 15 years of age. Int J Paediatr Dent 2008;18(3):189–96.

28. Sohn WW. Carbonated soft drinks and dental caries in the primary dentition. J Dent Res 2006;85(3):262–6.

29. Vieira C, Caramelli B. The history of dentistry and medicine relationship: could the mouth finally return to the body? Oral Dis 2009;15:538–46.

30. Beltran-Aguilar ED, Beltran-Neira RJ. Oral diseases and conditions throughout the lifespan. II. Systemic diseases. Gen Dent 2004;52:107–14.

31. Clemmens DA, Kerr AR. Improving oral health in women: nurses' call to action. MCN Am J Matern Child Nurs 2008;33:10–4 [quiz: 15–6].

32. Cullinan MP, Ford PJ, Seymour GJ. Periodontal disease and systemic health: current status. Aust Dent J 2009;54(Suppl 1):S62–9.

33. Hollister MC, Weintraub JA. The association of oral status with systemic health, quality of life, and economic productivity. J Dent Educ 1993;57:901–12.
34. Kornman KS. Patients are not equally susceptible to periodontitis: does this change dental practice and the dental curriculum? J Dent Educ 2001;65:777–84.
35. Krejci CB, Bissada NF. Women's health issues and their relationship to periodontitis. J Am Dent Assoc 2002;133:323–9.
36. Meurman J, Odont D. Dental infections and general health. Quintessence Int 1997;28:807–11.
37. Page R. The pathobiology of periodontal diseases may affect systemic diseases: inversion of a paradigm. Ann Periodontol 1998;3:108–20.
38. Pihlstrom BL, Michalowicz BS, Johnson NW. Periodontal diseases. Lancet 2005; 366:1809–20.
39. American Dental Association Council on Access. Women's oral health issues; oral health care series. Chicago: American Dental Association Council on Access; 2006. p. 2009. Available at: http://www.ada.org/sections/professionalResources/pdfs/healthcare_womens.pdf. Accessed February 28, 2013.
40. Guncu GN, Tozum TF, Caglayan F. Effects of endogenous sex hormones on the periodontium–review of literature. Aust Dent J 2005;50:138–45.
41. Grossi SG, Genco RJ. Periodontal disease and diabetes mellitus: a two-way relationship. Ann Periodontol 1998;3(1):51–61.
42. Miller LS, Manwell M, Newbold D, et al. The relationship between reduction in periodontal inflammation and diabetes control: a report of 9 cases. J Periodontol 1992;63:843.
43. Taylor G, Burt B, Becker M, et al. Non-insulin dependent diabetes mellitus and alveolar bone loss progression over 2 years. J Periodontol 1998;69:76.
44. Assael LA. The oral systemic link: now a task for health care policy. J Oral Maxillofac Surg 2007;65:1445–6.
45. D'Aiuto F, Parkar M, Nibali L, et al. Periodontal infections cause changes in traditional and novel cardiovascular risk factors: results from a randomized controlled clinical trial. Am Heart J 2006;151:977–84.
46. Desvarieux M, Demmer RT, Rundek T, et al. Relationship between periodontal disease, tooth loss, and carotid artery plaque. Stroke 2003;34:2120–5.
47. Engebretson SP, Lamster IB, Elkind MS, et al. Radiographic measures of chronic periodontitis and carotid artery plaque. Stroke 2005;36:561–6.
48. Marin C, Segura-Egea JJ, Martinez-Sahuquillo A, et al. Correlation between infant birth weight and mother's periodontal status. J Clin Periodontol 2005;32: 299–304.
49. Bosnjak A, Relja T, Vucicevic-Boras V, et al. Pre-term delivery and periodontal disease: a case-control study from Croatia. J Clin Periodontol 2006;33:710–6.
50. US Department of Health, Human Services. Oral health—healthy people. Washington, DC: US Department of Health and Human Services; 2010. p. 2009.
51. Centers for Disease Control, Prevention. National diabetes fact sheet: national estimates and general information on diabetes and prediabetes in the United States. Atlanta (GA): Centers for Disease Control and Prevention; 2011.
52. Schmandt RE, Iglesias DA, Na Co N, et al. Understanding obesity and endometrial cancer risk: opportunities for prevention. Am J Obstet Gynecol 2011;12:518–25.
53. Flegal KM, Graubard BI, Williamson DF, et al. Cause-specific excess deaths associated with underweight, overweight, and obesity. JAMA 2007;298: 2028–37.
54. Narayan KM, Boyle JP, Thompson TJ, et al. Lifetime risk for diabetes mellitus in the United States. JAMA 2003;290:1884–90.

55. Taylor GW, Borgnakke WS. Periodontal disease: associations with diabetes, glycemic control and complications. Oral Dis 2008;14:191–203.
56. Preshaw PM, Foster N, Taylor JJ. Cross-susceptibility between periodontal disease and type 2 diabetes mellitus: an immunobiological perspective. Periodontol 2000 2007;45:138–57.
57. Salvi GE, Carollo-Bittel B, Lang NP. Effects of diabetes mellitus on periodontal and peri-implant conditions: update on associations and risks. J Clin Periodontol 2008;35:398–409.
58. Skamagas M, Breen TL, LeRoith D. Update on diabetes mellitus: prevention, treatment, and association with oral diseases. Oral Dis 2008;14(2):105–14.
59. Gurav A, Jadhav V. Periodontitis and risk of diabetes mellitus. J Diabetes 2011; 3:21–8.
60. Emrich LJ, Shlossman M, Genco RJ. Periodontal disease in non-insulin-dependent diabetes mellitus. J Periodontol 1991;62:123–31.
61. Shlossman M, Knowler W, Pettitt D, et al. Type 2 diabetes mellitus and periodontal disease. J Am Dent Assoc 1990;121:532–6.
62. Nelson RG, Shlossman M, Budding LM, et al. Periodontal disease and NIDDM in Pima Indians. Diabetes Care 1990;13:836–40.
63. Nishimura F, Takahashi K, Kurihara M, et al. Periodontal disease as a complication of diabetes mellitus. J Periodontol 1998;3:20–9.
64. Novaes AB Jr, Gutierrez FG, Novaes AB. Periodontal disease progression in Type II non-insulin-dependent diabetes mellitus patients (NIDDM). Part I—Probing pocket depth and clinical attachment. Braz Dent J 1996;7(2):65–73.
65. Oliver R, Tervonen T. Periodontitis and tooth loss: comparing diabetics with the general population. J Am Dent Assoc 1993;124:71.
66. Jansson H, Lindholm E, Lindh C, et al. Type 2 diabetes and risk for periodontal disease: a role for dental health awareness. J Clin Periodontol 2006;33:408–14.
67. Grossi SG, Zambon JJ, Ho AW, et al. Assessment of risk for periodontal disease. I. Risk indicators for attachment loss. J Periodontol 1994;65:260–7.
68. Albrecht M, Bánóczy J, Tamás G Jr. Dental and oral symptoms of diabetes mellitus. Community Dent Oral Epidemiol 1988;16:378–80.
69. Soysa NS, Samaranayake LP, Ellepola ANB. Diabetes mellitus as a contributory factor in oral candidosis. Diabet Med 2006;23:455–9.
70. Kawamura M, Fukuda S, Kawabata K, et al. Comparison of health behaviour and oral/medical conditions in non-insulin-dependent (type II) diabetics and non-diabetics. Aust Dent J 1998;43:315–20.
71. Rees TD. Periodontal management of the patient with diabetes mellitus. Periodontol 2000 2000;23:63–72.
72. Manfredi M, McCullough MJ, Vescovi P, et al. Update on diabetes mellitus and related oral diseases. Oral Dis 2004;10:187–200.
73. Cowie CC, Rust KF, Byrd-Holt DD, et al. Prevalence of diabetes and impaired fasting glucose in adults in the US population. Diabetes Care 2006;29:1263–8.
74. Tsai C, Hayes C, Taylor GW. Glycemic control of type 2 diabetes and severe periodontal disease in the US adult population. Community Dent Oral Epidemiol 2002;30:182–9.
75. Lim L, Tay F, Sum C, et al. Relationship between markers of metabolic control and inflammation on severity of periodontal disease in patients with diabetes mellitus. J Clin Periodontol 2007;34:118–23.
76. Collin HL, Niskanen L, Uusitupa M, et al. Oral symptoms and signs in elderly patients with type 2 diabetes mellitus. Oral Surg Oral Med Oral Pathol Oral Radiol Endod 2000;90:299–305.

77. Sreebny LM, Yu A, Green A, et al. Xerostomia in diabetes mellitus. Diabetes Care 1992;15:900–4.
78. Thorstensson H, Falk H, Hugoson A, et al. Some salivary factors in insulin-dependent diabetics. Acta Odontol Scand 1989;47:175–83.
79. Guggenheimer J, Moore PA, Rossie K, et al. Insulin-dependent diabetes mellitus and oral soft tissue pathologies. II. Prevalence and characteristics of Candida and candidal lesions. Oral Surg Oral Med Oral Pathol Oral Radiol Endod 2000;89:570–6.
80. Finney L, Finney M, Gonzalez-Campoy J. What the mouth has to say about diabetes. Careful examinations can avert serious complications. Postgrad Med 1997;102:117.
81. Lamey PJ, Darwazeh A, Frier B. Oral disorders associated with diabetes mellitus. Diabet Med 1992;9:410–6.
82. Janket SJ, Wightman A, Baird AE, et al. Does periodontal treatment improve glycemic control in diabetic patients? A Meta-analysis of Intervention Studies. J Dent Res 2005;84:1154–9.
83. Witt BJ, Roger VL. Sex differences in heart disease incidence and prevalence: implications for intervention. Expert Opin Pharmacother 2003;4:675–83.
84. Mattila KJ, Nieminen MS, Valtonen VV, et al. Association between dental health and acute myocardial infarction. BMJ 1989;298:779–81.
85. Offenbacher S. Periodontal diseases: pathogenesis. Ann Periodontol 1996;1: 821–78.
86. DeStefano F, Anda RF, Kahn HS, et al. Dental disease and risk of coronary heart disease and mortality. BMJ 1993;306:688–91.
87. Higashi Y, Goto C, Hidaka T, et al. Oral infection-inflammatory pathway, periodontitis, is a risk factor for endothelial dysfunction in patients with coronary artery disease. Atherosclerosis 2009;206:604–10.
88. Humphrey LL, Fu R, Buckley DI, et al. Periodontal disease and coronary heart disease incidence: a systematic review and meta-analysis. J Gen Intern Med 2008;23:2079–86.
89. Hung HC, Willett W, Merchant A, et al. Oral health and peripheral arterial disease. Circulation 2003;107:1152–7.
90. Morrison HI, Ellison LF, Taylor GW. Periodontal disease and risk of fatal coronary heart and cerebrovascular diseases. J Cardiovasc Risk 1999;6:7–11.
91. Willershausen B, Kasaj A, Willershausen I, et al. Association between chronic dental infection and acute myocardial infarction. J Endod 2009;35: 626–30.
92. Bahekar AA, Singh S, Saha S, et al. The prevalence and incidence of coronary heart disease is significantly increased in periodontitis: a meta-analysis. Am Heart J 2007;154:830–7.
93. Janket SJ, Baird AE, Chuang SK, et al. Meta-analysis of periodontal disease and risk of coronary heart disease and stroke. Oral Surg Oral Med Oral Pathol Oral Radiol Endod 2003;95:559–69.
94. Khader YS, Albashaireh ZS, Alomari MA. Periodontal diseases and the risk of coronary heart and cerebrovascular diseases: a meta-analysis. J Periodontol 2004;75:1046–53.
95. Meurman JH, Sanz M, Janket SJ. Oral health, atherosclerosis, and cardiovascular disease. Crit Rev Oral Biol Med 2004;15:403–13.
96. Mustapha IZ, Debrey S, Oladubu M, et al. Markers of systemic bacterial exposure in periodontal disease and cardiovascular disease risk: a systematic review and meta-analysis. J Periodontol 2007;78:2289–302.

97. Scannapieco FA, Bush RB, Paju S. Associations between periodontal disease and risk for atherosclerosis, cardiovascular disease, and stroke. A Systematic Review. Ann Periodontol 2003;8:38–53.
98. Beck JD, Eke P, Heiss G, et al. Periodontal disease and coronary heart disease: a reappraisal of the exposure. Circulation 2005;112:19–24.
99. Hujoel PP, Drangsholt M, Spiekerman C, et al. Periodontal disease and coronary heart disease risk. JAMA 2000;284:1406–10.
100. Joshipura KJ, Rimm EB, Douglass CW, et al. Poor oral health and coronary heart disease. J Dent Res 1996;75:1631–6.
101. Seymour GJ, Ford PJ, Cullinan MP, et al. Relationship between periodontal infections and systemic disease. Clin Microbiol Infect 2007;13(Suppl 4):3–10.
102. Manson JE, Colditz GA, Stampfer MJ, et al. A prospective study of obesity and risk of coronary heart disease in women. N Engl J Med 1990;322:882–9.
103. Little J, Falace D, Miller C, et al. Dental management of the medically compromised patient. St Louis (MO): Mosby; 1997.
104. Bartlett D. Intrinsic causes of erosion. Monogr Oral Sci 2006;20:119–39.
105. Al Habashneh R, Guthmiller JM, Levy S, et al. Factors related to utilization of dental services during pregnancy. J Clin Periodontol 2005;32:815–21.
106. Christensen K, Gaist D, Jeune B, et al. A tooth per child? Lancet 1998;352:204.
107. Scheutz F, Baelum V, Matee M, et al. Motherhood and dental disease. Community Dent Health 2002;19:67–72.
108. Offenbacher S, Jared HL, O'Reilly PG, et al. Potential pathogenic mechanisms of periodontitis associated pregnancy complications. Ann Periodontol 1998;3: 233–50.
109. Jeffcoat M, Geurs N, Reddy M, et al. Periodontal infection and preterm birth: results of a prospective study. J Dent Res 2001;132(7):875–80.
110. Lopez NJ, Smith PC, Gutierrez J. Higher risk of preterm birth and low birth weight in women with periodontal disease. J Dent Res 2002;81:58–63.
111. Lopez NJ, Smith PC, Gutierrez J. Periodontal therapy may reduce the risk of preterm low birth weight in women with periodontal disease: a randomized controlled trial. J Periodontol 2002;73:911–24.
112. Offenbacher S, Lin D, Strauss R, et al. Effects of periodontal therapy during pregnancy on periodontal status, biologic parameters, and pregnancy outcomes: a pilot study. J Periodontol 2006;77:2011–24.
113. Moreu G, Tellez L, Gonzalez-Jaranay M. Relationship between maternal periodontal disease and low-birth-weight pre-term infants. J Clin Periodontol 2005;32:622–7.
114. Riche EL, Boggess KA, Lieff S, et al. Periodontal disease increases the risk of preterm delivery among preeclamptic women. Ann Periodontol 2002;7:95–101.
115. Mobeen N, Jehan I, Banday N, et al. Periodontal disease and adverse birth outcomes: a study from Pakistan. Am J Obstet Gynecol 2008;198:514.e1–8.
116. Boggess KA, Lieff S, Murtha AP, et al. Maternal periodontal disease is associated with an increased risk for preeclampsia. Obstet Gynecol 2003;101:227–31.
117. Canakci V, Canakci CF, Canakci H, et al. Periodontal disease as a risk factor for pre-eclampsia: a case control study. Aust N Z J Obstet Gynaecol 2004;44: 568–73.
118. Contreras A, Herrera JA, Soto JE, et al. Periodontitis is associated with preeclampsia in pregnant women. J Periodontol 2006;77:182–8.
119. Cota LO, Guimaraes AN, Costa JE, et al. Association between maternal periodontitis and an increased risk of preeclampsia. J Periodontol 2006;77: 2063–9.

120. Oettinger-Barak O, Barak S, Ohel G, et al. Severe pregnancy complication (preeclampsia) is associated with greater periodontal destruction. J Periodontol 2005;76:134–7.
121. Boggess KA, Beck JD, Murtha AP, et al. Maternal periodontal disease in early pregnancy and risk for a small-for-gestational-age infant. Am J Obstet Gynecol 2006;194:1316–22.
122. Pitiphat W, Joshipura KJ, Gillman MW, et al. Maternal periodontitis and adverse pregnancy outcomes. Community Dent Oral Epidemiol 2008;36:3–11.
123. Xiong X, Buekens P, Vastardis S, et al. Periodontal disease and gestational diabetes mellitus. Am J Obstet Gynecol 2006;195:1086–9.
124. Xiong X, Elkind-Hirsch KE, Vastardis S, et al. Periodontal disease is associated with gestational diabetes mellitus: a case-control study. J Periodontol 2009;80:1742–9.
125. Khader Y, Ta'ani Q. Periodontal diseases and the risk of preterm birth and low birthweight: a meta-analysis. J Periodontol 2005;76:161–5.
126. Vergnes JN, Sixou M. Preterm low birth weight and maternal periodontal status: a meta-analysis. Am J Obstet Gynecol 2007;196:135.e1–7.
127. Xiong X, Buekens P, Fraser WD, et al. Periodontal disease and adverse pregnancy outcomes: a systematic review. BJOG 2006;113:135–43.
128. Wimmer G, Pihlstrom BL. A critical assessment of adverse pregnancy outcome and periodontal disease. J Clin Periodontol 2008;35:380–97.
129. Polyzos NP, Polyzos IP, Mauri D, et al. Effect of periodontal disease treatment during pregnancy on preterm birth incidence: a metaanalysis of randomized trials. Am J Obstet Gynecol 2009;200:225–32.
130. Polyzos NP, Polyzos IP, Zavos A, et al. Obstetric outcomes after treatment of periodontal disease during pregnancy: systematic review and meta-analysis. BMJ 2010;341:c7017.
131. Scannapieco FA, Bush RB, Paju S. Periodontal disease as a risk factor for adverse pregnancy outcomes. A systematic review. Ann Periodontol 2003;8:70–8.
132. Genco RJ, Grossi SG. Is estrogen deficiency a risk factor for periodontal disease? Compend Contin Educ Dent Suppl 1998;(22):S23–9.
133. Tezal M, Wactawski-Wende J, Grossi SG, et al. The relationship between bone mineral density and periodontitis in postmenopausal women. J Periodontol 2000;71:1492–8.
134. Jeffcoat MK, Lewis CE, Reddy MS, et al. Post-menopausal bone loss and its relationship to oral bone loss. Periodontol 2000 2000;23:94–102.
135. Buencamino MC, Palomo L, Thacker HL. How menopause affects oral health, and what we can do about it. Cleve Clin J Med 2009;76:467–75.
136. Castro LC, Avina RL. Maternal obesity and pregnancy outcomes. Curr Opin Obstet Gynecol 2002;14:601–6.
137. Kumari AS. Pregnancy outcome in women with morbid obesity. Int J Gynaecol Obstet 2001;73:101–7.
138. Baeten J, Bukusi E, Lambe M. Pregnancy complications and outcomes among overweight and obese nulliparous women. Am J Public Health 2001;91:436–40.
139. Sebire NJ, Jolly M, Harris JP, et al. Maternal obesity and pregnancy outcome: a study of 287,213 pregnancies in London. Int J Obes Relat Metab Disord 2001;25:1175–82.
140. Michlin R, Oettinger M, Odeh M, et al. Maternal obesity and pregnancy outcome. Isr Med Assoc J 2000;2:10–3.
141. Weiss JL, Malone FD, Emig D, et al. Obesity, obstetric complications and cesarean delivery rate–a population-based screening study. Am J Obstet Gynecol 2004;190:1091–7.

142. Robinson HE, O'Connell CM, Joseph KS, et al. Maternal outcomes in pregnancies complicated by obesity. Obstet Gynecol 2005;106:1357–64.
143. Wall PD, Deucy EE, Glantz JC, et al. Vertical skin incisions and wound complications in the obese parturient. Obstet Gynecol 2003;102:952–6.
144. Bays RA, Weinstein RS. Systemic bone disease in patients with mandibular atrophy. J Oral Maxillofac Surg 1982;40:270–2.
145. Bras J. Mandibular atrophy and metabolic bone loss. Int Dent J 1990;40:298–302.
146. Jeffcoat MK, Chesnut CH 3rd. Systemic osteoporosis and oral bone loss: evidence shows increased risk factors. J Am Dent Assoc 1993;124:49–56.
147. Payne JB, Reinhardt RA, Nummikoski PV, et al. Longitudinal alveolar bone loss in postmenopausal osteoporotic/osteopenic women. Osteoporos Int 1999;10:34–40.
148. von Wowern N, Klausen B, Kollerup G. Osteoporosis: a risk factor in periodontal disease. J Periodontol 1994;65:1134–8.
149. Hart DJ, Spector TD. The relationship of obesity, fat distribution and osteoarthritis in women in the general population: the Chingford Study. J Rheumatol 1993;20:331–5.
150. Ruggiero SL, Mehrotra B, Rosenberg TJ, et al. Osteonecrosis of the jaws associated with the use of bisphosphonates: a review of 63 cases. J Oral Maxillofac Surg 2004;62:527–34.
151. Amar S, Chung KM. Influence of hormonal variation on the periodontium in women. Periodontol 2000 1994;6:79–87.
152. Cobb KL, Bachrach LK, Greendale G, et al. Disordered eating, menstrual irregularity, and bone mineral density in female runners. Med Sci Sports Exerc 2003;35:711–9.
153. Powers PS. Osteoporosis and eating disorders. J Pediatr Adolesc Gynecol 1999;12:51–7.
154. Misra M. Long-term skeletal effects of eating disorders with onset in adolescence. Ann N Y Acad Sci 2008;1135:212–8.
155. Grocholewicz K, Bohatyrewicz A. Oral health and bone mineral density in postmenopausal women. Arch Oral Biol 2012;57:245–51.
156. Neumark-Sztainer D, Falkner N, Story M, et al. Weight-teasing among adolescents: correlations with weight status and disordered eating behaviors. Int J Obes 2002;26:123–31.
157. Striegel-Moore RH, Silberstein LR, Frensch P, et al. A prospective study of disordered eating among college students. Int J Eat Disord 1989;8:499–509.
158. Castonguay LG, Eldredge KL, Agras WS. Binge eating disorder: Current state and future directions. Clin Psychol Rev 1995;15:865–90.
159. Hoek HW, van Hoeken D. Review of the prevalence and incidence of eating disorders. Int J Eat Disord 2003;34:383–96.
160. Hoek HW. Incidence, prevalence and mortality of anorexia nervosa and other eating disorders. Curr Opin Psychiatry 2006;19:389–94.
161. Hudson JI, Hiripi E, Pope HG, et al. The prevalence and correlates of eating disorders in the national comorbidity survey replication. Biol Psychiatry 2007;61:348–58.
162. Bulik CM, Sullivan PF, Carter FA, et al. Initial manifestations of disordered eating behavior: dieting versus binging. Int J Eat Disord 1997;22:195–201.
163. Haines J, Neumark-Sztainer D. Prevention of obesity and eating disorders: a consideration of shared risk factors. Health Educ Res 2006;21:770–82.
164. Field A, Camargo C, Taylor C, et al. Relation of peer and media influences to the development of purging behaviors among preadolescent and adolescent girls. Arch Pediatr Adolesc Med 1999;153:1184.

165. Killen J, Taylor C, Hayward C, et al. Weight concerns influence the development of eating disorders: a 4-year prospective study. J Consult Clin Psychol 1996;64:936.

166. Stice E. A prospective test of the dual pathway model of bulimic pathology: mediating effects of dieting and negative affect. J Abnorm Psychol 2001;110:124.

167. Santonastaso P, Friederici S, Favaro A. Full and partial syndromes in eating disorders: a 1-year prospective study of risk factors among female students. Psychopathology 1999;32:50–6.

168. Lo Russo L, Campisi G, Fede OD, et al. Oral manifestations of eating disorders: a critical review. Oral Dis 2008;14:479–84.

169. Grilo CM, White MA, Masheb RM. DSM-IV psychiatric disorder comorbidity and its correlates in binge eating disorder. Int J Eat Disord 2009;42:228–34.

170. Milosevic A, Slade PD. The Orodental status of anorexics and bulimis. Br Dent J 1989;167:66–7.

171. Robb ND, Smith BG, Geidrys-Leeper E. The distribution of erosion in the dentitions of patients with eating disorders. Br Dent J 1995;178:171–5.

172. Johansson A, Norring C, Unell L, et al. Eating disorders and oral health: a matched case-control study. Eur J Oral Sci 2012;120(1):61–8.

173. Pereira R, Alvarenga M. Disordered eating: identifying, treating, preventing, and differentiating it from eating disorders. Diabetes Spectrum 2007;20:141–8.

174. Ackard DM, Fulkerson JA, Neumark-Sztainer D. Prevalence and utility of DSM-IV eating disorder diagnostic criteria among youth. Int J Eat Disord 2007;40:409–17.

175. Boutelle K, Neumark-Sztainer D, Story M, et al. Weight control behaviors among obese, overweight, and nonoverweight adolescents. J Pediatr Psychol 2002;27:531–40.

176. Fairburn CG, Welch SL, Doll HA, et al. Risk factors for bulimia nervosa: a community-based case-control study. Arch Gen Psychiatry 1997;54:509–17.

177. Neumark-Sztainer D, Wall M, Guo J, et al. Obesity, disordered eating, and eating disorders in a longitudinal study of adolescents: how do dieters fare 5 years later? J Am Diet Assoc 2006;106:559–68.

178. Johansson AK, Nohlert E, Johansson A, et al. Dentists and eating disorders–knowledge, attitudes, management and experience. Swed Dent J 2009;33(1):1–9.

179. Willumsen T, Graugaard PK. Dental fear, regularity of dental attendance and subjective evaluation of dental erosion in women with eating disorders. Eur J Oral Sci 2005;113(4):297–302.

180. DeBate RD, Plichta SB, Tedesco LA, et al. Integration of oral health care and mental health services: dental hygienists' readiness and capacity for secondary prevention of eating disorders. J Behav Health Serv Res 2006;33:113–25.

181. Satcher D. Oral health in America: a report of the surgeon general. 2000. Available at: http://www.surgeongeneral.gov/library/reports/oralhealth/index.html. Accessed February 28, 2013.

182. US Department of Health and Human Services. Oral health—healthy people 2020. Available at: http://www.healthypeople.gov/2020/topicsobjectives2020/overview.aspx?topicid=32. Accessed October 15, 2012.

183. US Department of Health and Human Services. Promoting and Enhancing the Oral Health of the Public. 2010. Available at: http://www.hrsa.gov/publichealth/clinical/oralhealth/hhsinitiative.pdf. Accessed October 15, 2012.

184. Johnston LD. Soft drink availability, contracts, and revenues in American secondary schools. Am J Prev Med 2007;33(4):209.

185. Turner LL. Wide availability of high-calorie beverages in US elementary schools. Arch Pediatr Adolesc Med 2011;165(3):223.

186. Stallings V. Nutrition standards for foods in schools: leading the way toward healthier youth. Washington, DC: National Academies Press; 2007.
187. Wiecha JJ. School vending machine use and fast-food restaurant use are associated with sugar-sweetened beverage intake in youth. J Am Diet Assoc 2006; 106:1624–30.
188. Cullen KK. Improving the school food environment: results from a pilot study in middle schools. J Am Diet Assoc 2007;107(3):484–9.
189. Wootan MG, et al. State school foods report card 2007. Center for science in the public interest. Available at: http://www.cspinet.org/2007schoolreport.pdf. Accessed October 15, 2012.
190. Taber DD. Banning all sugar-sweetened beverages in middle schools: reduction of in-school access and purchasing but not overall consumption. Arch Pediatr Adolesc Med 2012;166(3):256–62.
191. Farley T. The role of government in preventing excess calorie consumption: the example of New York City. JAMA 2012;308(11):1093.
192. Alcorn T. Redefining public health in New York City. Lancet 2012;379(9831): 2037–8.
193. Greenberg BL, Glick M, Frantsve-Hawley J, et al. Dentists' attitudes toward chairside screening for medical conditions. J Am Dent Assoc 2010;141:52–6.
194. Esmeili T, Ellison J, Walsh MM. Dentists' attitudes and practices related to diabetes in the dental setting. J Public Health Dent 2010;70:108–14.
195. American Dietetic Association. Position of the American Dietetic Association: oral health and nutrition. J Am Diet Assoc 2007;107:1418–28.
196. Hornick B. Diet and nutrition: implications for oral health. J Dent Hyg 2002;76: 67–82.
197. Hazelton L, Faine M. Diagnosis and dental management of eating disorder patients. Int J Prosthodont 1996;9:65–72.
198. Sandstead H, Koehn C, Sessions S. Enlargement of the parotid gland in malnutrition. Am J Clin Nutr 1955;3:198–214.
199. Mandel L, Kaynar A. Bulimia and parotid swelling: a review and case report. J Oral Maxillofac Surg 1992;50:1122–5.
200. Mandel L, Surattanont F. Bilateral parotid swelling: a review. Oral Surg Oral Med Oral Pathol Oral Radiol Endod 2002;93:221–37.
201. Reamy B, Derby R, Bunt C. Common tongue conditions in primary care. Am Fam Physician 2010;81:627–34.
202. Tyler I, Wiseman M, Crawford R, et al. Cutaneous manifestations of eating disorders. J Cutan Med Surg 2002;6:345–53.
203. Strumia R. Dermatologic signs in patients with eating disorders. Am J Clin Dermatol 2005;6:165–73.
204. Strumia R. Skin signs in anorexia nervosa. Dermatoendocrinol 2009;1:268–70.
205. Neiva R, Steigenga J, Al-Shammari K, et al. Effects of specific nutrients on periodontal disease onset, progression and treatment. J Clin Periodontol 2003;30: 579–89.
206. Lundgren J, Allison K, Crow S, et al. Prevalence of the night eating syndrome in a pyschiatric population. Am J Psychiatry 2006;163:156–8.
207. Farah C, Lynch N, McCullough M. Oral fungal infections: an update for the general practitioner. Aust Dent J 2010;55:48–54.
208. Cashman M, Sloan S. Nutrition and nail disease. Clin Dermatol 2010;28:420–5.
209. Dynesen A, Bardow A, Petersson B, et al. Salivary changes and dental erosion in bulimia nervosa. Oral Surg Oral Med Oral Pathol Oral Radiol Endod 2008;106: 696–707.

210. Porto I, Andrade A, Montes M. Diagnosis and treatment of dentinal hypersensitivity. J Oral Sci 2009;51:323–32.
211. Mitchell J. Medical complications of bulimia nervosa. In: Brownell K, Fairburn C, editors. Eating disorders and obesity: a comprehensive handbook. New York: The Guilford Press; 1995. p. 271–8.
212. Ritchie C, Joshipura K, Hung H, et al. Nutrition as a mediator in the relatin betweeen oral and systemic disease: associations between specific measures of adult oral health and nutrition outcomes. Crit Rev Oral Biol Med 2002;13: 291–300.
213. Petersen P. The World Oral Health Report 2003: Continuous improvement of oral health in the 21st century–the approach of the WHO Global Oral Health Programme. Community Dent Oral Epidemiol 2003;31:3–24.
214. Naidoo S, Myburgh N. Nutrition, oral health and the young child. Matern Child Nutr 2007;3:312–21.
215. Touger-Decker R. Nutrition education of medical and dental students: innovation through curricular integration. Am J Clin Nutr 2004;79:198–203.
216. Fisher J, Fisher W. The information-motivation-behavioral skills model. In: DiClemente R, Crosby R, Kegler M, editors. Emerging Theories in Health Promotion Practice and Research: strategies for Improving Public Health. San Francisco (CA): Joseey-Bass; 2002. p. 40–7.
217. Dovey S. The ecology of medical care for children in the United States. Pediatrics 2003;111(5):1024.
218. Vann WF, Bouwens TJ, Braithwaithe AS, et al. The childhood obesity epidemic: a role for pediatric dentists? Pediatr Dent 2005;27:271–6.
219. American Academy of Pediatric Dentistry. Policy on dietary recommendations for infants, children, and adolescents. Reference Manual 2006-07. Pediatr Dent 2007;29(Suppl):45–6.
220. Medical Home Initiatives for Children With Special Needs Project Advisory Committee. American Academy of Pediatrics. The medical home. Pediatrics 2002;110(1 Pt 1):184–6.
221. Muller CF. Health care and gender. New York: Russell Sage Foundation; 1990. p. 99.

Pain and Temporomandibular Disorders: A Pharmaco-Gender Dilemma

Jeffry R. Shaefer, DDS, MS, MPH[a],*, Nicole Holland, DDS, MS[b],
Julia S. Whelan, MS[c], Ana Miriam Velly, DDS, MS, PhD[d,e]

KEYWORDS

- TMD • Gender • Pharmacokinetics • Orofacial pain • Bruxism

KEY POINTS

- Genetic studies indicate that the genetic contribution to the development of temporomandibular disorders (TMD) and orofacial pain is a small part of the overall risk for these disorders. However, gender is the most significant risk factor.
- Gender differences in pain thresholds, temporal summation, pain expectations, and somatic awareness can exist in patients with chronic TMD or orofacial pain.
- A better understanding of the mechanisms that contribute to the increased incidence and persistence of chronic pain in females is needed. Future research needs to elucidate the sex effects on factors that protect against developing pain or prevent pain from becoming debilitating pain.
- Gender-based treatments for TMD and orofacial pain treatment will evolve from the translational research stimulated from understanding the gender differences in pain modulation and perception.

INTRODUCTION

A clinician must understand the cause of the problem that they are treating. Does the patient fit into a normal pattern of presentation for the disorder in terms of age, sex, race, and so forth? Epker and colleagues'[1] assessment of masticatory muscle pain found that individuals with a pain intensity of 7 out of 10 or greater remain symptomatic despite treatment. Is this poor prognosis related to sex/gender differences or comorbidities? Is an innate pain-processing problem responsible? This article provides an evidence-based review of temporomandibular disorders (TMD) and pain in relation to:

1. Gender-based effects on musculoskeletal disorders
2. Pain-processing disorders leading to TMD and its comorbidities

[a] Department of Oral and Maxillofacial Surgery, Harvard School of Dental Medicine, 188 Longwood Avenue, Boston, MA 02215, USA; [b] Massachusetts General Hospital, MGH Dental Group, Suite 401, 165 Cambridge Street, Boston, MA 02043, USA; [c] Countway Library of Medicine, Harvard Medical School, 10 Shattuck Street, Boston MA 02115, USA; [d] Faculty of Dentistry, McGill University, 3755 Cote Ste Catherine, Suite H 4.16.2, Montreal, Quebec H3T 1E2, Canada; [e] Division of Clinical Epidemiology, Department of Dentistry, Jewish General Hospital, McGill University, 3755 Cote Ste Catherine, Suite H 4.16.2, Montreal, Quebec H3T 1E2, Canada
* Corresponding author. 4 Monument Circle, Hingham, MA 02043.
E-mail address: jeffry_shaefer@hsdm.harvard.edu

Dent Clin N Am 57 (2013) 233–262
http://dx.doi.org/10.1016/j.cden.2013.02.005
0011-8532/13/$ – see front matter © 2013 Elsevier Inc. All rights reserved.

3. Neuropathic pain affecting the trigeminal distribution: is this process gender specific?
4. Genetic influences on orofacial pain
5. Pharmacokinetics/pharmacodynamics of medications for orofacial pain

EPIDEMIOLOGY OF GENDER AND TMD/OROFACIAL PAIN

TMD is a collection of musculoskeletal disorders of the head and neck. Epidemiologic studies have shown that 40% to 70% of individuals can show signs and symptoms of TMD, whereas 80% have or have had facial pain.[2] Approximately 6% of these persons have symptoms severe enough to require treatment. Community studies show there is a 2:1 to 3:1 predilection in favor of women, and women seek care at an 8:1 ratio over men. The pain characteristics of men who present for treatment are similar to women in treatment.[3,4]

Gender Differences in Pain

The pain field has moved from debating whether sex differences in pain exist to recognizing the importance of these differences (**Table 1**). Attention is now directed toward understanding (1) which conditions lead to the sex and gender difference, (2) which mechanisms are responsible, and (3) should these differences inform clinical management of pain.[5–7]

Shinal and Fillingim's study[2] of gender differences in orofacial pain states "Orofacial pain refers to a large group of disorders, including TMDs, headaches, neuralgia, pain arising from dental or mucosal origins such as burning mouth syndrome (BMS), and idiopathic pain affecting 10% of adults and up to 50% of the elderly." There is a higher prevalence of clinical pain conditions in women than in men (see **Tables 3** and **4**).[8] The prevalence in females increases during the pubertal period.[9] Pereira and colleagues[10] assessed TMD in 508 12-year-olds (330 girls and 228 boys) and found that gender was related to TMD but menarche, malocclusion, and oral habits were not.

We consider the target group for TMD to be women of childbearing age (20–40 years old).[11] Other pain conditions that present as TMD comorbidities, such as migraine headaches, decline in prevalence after the fourth decade of life. Interstitial cystitis, joint pain, and fibromyalgia (FM) seem to persist until later ages.[6] The OPPERA (Orofacial Pain Prospective Evaluation and Risk Assessment) study (**Box 1**) identified which TMD risk factors influence the incidence of TMD/orofacial pain.[12]

Gender Differences in Musculoskeletal Function

Cause of TMD

Manfredini and colleagues' meta-analysis on TMD diagnosis had 3463 clinical subjects (female/male ratio 3.3), including 45.3% with muscle disorders (group [Gp] I diagnoses), 41.1% with DD (Gp II), and 30.1% with joint disorders (Gp III). Studies from the community studied 2491 individuals, with an overall 9.7% prevalence for Gp I, 11.4% for Gp IIa, and 2.6% for Gp IIIa diagnoses. Myofascial pain (MFP) was the most common diagnosis in TMD patient populations, and DD with reduction in community samples.[13]

The diagnostic discrepancy between a clinical and community TMD population could indicate the chronicity of muscle pain. It seems that joint sounds, which identify a community-based patient with TMD, often are asymptomatic, thus reserving the clinic visit for the female patient with chronic muscle pain. In contrast, recent OPPERA (see **Box 1**) data showed that the most common patient with TMD was age 60 years, female, and had osteoarthritis (OA) of the temporomandibular joint (TMJ). The

Table 1
Sex prevalence in pain disorders

Female Prevalence	Male Prevalence	No Sex Prevalence
Head and Neck Pain		
Migraine headache with aura	Migraine without aura	Acute tension headache
Chronic tension headache	Cluster headache	Cluster-tic syndrome
Postdural puncture headache	Posttraumatic headache	Jabs and jolts syndrome
Hemicrania continua	SUNCT syndrome	Secondary trigeminal neuralgia
Cervicogenic headache	Raeder paratrigeminal syndrome	Nervus intermedius neuralgia
Tic douloureux		Painful ophthalmoplegia
Temporomandibular joint disorder		Toothache caused by pulpitis
Occipital neuralgia		Cracked tooth syndrome
Periapical periodontitis and abscess		Dry socket
Atypical odontalgia		Vagus nerve neuralgia
Burning tongue		Stylohyoid process syndrome
Carotidynia		
Chronic paroxysmal hemicrania		
Temporal arteritis		
Generalized Syndromes		
Carpal tunnel syndrome	Ankylosing spondylitis	Thoracic outlet syndrome
Raynaud disease	Pancreatic disease	Familial Mediterranean fever
Chilblains	Lateral femoral cutaneous neuropathy	Acute herpes zoster
Causalgia	Postherpetic neuralgia	
Reflex sympathetic dystrophy	Hemophilic arthropathy	
Multiple sclerosis	Brachial plexus avulsion	
Rheumatoid arthritis	Lateral femoral cutaneous neuropathy	
Pain of psychological origin		
Visceral Pain		
Irritable bowel syndrome	Abdominal migraine	Esophageal motility disorders
Interstitial cystitis	Duodenal ulcer	Chronic gastric ulcer
Twelfth rib syndrome		Crohn disease
Gallbladder disease		Diverticular disease of colon
Chronic constipation		Carcinoma of the colon
Pyriformis syndrome		

Data from Berkley KJ. Sex differences in pain. Behav Brain Sci 1997;20:371–80; and Dao TT. Pain and gender. In: Lund J, Lavingne G, Dubner R, et al, editors. Orofacial pain: from basic science to clinical management. Chicago: Quintessence; 2001. p. 131.

> **Box 1**
> **The OPPERA study**
>
> Recently, the OPPERA study published its first findings from the baseline case-control study of the OPPERA program,[12] a series of studies designed to identify risk factors for the onset and persistence of painful TMD. Phenotypic and genotypic data were collected for TMD arthralgia, myalgia, or both cases (TMD) and people who were found not to have TMD (controls). The basic premise of OPPERA hypothesizes that clinical manifestation of TMD is driven by 2 global intermediate phenotypes: psychological distress and pain amplification, which are both influenced by genetic factors and environmental exposures.[6,12] Phenotypic data were collected across multiple domains: sociodemographic, clinical, psychosocial, pain sensitivity, and autonomic function risk factors were associated with increased odds of TMD. Genetic associations to biological pathways that may contribute to TMD pathophysiology were also identified. The strongest associations with TMD were measures related to bodily tenderness (eg, pressure pain thresholds) and salience of symptoms (eg, somatic awareness). Odds ratios (ORs) were smaller for measures of other phenotypes, to include mood, autonomic function, impaired temporal regulation of pain, and genetic variants (8 gene single nucleotide polymorphism [SNPs] had an allele frequency of 20% and OR at 1.5 or 0.6 [protective]).[12]

OPERRA investigators found that greater age, female gender, and white racial/ethnic group were all associated with increased odds of TMD, whereas higher educational achievement was just modestly associated.[12]

Chronic dull aching pain in TMD is associated with MFP and the presence of myofascial trigger points (MTrPs).[14] MTrPs develop through local afferent nerve sensitization from inflammatory mediators such as calcitonin gene-related peptide, bradykinin, and substance P.[14]

TMJ dysfunction

TMJ disk displacement (DD) occurs more often in women.[15] This has been attributed to gender differences in joint laxity,[10] type of collagen in TMJ retrodiskal tissues,[16] and increased intra-articular pressure.[17] Women have more hypermobility, and hypermobile TM joints have more DD, which leads to more TMJ dysfunction. A difference in collagen type exists in people with painful versus asymptomatic DD.[18]

Abubaker and colleagues[19] suggest that sex steroids influence the content of collagen and protein in the rat TMJ disk. Type III collagen, a more easily distorted type of collagen, was identified in the posterior disk attachments of humans. It has been speculated[20] that women have more type III collagen in the posterior TMJ disk attachment than men because women have more DD.

The association between joint laxity and TMD symptoms has been evaluated. Wang and colleagues[21] measured the function of multiple joints in 66 young female patients with TMJ internal derangement (ID) evident on magnetic resonance imaging (MRI) and in 30 age-matched female controls. The Beighton score (a measure of joint laxity) did not differentiate between individuals with and without TMJ ID. Perrini evaluated 32 asymptomatic volunteers and 62 symptomatic patients. Joint laxity was diagnosed if the Beighton test was greater than 4. Thirteen percent of controls and 37% of patients with TMD had joint laxity. There was no difference in the ratio of women compared with men who had TMD and an increased Beighton score.[22]

Yamada and colleagues[23] found decreased steepness in the articular eminence associated with DD without red, whereas a steeper posterior slope was associated with DD with red.

The significance of occlusal factors in cause of TMD will forever be debated. However, it is generally accepted that occlusal instability can lead to an unequal distribution of functional forces, thereby increasing the risk for arthralgia, myalgia, or increased trigeminal stimulation affecting neuropathic pain.

There is evidence that loss of posterior support can contribute to changes in TMJ structure and symptoms of TMD.[24–27] Localized pressure in the TMJ potentially affects its adaptive capabilities, leading to signs and symptoms of TMJ arthralgia.

Huber and Hall[28] found no significant gender differences in TMJ dysfunction and occlusal discrepancies. Warren and Fried[29] states that an equal number of men and women have joint morphology changes, but women still report having more pain, report pain more frequently, and seek care more than men. Is this related to hormonal factors?

Li and colleagues[30] found a role for sex hormones in the TMJD inflammatory cascade. Estradiol increased the synthesis of interleukin 1 and interleukin 6, but testosterone did not.[31] Estrogen coupled with changes in dietary loading affected cartilage degradation with increased TMJ pain and swelling in females, whereas testosterone increased inflammation-sparing plasma extravasation in males.[32,33] Rats treated with estrogen replacement experienced excitability of afferent innervations of the TMJ and masticatory muscles.[31] Gender differences in TMJ nociception were established further when levels of C-Fos, an early response transcription factor in neural tissue, in the brainstem were most increased after TMJ stimulation in female rats with high hormone levels.[34,35] Prolactin induces the release of estradiol in female mice to exacerbate collagen-induced arthritis.[31]

Human studies also support gender-based risk factors for TMJ arthralgia. Wiese and colleagues[36] found gender differences in the clinical presentation of TMD. Age, gender (OR $\geq$2.36), and coarse crepitus, but no pain-related variables, were associated with an increased risk of degenerative findings in TMJ tomograms. Cadaver studies indicate that more DD exists in women compared with men, that there are more estrogen receptors (ER) in the TMJs of women, and that cartilage and bone metabolism are affected by estrogen and progesterone.[31] Relaxin, a female hormone associated with joint laxity during pregnancy and the last days of the menstrual cycle, is believed to affect cartilage-degrading enzymes.[37] Prolactin was associated with accelerated condylysis in pregnant women.[38]

LaResche and colleagues[37] found that low estrogens levels during the menstrual cycle were related to TMD pain and TMD symptoms during pregnancy decreased at the end of pregnancy when hormone levels are high.[39] The influence of estrogen may depend on the particular type of ER that a woman expresses at the genetic level. Milam[37] proposes that ER polymorphisms may be associated with a higher prevalence of osteophoresis, rheumatoid arthritis (RA), and breast cancer in women.

A gender difference has not been established in polymorphisms affecting how types of collagen maintain articular surface integrity.

Parafunctional habits
Parafunctional habits are routinely considered a cause associated with TMD.[20,40] Michelotti and colleagues[41] identified female gender as a significant risk factor for MFP (OR = 3.8) but not arthralgia/arthritis/arthrosis when assessing the frequency of diurnal clenching or grinding and nail-biting habits.

Bruxism, defined as nonfunctional contact of the teeth, is considered by many to be the major cause triggering expression of orofacial disease in susceptible individuals. In the general population, the awareness of night-time bruxism is 8%, clenching 20%, with no evident gender differences; however, there does seem to be a genetic predisposition for nocturnal parafunctions such as sleep bruxism or restless legs syndrome.[42,43] The phenotypic variance of bruxism attributed to genetic influences is estimated to be 39% in males and 53% in females.[44]

TMJ arthridites

There is a genetic predisposition for the development of arthridites. Certain systemic arthridites affect men more than women (**Table 2**). Ankylosing spondylitis is twice as common in men as in women and presents in the third to fifth decades as lower back pain.[45]

Women are more likely than men to develop RA and suffer greater disability from it.[37] The reasons for this sexually dimorphic pattern of disease is unknown; however, women may be more susceptible to RA because of sex-specific differences in body composition and structure. Lupus affects women more than men, affecting 1.8 to 7.6 per 100,000 persons. In patients with systemic lupus erythematosus (SLE), 33% have TMJ symptoms, 22% clinical signs, and 11% radiographic signs of TMJ arthopathy.[45]

Hallert and colleagues[46] and Jawaheer and colleagues[47] found differences in disease progression and response to treatment in females compared with men in early versus chronic RA.

These results are consistent with the OPPERA findings of increased arthritis in older women, pointing to a gender difference in the disability associated with chronic TMJ symptoms from both types of arthritis.

Idiopathic condylar resorption

Those who manage adolescent females with idiopathic condylar resorption (ICR) recognize it as a gender disability. This problem is generally found in women in their

Table 2
Clinical conditions presenting with polyarthralgia that may accompany TMJ arthritis and screening evaluation for them

Illness/Condition	Screening	Appropriate Test
Rheumatic disease		
Systematic lupus erythematosus	Hx and Px	ANA, ESR
Rheumatoid arthritis	Hx and Px	RF, ESR
Sjögren syndrome	Hx and Px	ANA, ASSA, ASSB
Polymyositis	Hx and Px	CPK, EMG, Bx
Chronic infection/inflammation		
Tuberculosis	Hx and Px	PPD, ESR
Chronic syphilis	Hx and Px	VDRL, FTA
Bacterial endocarditis	Hx and Px	Blood culture, ESR
Lyme disease	Hx and Px	Lyme serology, PCR
Acquired immunodeficiency	Hx and Px	AIDS serology, CD_4
Breast implantation	Hx and Px	Possible serology
Endocrine disorders		
Hypothyroidism	Hx and Px	T_4, TSH, CPK
Hypopituitary	Hx and Px	Prolactin, others

Abbreviations: ANA, antinuclear antibody; ASSA, antibody to SSA; ASSB, antibody to SSB; Bx, biopsy of labial minor salivary glands; CD4, lymphocytes positive for the CD4 surface antigen; CPK, creatine phosphokinase; EMG, electromyography; ESR, erythrocyte sedimentation rate; FTA, fluorescent treponemal antibody; Hx and Px, insightful medical history and physical examination; PCR, polymerase chain reaction; PPD, delayed hypersensitivity skin test for tuberculosis; RF, rheumatoid factor; T4, thyroid hormone; TSH, thyroid-stimulating hormone; VDRL, serologic test for syphilis.

Data from Mense S, Simons D, Russel IJ, editors. Muscle pain: understanding its nature, diagnosis and treatment. Philadelphia: Lippincott Williams & Wilkins; 2001. p. 302; and Russell IJ. Fibromyalgia syndrome: approach to management. Bull Rheum Dis 1996;45(3):1–4.

second and third decades or as they reach puberty. A common initial sign of ICR is a changing bite, with the sensation of biting posteriorly. Retrognathism, clockwise rotation of the mandible, and an anterior open bite eventually develop. Risk factors include long-faced females with large mandibular plane angles, history of steroid use, RA, SLE, and sclerodema.[48] History of orthognathic surgery is also a risk factor; these surgical patients have a 7% to 12.2% chance of developing ICR, especially if it is advanced more than 10 mm.[48] Activation of ERs promoting TMJ arthritis may also be a risk factor.[45] Alternatively, some suggest that ICR is a problem of osteonecrosis caused by disruption of the blood supply to the condyle.[48] Previous orthodontic appliance therapy promoting a posterior force on the condyles may be an initiating factor.[20] Collaboration of the ICR diagnosis is aided by testing for RA factor (80% positive in patients with RA, 33% in patients with scleroderma).[48]

Summary: TMD musculoskeletal pain

TMJD and MFP both have complex causes with many risk factors. Most patients (80%) respond to nonoperative therapy targeting jaw or orofacial dysfunction. However, many (5%–20%) remain refractive to treatment. Does a gender-based problem explain the poor response? Recent studies suggest that the most important factors in identifying whether a person has a long-term problem with TMJ arthralgia or TMD MFP are psychosocial and affected by gender, such as catastrophizing, depression, anxiety, sleep quality, and pain-coping mechanisms.[12,40] Prolonged nociception in such patients could lead to peripheral or central nervous system (CNS) sensitization, resulting in pain perception long after the physical findings initiating the pain have disappeared.

GENDER DIFFERENCES IN PAIN PROCESSING

Widespread pain is a risk indicator for painful TMD, and predicts treatment response.[40,49]

Central Sensitivity Syndrome

Evidence points to the conclusion that MFP and TMJD are different but related disorders under the heading TMD. Recently, Woolf[50] reviewed research findings indicating that OA in the TMJ and other joints, rather than being primarily a degenerative disease associated with morphologic and functional factors, has characteristics of a central sensitization syndrome (CSS)[51] much like TMD muscular pain and its associated comorbidities.

Box 2 reviews TMD and orofacial pain comorbidities.

There are gender differences in peripheral pain perception. Riley and colleagues' meta-analysis[63] found that females have higher threshold and tolerance measures to pressure pain and electrical stimulation, but not to thermal stimuli. As for deep tissue pain, females did show a lower pain threshold in visceral pain tests measuring esophageal distension but not for mechanical thresholds in rectal stimulation studies.[6]

Gender Differences in Experimentally Induced Hyperalgesia

Studies of experimentally induced hyperalgesia have found robust sex differences.[6,64] In animals, the sex differences found in acute pain models depend on the type of animals tested.[6] This finding also applies to chronic pain models used in nerve ligation and arthritis studies.[6]

It is clear that more than morphologic differences exist between patients with and without TMD pain and that females commonly experience more pain than males.[65]

Box 2
Comorbidity, CSS, and TMD

Comorbidity is defined as the co-occurrence of 2 or more diseases at a rate higher than expected by chance.[52] A large population-based cross-sectional study, which included 189, 977 people, showed that 83% of 8964 individuals suffering from TMD pain reported a comorbid pain condition. Females were 1.4 times more likely than males to report at least comorbid pain conditions.[40] Hispanics and Afro-Americans report more comorbidities and have the greatest risk for developing chronic TMD.[53] Recent OPERRA data contradict this assumption, pointing toward a higher TMD prevalence in older white women rather than in minority populations.

Headaches/migraine are common among people with TMD and all 3 are more common in women.[40] Marcus[54] found that 14% of women with migraine have it only with their menses. Estrogen replacement therapy increases migraine and TMD prevalence by 30% and oral contraceptives also increase TMD and migraine prevalence.[39,40,53] Gupta and colleagues[55] reviewed the mechanisms through which female sex steroids might influence the trigeminal nociceptive pathways involved with migraine. There has been only 1 study evaluating the prevalence of various comorbid conditions with TMD at the same time.[53,56] Hoffman and colleagues' study[56] surveyed 1511 people with TMD and found that 70% had tension headaches, 60% had allergies, 50% had migraines, 50% had tinnitus, 40% had chronic fatigue syndrome, 25% had irritable bowel syndrome (IBS), and 20% had FM. MFP seems to have a higher rate of comorbidities than TMJD.

MFP can be more difficult to treat than TMJD,[57–61] and poor response to treatment is a consistent factor in other CSS disorders. Patients with MFP are known to have higher levels of somatization, depression, and anxiety than TMJD.[62] Such risk factors associated with MFP also have a higher prevalence in women than men.[40]

The fact that imaging findings of TMJ disease do not always correlate with symptoms points to a difference in how symptomatic and asymptomatic patients process pain. Chronically symptomatic patients have signs and symptoms consistent with a neuropathic pain presentation.

Neuropathic Pain

Neuropathic pain is pain that arises after injury to nerves or to sensory transmitting systems in the spinal cord and brain.[66] A key feature of neuropathic pain is the combination of sensory loss with hypersensitivity. After mandibular osteotomy, only 10% of patients with severe intraoperative nerve damage developed clinically significant neuropathic pain.[66,67] Nerve damage seems necessary for the initiation of postsurgical persistent pain, but is not always sufficient by itself to cause neuropathic pain development. There exists genetic susceptibility to the experience of neuropathic pain, elucidated by high pain levels and response to analgesics.[66] An example is postherpetic neuralgia preceded by severe zoster pain. Findings of several studies[66] show that women have higher postoperative pain than men. Cairns[68] offers evidence for sex-related differences in the response of afferent fibers and second-order trigeminal sensory neurons that innervate tissues associated with chronic pain conditions. Further, pain modulation by opioidergic receptor mechanisms seems dependent on gender.[68]

Tables 3 and **4** list gender-based differences in pain affecting ion channels and neurotransmitters, respectively.

There are indications that patients can be tested and then their susceptibility for chronic pain symptoms predicted. Studies have noted a positive correlation between preoperative pain response and degree of early postoperative pain. Preoperative

Table 3
Pain-related genes associated with ion channel and receptor function

Gene Name	Channel Type Affected	Phenotype	Locus
SCN9A	Voltage-gated Na⁺ channels	↑ Chronic pain in mixed cohort (sciatica, OA, pancreatitis, lumbar diskectomy, and phantom limb) ↑ Sensitivity for experimental pain	
OPRD1	Opioid receptor		1p35.3
OPRM1	Opioid receptor		6q25.2
ATP1A2	Na and K channels at plasma membrane	Maintains electrochemical gradient	1q23.3
MC1R	κ opioid receptor	Receptor protein for melanocyte stimulating hormone	16q24.3
KCNS1	Voltage-gated K⁺ channels	↑ Chronic pain in 5 cohorts (sciatica, lumbar pain, amputation, phantom limb) ↑ Sensitivity for experimental pain	
CACNA2D3	Voltage-gated Ca²⁺ channels	↑ Sensitivity to thermal pain ↑ Chronic postsurgical pain (diskogenic)	
CACNG2	Voltage-gated Ca²⁺ channels	↑ Chronic postsurgical pain (mastectomy)	
CACNA1A	Voltage-gated Ca channels	Mediates entry of Ca into neuronal tissue cells	19p13.13

Data from Oakley M, Vieira AR. The many faces of genetics contribution to temporomandibular joint disorder. Orthod Craniofac Res 2008;11:125–35; and Young EE, Lariviere WR, Belfer I. Genetic basis of pain variability: recent advances [review]. J Med Genet 2012;49:1–9.

catastrophizing has been correlated with acute but not postoperative pain intensity.[66] Pinto and colleagues[69] found that presurgical anxiety, emotional illness representation, and pain catastrophizing predicted persistent postsurgical pain 4 months after hysterectomy.

Wind-up pain
Postsurgical neuropathic pain that develops because of nerve damage is often attributed to receptor field spreading involving interneurons at the second-order neuron level in the CNS. The resulting CNS sensitization is referred to as wind-up pain. Wind-up is a transient upregulation, whereas central sensitization is a long-term upregulation, of postsynaptic response to a wider range of inputs.[6] Wind-up could be considered as a gateway to central sensitization.[6,12] The psychophysical correlate of wind-up is believed to be temporal summation (TS) of pain.[6,12] Like wind-up pain, TS requires 3 factors: C-fiber stimulation, short interstimulus intervals, and N-methyl-D-aspartate (NMDA) receptor activation.[70]

Greater TS was found in women with chronic pain conditions such as FM and TMD[6,12,71] and was observed even in asymptomatic body sites, pointing toward a central pain-processing problem.[6]

Stress reaction
Reaction to stress is credited with causing enhanced pain perception in many patients with chronic pain. The cause for this connection is dysfunction in the hypothalamus-pituitary-adrenal (HPA) axis.[72] Support for this concept exists: 40% to 70% of patients

Table 4
Pain-related genes associated with neurotransmitter systems and inflammation

Gene Name	Neurotransmitter System Affected	Phenotype	Locus
GCH1	Serotonin, dopamine, norepinephrine and epinephrine, NO	↓ Sensitivity to pain ↓ postsurgical pain	
SLC6A4	Serotonin	↑ Risk for CWP ↑ facilitation	17q11
ADRB2	Epinephrine	↑ Risk for CWP	5q33.1
HTR2A	Serotonin	↑ Risk for CWP ↑ postsurgical pain	13q14.2
PTGS2	Prostaglandin	↑, ↓ prostaglandin biosynthesis	1q25.2-q25.3
IL10	Cytokine	Immunoregulation and inflammation	1q32.1
IL1B	Cytokine	Mediates cell proliferation, differentiation	2q13
IL1RN	Cytokine	Inhibits interleukin 1A activity	2q13
IL1A	Cytokine	Immune response, inflammation, hematopoiesis	2q13
CYP19A1	Isoenzyme	Cholesterol, steroid metabolism and synthesis	15q21.1
CYP2D6	Isoenzyme	Cholesterol, steroid metabolism and synthesis	22q13.1
CCL7		Attracts macrophages	17q12
CCF3		Controls differentiation/function of granulocytes	17q21.1

Abbreviation: CWP, chronic widespread pain.
Data from Oakley M, Vieira AR. The many faces of genetics contribution to temporomandibular joint disorder. Orthod Craniofac Res 2008;11:125–35; and Young EE, Lariviere WR, Belfer I. Genetic basis of pain variability: recent advances [review]. J Med Genet 2012;49:1–9.

with chronic pain have a history of abuse. In these patients, emotions and thoughts create a physiologic response just like a real stressor. These deep-seated memories upregulate the autonomic nervous system, resulting in a state of hypervigilance with corresponding secretion of norepinephrine and epinephrine targeting nociceptors so as to heighten pain perception.[72] Studies examining the stress response in women with TMD and FM support the concept of a turned-on HPA axis in these patients.[73–75]

Martenson and colleagues[76] give a neural-based explanation for stress-induced hyperalgesia, whereas King and colleagues[57] show similar dysfunctional pain responses in patients with both TMD and IBS.

Milam[37] points toward a gender difference in stress response for the antinociception discrepancy between sexes. One difference involves an increase in nerve growth factor (NGF) levels in times of stress. NGF levels are associated with muscle, neuropathic, sympathetically maintained pain, and reflex sympathetic dystrophy pain. Females are more sensitive to NGF than males,[37,77] and the difference is believed to involve NGF and its primary tyrosine kinase A (TRKA) receptor. These receptors respond to estrogen. Women produce more TRKA receptors than men, which can account for women's increased sensitivity to NGF.[37]

Stress turns on the HPA axis,[78] which is sustained in patients with a history of physical abuse (predominantly females). Such prolonged HPA activity in times of stress has also been correlated to increased rates of obesity, depression, and memory loss.[79]

Pain processing in patients with TMD

Dysregulation of cortisol and adrenaline levels seems to be associated with heightened pain awareness[73,74] and limited pain modulation abilities[80] in individuals with TMD. This difference could be genetically programmed and in some cases gender based.[81] Through the human genome project, more than 13 million polymorphisms have been identified that can affect the absorption, distribution, metabolism, and excretion of enzymes and medications. Specifically, some women have an SNP, resulting in a 40% increase in metabolism of endogenous opioids. Also, the catechol-O-methyltransferase (COMT) enzyme, which affects catecholamine metabolism via adrenergic and dopaminergic pathways, is reduced 3 to 4 times in those persons with an SNP at the Val158Met COMT gene.[81] Zubieta and colleagues[75] showed that the pain response of individuals whose TMJs were injected with saline was related to levels of COMP activity. The relative risk for developing TMD after orthodontic treatment was associated to a variant of the COMT gene.[83,84] Diatchenko and colleagues[82] identified 3 genetic COMT variants (haplotypes). These investigators designated them as low pain sensitivity (LPS), average pain sensitivity, and high pain sensitivity. They found that the presence of a single LPS haplotype diminished the risk of developing myogenous TMJ disorder (MFP).

Others found an association between pain and epinephrine metabolism in response to a polymorphism at the β_2 adrenergic ADRB2 receptor.[67] Rogers found that differences in pain tolerance can explain women's overall response to treatment when compared with men, whereas catastrophizing seems important in understanding sex differences in daily pain levels.[85] Possibly, these studies explain why women with TMJD, TMD, or FM can have a heightened response to painful stimuli that indicates hyperalgesia; these studies also highlight the role that neuropathic pain mechanisms play in the development of chronic TMJ arthralgia and TMD.[86,87] In addition to understanding how nociception develops in TMJ arthritis and MFP of the masticatory muscles, development of neuropathic pain must be understood to diagnose and treat chronic TMD effectively.

PAIN MODULATION

Research indicates that a difference in gender-based coping strategies leads to a tendency to catastrophize and higher pain levels in women[6] Expectations of this pain response may explain why certain pain conditions persist until later ages.[40] Litt and colleagues[88] showed that low somatization scores, self-efficacy, and readiness for treatment in patients with TMD identified responders to treatment by cognitive behavioral training. The increased expectation of TMD pain in women could be attributed to the exaggerated TS of pain that has been documented for women with TMD, but not for men.[6,71] Fillingim and colleagues[12] found that somatic awareness was the key difference in women compared with men with chronic TMD. Such findings point to a physiologic (biological) cause, whereas the findings of increased catastrophizing, anxiety, and depression in women point to a psychosociologic explanation for higher numbers of women with TMD.[40]

Nonpharmacologic treatment studies have shown a potential for sex differences in response to TMD treatment,[6] pointing to psychological and social variables being more important than biological variables in explaining the variance in pain conditions between the sexes. Women have higher levels of anxiety than men, but some studies suggest that anxiety and pain may be more closely related to pain conditions in men than in women.[6] Although increased pain in women explains the higher numbers of women in clinical pain studies, there are indications that pain characteristics of men in treatment settings are not different.[3,4] Providers should approach both male and female patients presenting with chronic pain similarly. LeResche[65] proposes that the clinician's gender stereotypes, as well as the clinician's own gender, influence diagnostic and treatment decisions for chronic pain. She concludes that gender-specific treatment may be appropriate for certain orofacial pain presentations.

Placebo Response: the Endogenous Opioids

The difference in response to behavioral therapy between women and men may indicate a deficiency in the female endogenous opioid system and an inability to modulate pain.[6]

Rhudy and colleagues,[89] examining whether sex differences in emotion lead to sex differences in pain modulation, found that affective processes may not contribute to sex differences in pain in healthy individuals.

Davis and colleagues[90] looked at the disability in patients with chronic pain from RA. These investigators' findings support that the effect of stress on symptoms in men and women with chronic pain is similar, but better pacing of activity in women on good days may reduce their overall symptoms and disability. These findings can help clinicians target psychosocial factors to reduce patients' experience of fatigue.

Dysfunction of descending pain modulatory mechanisms can be measured via conditioned pain modulation (CPM). CPM refers to the inhibition of 1 source of pain by a second noxious stimulus (ie, the conditioning stimulus). Patients with FM, IBS, and TMD show reduced effect of CPM.[91] Females show greater reactivity to unpleasant stimuli and less reactivity to pleasant stimuli compared with males.[91]

Previous studies[91] have observed better placebo analgesia in males, and coupling expectations with active treatment can influence this response. Bjørkedal and Flaten[91] investigated sex differences in expectations and response to conditioning stimulation. Their results suggest that reduced inhibitory CPM is related to cognitive and emotional factors and not necessarily a dysfunction of descending inhibitory pathways.

Gender Differences in Opioid Efficacy

Animal studies reveal sex differences in stress-induced analgesia, which tests endogenous pain modulation.[2,92] Study of opioid response in humans is less consistent, indicating greater morphine analgesia in women and no sex difference in morphine analgesia.[2] More consistent sex differences are found with mixed action κ opioids.[92] Measuring postoperative pain after third molar extraction, Gear and colleagues[93] found that pentazocine and butorphanol produced better and longer-lasting analgesia among women versus men, but nalbuphine had antianalgesic effects in men.

Some studies[2,94] do not support that these sex differences in mixed action analgesics exist. Niesters and colleagues' 2011 meta-analysis of opioid efficacy in humans[94] examines this discrepancy. Reviewing 25 studies on acute and experimental pain, these investigators found that gender differences in opioid efficacy were limited to morphine, a natural opioid, and only when administered by patient-controlled anesthesia. These investigators' explanation for the differences in animal versus human studies is that, although genetics does affect analgesia in rodent studies, the variability in responses depends on the way nociception is tested (pain thresholds in animals vs opioid consumption in humans), age and the sex of the subjects, and type of opioid.[94] Niesters and colleagues also found that morphine was more potent in women but had a slower onset of action, and there was no sex difference in the pharmacokinetics of morphine. The slower onset of morphine in women caused greater analgesic effect in men directly after injection, despite greater morphine potency in women. Only at later times is the analgesic efficacy in women greater than that in men.[94] Sex differences in body mass index (BMI, calculated as weight in kilograms divided by the square of height in meters) can affect the volume of distribution (Vd) for lipophilic opioids, postponing their onset and prolonging their effect in women. In human studies, efficacy is determined via opioid consumption without reporting plasma levels of the opioids administered, leading to underestimating sex differences in opioid analgesia, because most studies involve healthy young women with low BMIs.[94]

Sex differences in the pharmacodynamics of opioids exist. In addition to increased potency, women report a higher incidence in opioid-induced emesis and respiratory depression.[94,95]

Niesters and colleagues observed that study duration has a significant influence on study outcome, a sign that opioid pharmacokinetics can play a significant role in the development of sex differences.

Most studies do not take into account possible sex differences in pharmacokinetics or pharmacodynamics of the tested opioid.[96] Knowledge of pharmacodynamic factors is critical for gender-based tailoring of opioid prescribing.[97]

The role of pain and the interaction of opioid analgesics with selective serotonin reuptake inhibitors (SSRIs) and NMDA inhibitors, which have been used to prevent opioid tolerance, need better understanding.[98] Snijdelaar and colleagues' study[99] shows promise in the therapeutic use of NMDA inhibitors, such as the noncompetitive antagonist amantadine, to prevent opioid tolerance and opioid-induced hyperesthesia.

Pharmacotherapeutics by Gender

Tanaka[100] summarized gender differences in pharmacokinetics involving the cytochrome P450 (CYP) isozymes. CYP3A4, responsible for the metabolism of more than 50% of therapeutic drugs, shows higher activity in women than in men, and its function is related to steroid hormone levels.

Drug metabolism in women is also affected by sex-related factors such as menopause, pregnancy, and menstruation, in addition to cigarette smoking, drug ingestion, and alcohol consumption.[100] Furthermore, women are affected by physiologic factors such as drug absorption, protein binding, and elimination. Thus, careful attention should be paid to the side effects and toxicity arising from sex differences in drug metabolism in clinical situations. The activity of several other CYP (CYP2C19, CYP2D6, CYP2E1) isozymes and the conjugation (glucuronidation) activity involved in drug metabolism may be higher in men than in women.[100] Specifically referring to medications used in orofacial pain management, enhanced medication clearance (metabolism and elimination) occurs in women with midazolam and methylprednisolone. Enhanced liver conjugation before kidney elimination occurs in males with acetaminophen and the benzodiazepines temazepam, and oxazepam. There seem to be pharmacokinetic gender differences in drug absorption, protein binding affecting Vd, and excretion.[101–103]

Although such differences can explain sex differences in drug efficacy, they best explain differences in side effects and patient compliance with medications.[100]

GENOMICS AND TMD

Research with animal studies and candidate gene testing in humans suggests that pain sensitivity and risk for chronic pain are complex polygenic traits. Oakley and Vieira[104] categorize the genetic contributions to TMD under pain perception, gender and ethnicity, proinflammatory cytokines, extracellular matrix breakdown, and syndromes. Referring to both pain perception and gender, genetic influences on COMT metabolism can explain as much as 30% of new TMD cases.[104] The application of the genome-wide association methodology offers a new tool for better understanding the genetic contribution to pain in the clinical patient. (**Fig. 1**(A, B) compares gene candidate testing and genome-wide association methodology techniques.) Young and colleagues'[105] review updates the most recent findings associating genetic variation with variability in pain and provides an overview of the candidate genes with the highest translational potential.

The high points of Young and colleagues' review are listed in **Tables 3** and **4**, depicting genes that affect neurotransmitter systems to determine how a pain message is sent or received and ion channel functions that change nerve excitability to augment or depress a pain message. **Table 5** lists pain syndrome phenotypes, whereas **Table 6** lists genotypes for differences in efficacy of analgesic medications. Palmer and colleagues[81] places these SNPs into 3 categories: pain-facilitating alleles, pain-protective alleles, and alleles related to anesthesia.

Gender-Based Treatment of TMD and Orofacial Pain

There has been great progress in associating genetic polymorphisms to musculoskeletal disorders such as FM and low back pain, but family-aggregation studies have not yet found a genetic influence on TMD.[83] TMD is a complex, multifactorial musculoskeletal disorder influenced by environmental factors on an array of prevalent genetic polymorphisms (SNPs). The interaction of these SNPs is best identified by looking at the risk of disease in subgroups with common allelic variants.[83]

Only 3 genetic variants show promise for tailored treatments based on genetic profiles.

The function of serotonin, a key neurotransmitter in modulation of pain, influences TMD and its comorbidities such as sleep disorders, headaches, fatigue, and depression; however, only 1 TMD study found a polymorphism at the human serotonin transporter gene promoter region (5HTTLPR) in its subjects.[83]

Tchivileya and colleagues[106] had success in treating patients with TMD with propranolol after genotyping them for COMT haplotypes affecting catecholamine physiology.

Most encouraging could be the potential for genetic profiling in identifying alleles for ERs. Possibly ER modulators such as raloxifene and tamoxifen used in breast cancer

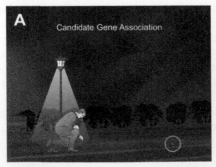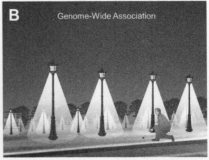

Fig. 1. Comparison of the nature of the restrictive candidate gene association (*A*) testing with that of the more productive genome-wide association (*B*) testing technique, which gives a better understanding of the effect of gender on TMD and orofacial pain. (*Courtesy of* Dr Francis Collins, National Institutes of Health.)

Table 5
Mendelian heritable pain conditions

Pain Syndrome	Gene Affected	Transmission	Gene Product Effect	Phenotype
HSAN-I[a]	A: *SPTLC1*	Dominant	Disrupted sphingolipid synthesis	Pain and heat loss
	C: *SPTLC2*	Dominant	Disrupted sphingolipid synthesis	Sensory loss
	D: *ATL1*	Dominant	Reduced GTPase activity; disrupted sensory neuron function	Sensory loss
	E: *DNMT1*	Dominant	Disrupted DNA methylation resulting in neurodegeneration	Sensory loss; hearing loss; early-onset dementia
Channelopathy-associated insensitivity to pain	*SCN9A*	Recessive	Loss of function in $Na_v1.7$ channel	Congenital insensitivity to pain without anhydrosis
Erythromelalgia	*SCN9A*	Dominant	Decreased threshold in $Na_v1.7$ channel	Chronic inflammation/burning pain
PEPD	*SCN9A*	Dominant	Impaired $Na_v1.7$ channel inactivation	Mandibular, ocular, and rectal pain
FHM-I	*CACNA1A*	Dominant	Increased $Na_v1.7$ channel inactivation at negative potentials	Migraine (with or without aura/hemiparesis) and cellular degeneration
FHM-II	*ATP1A2*	Dominant	Loss of function/reduced Na^+/K^+	Migraine (with or without aura/hemiparesis) adenosine triphosphatase activity
FHM-III	*SCN1A*	Dominant	Loss of $Na_v1.7$ subunit	Migraine (with or without aura/hemiparesis) neuronal hyperexcitability

Abbreviations: FHM, familial hemiplegic migraine (types I–III); HSAN, hereditary sensory and autonomic neuropathy (types I–V); PEPD, paroxysmal extreme pain disorder.

[a] Also referred to as hereditary sensory radicular neuropathy and familial syringomyelia.

Data from Young EE, Lariviere WR, Belfer I. Genetic basis of pain variability: recent advances [review]. J Med Genet 2012;49:1–9.

can be used to prevent gender-based functional TMJ disturbances or control estrogen-related modulation of TMJ arthralgia.[83]

Findings of an enhanced female response to ketamine, the NMDA receptor blocker, gives hope for a gender-based treatment of chronic TMJ arthralgia.[83] SSRIs are more effective for women than men for depression[107,108]; but it is not known if this difference occurs when SSRIs are used for pain. **Table 7** provides a review of gender-based drug interactions.

Boxes 3–5 provide treatment recommendations for pregnant and lactating patients.

Table 6
Example genotypes linked to individual differences in the metabolism, efficacy, and side effects of commonly used anesthetic agents

Drug Associated with Allele[a]	Gene	Allele	Effect
Diazepam	CYP2C19	G681A	Increased half-life, prolonged sedation, greater likelihood of unconsciousness
Midazolam	CYP3A4	A290G (*1B)	Reduced clearance of systematic (but not oral) midazolam
Midazolam	CYP3A5	A22893G (*3)	Reduced clearance of systematic (but not oral) midazolam
Morphine, morphine-6-glucuronide	μ-Opioid receptor	A118G	Reduced nausea, vomiting, sedation, drowsiness
Morphine	Uridine disphosphate glycoslytransferase	C-161T and C802T	More rapid glucuronidation
Codeine	CYP2D6	G1846A (*4) Deletion of gene (*5) 1707T>del (*6)	Slower conversion of codeine to morphine; reduction in analgesic effect (but not adverse effects)
Tramadol	CYP2D6	G1846A (*4) Deletion of gene (*5)	Slower conversion to O-demethytramadol and N-demethytramadol; greater need to rescue analgesics after surgery
Methadone	CYP2D6	G1846A (*4) 1707T>del (*6)	Slower metabolic clearance (although not consistently)
Celecoxib, naproxen, piroxicam, ibuprofen, flurbiprofen	CYP2D6	A1075C (*3)	Slower metabolism
Acetominophen	CYP2EI	c2	Accelerated elimination rate
Acetominophen	Tumor necrosis factor β	B2	Lower risk of encephalopathy in patients with acetaminophen-induced acute liver failure
Various NSAIDs	HLA-DRB1	*11	Higher risk of anaphylactoid reaction

Abbreviations: CYP, cytochrome P450; HLA, human leukocyte antigen; NSAID, nonsteroidal antiinflammatory drug; RYR1, rynodine receptor.

[a] Effects described as those of the variant allele compared with the wild-type allele for each polymorphism.

Data from Palmer SN, Gieseche NM, Body SC, et al. Pharmacogenetics of anesthetic and analgesic agents. Anesthesiology 2005;102(3):663–71.

Table 7
Gender-related drug pharmacokinetic and pharmacodynamic effects

Drug	Action	Result	Pathway	Reference
Antiepileptics				
Carbamazepine	Decreased level of contraceptive steroids (OC)	Breakthrough bleeding Ovulation	Rapid inducer of P450 system known to decrease levels of OC	Davis et al,[114] 2011
Lamotrigine (LTG) and oxcarbazepine (OXC)	During pregnancy, clearance of LTG/OXC is altered	Increase in seizures	Increased excretion explained by steroid induction of hepatic N-2 glucuronidation	Wegner et al,[115] 2010
Muscle Relaxants				
Tizanidine	"Any possible effect of gender and smoking is largely outweighed by individual variability in CYP1A2 activity due to genetic and environmental factors and in body weight. Careful dosing of tizanidine is warranted in small females, whereas male smokers can require higher than average doses."	Mean values of C_{max} (the peak plasma concentration) and $AUC_{0-\infty}$ (the area under plasma concentrations from 0 to infinity) were 30% and 34% higher in women than in men, and in 5 of the 18 women, the C_{max} of tizanidine was higher than in any men. However, the mean elimination $t_{1/2}$ of tizanidine was 9% shorter in the nonsmoking women than nonsmoking men	Men have more CYP isoenzymes, e.g., CYP1A2 and CYP2E1, but less CYP3A4. Differences in the membrane transport of exogenous compounds exist, e.g. increased excretion of pravastatin in males (SNP in hepatic uptake transporter organic anion transporting polypeptide 1B1). Women have a lower glomerular filtration rate	Backman et al,[116] 2008
Tizanidine	Effect of combined OCs on CYP1A2 activity (inhibition)	OCs containing ethinyl estradiol and gestodene increase the plasma concentrations of tizanidine	CYP1A2. Care should be exercised when tizanidine is prescribed to OC users	Granfors et al,[117] 2005

(continued on next page)

Table 7
(continued)

Drug	Action	Result	Pathway	Reference
Tocolytic agents (prevention of premature birth)	Pharmacologic agents used to treat preterm labor (review) Includes beta-adrenergic agonists, NSAIDS, calcium channel blockers, magnesium sulfate, oxytocin agonists	During pregnancy: oral absorption decreased due to delayed stomach emptying and decreased intestinal motility. The volume of distribution of drugs increased. Liver metabolic activity increased, renal filtration increased. Result: reduced plasma concentration and reduced half-life of most drugs in pregnant women	NSAIDS (indomethacin specifically) was the number 1 choice to prevent preterm delivery. But 100% placental transfer, 7-fold increase in fetal half-life, and premature closure of the ductus arteriosus; no longer used as a tocolytic agent	Tsatsaris, Cabrol et al,[118] 2004
NSAIDS				
Keterolac (low dose)	Gender was not really a factor in this study; all subjects were women			Bendixen et al,[119] 2010
Ibuprofen	Can cause hypersensitivity reaction. The highest incidence of liver reaction is seen in women. Women over 50 y of age are at higher risk than men	Hypersensitivity reaction and liver damage	Ibuprofen inhibits COX-1 and COX-2 by 50% Variability in CYP, CYP2C9, and CYP2C8 can decrease metabolism of NSAIDs	Nanau & Neuman,[120] 2010
Opioids				
Methadone	Rate of clearance of methadone during pregnancy changes	As pregnancy progresses, patients who are addicted may need smaller or larger doses	The induction effect of liver enzymes CYP3A4 and CYP2D6, typically noninducible, affects metabolism	Wolff et al,[121] 2005

Drug				Reference
Tramadol	Pharmacokinetics of tramadol and its metabolites		No significant gender differences in pharmacokinetics of tramadol	Ardakani & Rouini,[122] 2007
Sedatives and Hypnotics				
Triazolam	CYP450 3A		Gender differences in triazolam kinetics were not apparent. There were age differences	Greenblatt et al,[123] 2004
Triptans	Numerous kinetic parameters of triptans vary according to gender. C_{max} and $AUC_{0-\infty}$ of frovatriptan, naratriptan, rizatriptan, and zolmitriptan are greater in males due to higher bioavailability in females and total body clearance is greater in males	Nonpharmacokinetic factors of variability of response to triptans: Genetic Polymorphisms Receptor adaptation Fluctuation of migraine Prophylactic treatments Previous therapies Time of medication Severity of migraine attack	Wide variance in response to explain triptan efficacy	Ferrari et al,[124] 2011
Sumatriptan	Studied times to response and therapeutic threshold with either response or no response to sumatriptan	Wide variability in plasma concentrations after oral dose in both sexes. Also high variability with fast-disintegrating formulation	Intersubject variability in plasma concentration after subcutaneous use clinically nonsignificant	Ferrari et al,[125] 2008
Frovitriptan	Women oral contraceptive users had 26–68% higher C_{max} and AUC	Twice daily lower dose recommended to maintain therapeutic levels and to prevent menstrual migraine		Wade et al,[126] 2009

(continued on next page)

Table 7
(continued)

Drug	Action	Result	Pathway	Reference
SSRIs				
Duloxetine	CYP2D6 enzyme is involved in the metabolism of duloxetine. CYP1A2 activity is higher in men and smokers than in women and nonsmokers	Other CYP enzymes implicated. Tested CYP1A2 enzymes involved in duloxetine metabolism	Duloxetine did not clinically affect CYP1A2 levels; but coadministration of duloxetine with potent CYP1A2 inhibitors should be avoided	Lobo et al,[127] 2008
Duloxetine	Reduced stress, urinary incontinence in women	All subjects were women		McCormack & Keating,[128] 2004

Box 3
Treating the pregnant and lactating patient with medications

Several factors can affect the efficacy of medication in the pregnant patient, and pregnancy can intensify gender differences in pharmacotherapeutics.[100] In addition, fetal drug exposure must be taken into account.

Despite the limited and nongeneralizable data regarding appropriate dosing and treatment schedules in pregnant and nursing women, several guidelines are available to assist providers in choosing appropriate pharmacotherapies for women in the perinatal period.[109] The US Food and Drug Administration (FDA) has created a drug classification system for guidance in weighing the risks and benefits of prescribing medications for pregnant women (see **Box 4**). In addition, electronic databases such as Teratogen Information System (TERIS) and Reprotox enable providers to perform risk assessments of potential teratogenic exposures.[110,111] A common list of drugs used in dental settings and their FDA classifications can be found in **Box 5**.

The risk/benefit ratio of pharmacotherapy during pregnancy differs from that while breast-feeding and can be another source of confusion for clinicians. LactMed and DailyMed, databases created by the National Library of Medicine, are sources that can assist providers in prescribing safe and effective medications to nursing mothers.[112,113] When prescribing medications to lactating patients, one should use a systemic drug with a short half-life or have the patient take it just after breastfeeding.

Box 4
FDA pregnancy category definitions

Category	Definition
A	Adequate and well-controlled studies (AWC) in pregnant women have failed to demonstrate a risk to the fetus in the first trimester of pregnancy (and there is no evidence of a risk in later trimesters).
B	Animal reproduction studies have failed to demonstrate a risk to the fetus and there are no AWC studies in humans, AND the benefits from the use of the drug in pregnant women may be acceptable despite its potential risks. OR animal studies have not been conducted and there are no AWC studies in humans.
C	Animal reproduction studies have shown an adverse effect on the fetus, there are no AWC studies in humans, AND the benefits from the use of the drug in pregnant women may be acceptable despite its potential risks. OR animal studies have not been conducted and there are no AWC in humans.
D	There is positive evidence of human fetal risk based on adverse reaction data from investigational or marketing experience or studies in humans, BUT the potential benefits from the use of the drug in pregnant women may be acceptable despite its potential risks.
X	Studies in animal or humans have demonstrated fetal abnormalities OR there is positive evidence of fetal risk based on adverse reaction reports from investigational or marketing experience, or both, AND the risk of the use of the drug in pregnant women clearly outweighs any possible benefit.

Adapted from U.S. Food and Drug Administration; Federal Register 1980; 44:37434–67.

Box 5
Risk classification for use of medications during pregnancy

Drug	FDA Classification
Analgesic	
Acetaminophen	Over-the-counter oral form not formally categorized by the FDA; however, acetaminophen is considered safe for use during pregnancy[a]
Piroxicam	C
Indomethacin	C
Etodolac	C
Meperidine	C
Naproxen	C
Nabumetone	C
Diclofenac	C
Antibiotics	
Penicillin	B
Amoxicillin	B
Cephalexin	B
Clindamycin	B
Erythromycin	B
Tetracycline	D
Ciprofloxacin	C
Clarithromycin	C
Muscle Relaxants	
Baclofen	C
Cyclobenzaprine	B
Methocarbamol	C
Tizanadine	C
Benzodiazepines	
Triazolam	X
Clonazepam	D
Temazepam	X
Diazepam	D
Anticonvulsants	
Gabapentin	C
Pregabalin	C
Oxcarbazepine	C
Carbamazepine	D
Topiramate	D
Opioids	
Codeine	C
Demerol (see analgesics)	
Fentanyl	C
Hydrocodone (+acetaminophen)	C
Ketamine	Not formally categorized by the FDA
Methadone	C
Morphine	C
Oxycodone	B
Oxycodone (+acetominophen)	C
Promethazine	C
Buprenorphine + naloxone	C
Tramadol	C
Triptans	
Sumatriptan	C
Rizatriptan	C
Zolmitriptan	C
Antidepressants	
Amitriptyline	C

Duloxetine	C
Doxepin	Not formally categorized by the FDA
Nortriptyline	Not formally categorized by the FDA
Trazodone	C
Local Anesthetics	
Articaine + epinephrine	C
Lidocaine	B
Bupivacaine + epinephrine	C
Mepivacaine	C
Prilocaine	B
Miscellaneous	
Chlorhexidine mouth rinse	B
Xylitol	Undetermined
Capsaicin	Not formally categorized by the FDA

[a] DailyMed Citation.
Data from Feldkamp ML, Meyer RE, Krikov S, et al. Acetaminophen use in pregnancy and risk of birth defects: findings from the National Birth Defects Prevention Study. Obstet Gynecol 2010;115(1):109–15.

SUMMARY

Genetic studies indicate that the genetic contribution to the development of TMD and orofacial pain is a small part of the overall risk for these disorders. However, gender is the single biggest risk factor.[5,6,65] It must be realized that gender differences in pain thresholds, TS, pain expectations, and somatic awareness can exist in patients with chronic TMD or orofacial pain.

A better understanding of the mechanisms that contribute to the increased incidence and persistence of chronic pain in females is needed, and this knowledge can then be used to improve pain management for both sexes. Future research needs to elucidate the sex effects on factors that protect against developing pain or prevent pain from becoming debilitating pain. Also, it is recommended that investigators performing medication trials report outcomes for each sex.[6] Further understanding is also needed of the impact of pain and trauma on infants, children, and adolescents and of pain sensitivity and response to reinjury in adulthood.[6,66]

Clinical interventions are proposed as the first phase of translational research to develop gender-based treatments for the management of TMD and orofacial pain. Outcomes will be measured from the implementation of the evidenced-based guidelines that will result from our research.

REFERENCES

1. Epker J, Gatchel RJ, Ellis E III. A model for predicting chronic TMD: practical application in clinical settings. J Am Dent Assoc 1999;130:1470–5.
2. Shinal RM, Fillingim RB. Overview of orofacial pain: epidemiology and gender differences. Dent Clin North Am 2007;51:1–18.
3. Bush FM, Harkins SW, Harrington WG, et al. Analysis of gender effects on pain perception and symptom presentation in temporomandibular pain. Pain 1993; 53:73–80.
4. Robinson ME, Gagnon CM, Riley JL, et al. Altering gender role expectations: effects on pain tolerance, pain threshold, and pain ratings. J Pain 2003;4:284–8.

5. Dao TT. Pain and gender. In: Lund J, Lavingne G, Dubner R, et al, editors. Orofacial pain; from basic science to clinical management. Chicago: Quintessence; 2001. p. 129–38.

6. Greespan JD, Craft RM, LeResche L, et al, the Consensus Working Group of the Sex, Gender, and Pain SIG of the IASP. Studying sex and gender differences in pain and analgesia: a consensus report. Pain 2007;132(Suppl 1): S26–45.

7. Becker JB, Arnold AP, Berkley KJ, et al. Strategies and methods for research on sex differences in brain and behavior. Endocrinology 2005;146:1650–73.

8. Berkley KJ. Sex differences in pain. Behav Brain Sci 1997;20:371–80.

9. LeResche L, Mancl LA, Drangsholt MT, et al. Relationship of pain and symptoms to pubertal development in adolescents. Pain 2005;118:201–9.

10. Pereira LJ, Pereira-Cenci T, Del Bel Cury AA, et al. Risk indicators of temporomandibular disorder incidences in early adolescence. Pediatr Dent 2010; 32(4):324–8.

11. Drangsholt MT, LeResche L. Temporomandibular disorder pain. In: Crombie IK, Croft PR, Linton SJ, et al, editors. Epidemiology of pain. Seattle (WA): IASP Press; 1999. p. 203–33.

12. Fillingim RB, Slade GD, Diatchenko L, et al. Summary of findings from the OPPERA baseline case-control study: implications and future directions. J Pain 2011;12(Suppl 11):T102–7.

13. Manfredini D, Guarda-Nardini L, Winocur E, et al. Research diagnostic criteria for temporomandibular disorders: a systematic review of axis I epidemiologic findings. Oral Surg Oral Med Oral Pathol Oral Radiol Endod 2011;112(4): 453–62.

14. Shah JP, Phillips TM, Danoff JV, et al. An in vivo microanalytical technique for measuring the local biochemical milieu of human skeletal muscle. J Appl Physiol 2005;99(5):1977–84.

15. Solberg WK, Hansson TL, Nordstrom B. The temporomandibular joint in young adults at autopsy: a morphological classification and evaluation. J Oral Rehabil 1985;12:303–21.

16. Gage JP, Virdi AS, Trippitt RG, et al. Presence of type III collagen in disk attachments of temporomandibular joints. Arch Oral Biol 1990;35:283–8.

17. Nitzan DW. Intraarticular pressure in the functioning human temporomandibular joint and its alteration by uniform elevation of the occlusal plane. J Oral Maxillofac Surg 1994;52(7):671–9 [discussion: 679–80].

18. Stegenga B, de Bont LG. TMJ disk derangements. In: Laskin DM, Greene CS, Hylander WL, editors. TMDs: an evidenced approach to diagnosis and treatment. Chicago: Quintessence; 2006. p. 129.

19. Abubaker AO, Raslan WF, Sotereanos GC. Estrogen and progesterone receptors in temporomandibular joint discs of symptomatic and asymptomatic persons: a preliminary study. J Oral Maxillofac Surg 1993;51:1096–100.

20. Mitchel RJ. Etiology of temporomandibular disorders. Curr Opin Dent 1991;1: 471–5.

21. Wang HY, Shih TT, Wang JS, et al. Temporomandibular joint structural derangement and general joint hypermobility. J Orofac Pain 2012;26(1):33–8.

22. Perrini F, Tallnets RH, Katzsburg RW. Generalized joint laxity and temporomandibular disorders. J Orofac Pain 1997;11(3):215–21.

23. Yamada KJ, Tsuruta A, Hanada K, et al. Morphology of the articular eminence in temporomandibular joints and condylar bone change. Oral Rehab 2004;31(5): 438–44.

24. Pullinger AG, Seligman DA. Quantification and validation of predictive values of occlusal variables in temporomandibular disorders using a multifactorial analysis. J Prosthet Dent 2000;83:66–75.

25. Christensen LV, Ziebert GJ. Effects of the experimental loss of teeth on the temporomandibular joint. J Oral Rehabil 1986;13:587–98.

26. Kopp S, Carlsson GE. The temporomandibular joint: problems related to occlusal function. In: Mohl ND, Zarb GA, Carlsson GE, et al, editors. A Textbook of Occlusion. Chicago: Quintessence; 1989. p. 255–68.

27. The American Academy of Orofacial Pain, de Leeuw R, editors. Orofacial pain: guidelines for assessment, diagnosis and management. 4th edition. Chicago: Quintessence; 2008. p. 137–8.

28. Huber MA, Hall EH. A comparison of the signs of temporomandibular joint dysfunction and occlusal discrepancies in a symptom-free population of men and women. Oral Surg Oral Med Oral Pathol 1990;70(2):180–3.

29. Warren MP, Fried JL. Temporomandibular disorders and hormones in women. Cells Tissues Organs 2001;169:187–92.

30. Li ZG, Danis VA, Brooks PM. Effect of gonadal steroids on the production of IL-1 and IL-6 by blood mononuclear cells in vitro. Clin Exp Rheumatol 1993;11:157–63.

31. Halpern LR, Levine M, Dodson TB. Sexual dimorphism and temporomandibular disorders. Oral Maxillofac Surg Clin North Am 2007;19(2):267–77.

32. Flake NM, Hermanstyne TO, Gold MS. Testosterone and estrogen have opposing actions on inflammation-induced plasma extravasation in the rat temporomandibular joint. Am J Physiol Regul Integr Comp Physiol 2006;291:343–8.

33. Oraijarvi M, Puijola E, Yu S, et al. Effect of estrogen and dietary loading on condylar cartilage. J Orofac Pain 2012;26:328–36.

34. Bereiter DA. Sex differences in brainstem neural activation after injury to the TMJ region. Cells Tissues Organs 2001;169:226–37.

35. Berieter DA, Bereiter DF. Morphine and NMDA receptor antagonism reduce c-fos expression in spinal trigeminal nucleus produced by acute injury to the TMJ region. Pain 2000;85:65–77.

36. Wiese M, Svensson P, Bakke M, et al. Association between temporomandibular joint symptoms, signs, and clinical diagnosis using the RDC/TMD and radiographic findings in temporomandibular joint tomograms. J Orofac Pain 2008; 22(3):239–51.

37. Milam S. TMJ osteoarthritis. In: Laskin DM, Greene CS, Hylander WL, editors. TMDs: an evidenced approach to diagnosis and treatment. Chicago: Quintessence; 2006. p. 105–25.

38. Chase DC. The Christensen prosthesis: a retrospective study. Oral Surg Oral Med Oral Pathol Oral Radiol Endod 1995;80:273–8.

39. LeResche L, Sherman JJ, Huggins KH, et al. Musculoskeletal orofacial pain and other signs and symptoms of temporomandibular disorders during pregnancy: a prospective study. J Orofac Pain 2005;19:193–201.

40. Velly AM, Fricton J. The impact of comorbid conditions on treatment of temporomandibular disorders. J Am Dent Assoc 2011;142:170–2.

41. Michelotti A, Cioffi I, Festa P, et al. Oral parafunctions as risk factors for diagnostic TMD subgroups. J Oral Rehabil 2010;37(3):157–62.

42. Huynh N, Manzini C, Rompre PH, et al. Weighing the potential effectiveness of various treatments for sleep bruxism. J Calif Dent Assoc 2007;73(8):727–30.

43. Ojima K, Watanabe N, Narita N, et al. Temporomandibular disorder is associated with a serotonin transporter gene polymorphism in the Japanese population. Biopsychosoc Med 2007;1:3.

44. Hublin C, Kaprio J, Partinen M, et al. Parasomnias: co-occurrence and genetics. Psychiatr Genet 2001;11(2):65–70.
45. Kononen M, Wenneberg B. Systemic conditions affecting the TMJ. In: Laskin DM, Greene CS, Hylander WL, editors. TMDs: an evidenced approach to diagnosis and treatment. Chicago: Quintessence; 2006. p. 137–46.
46. Hallert E, Björk M, Dahlström O, et al. Disease activity and disability in women and men with early rheumatoid arthritis (RA): an 8-year follow-up of a Swedish early RA project. Arthritis Care Res (Hoboken) 2012;64(8):1101–7.
47. Jawaheer D, Olsen J, Hetland ML. Sex differences in response to anti-tumor necrosis factor therapy in early and established rheumatoid arthritis–results from the DANBIO registry. J Rheumatol 2012;39(1):46–53.
48. Pogrel MA, Chigurupati R. Management of idiopathic condylar resorption. In: Laskin DM, Greene CS, Hylander WL, editors. TMDs: an evidenced approach to diagnosis and treatment. Chicago: Quintessence; 2006. p. 553–60.
49. John MT, Miglioretti DL, LeResche L, et al. Widespread pain as a risk factor for dysfunctional temporomandibular disorder pain. Pain 2003;102:257–63.
50. Woolf CJ. Central sensitization: implications for the diagnosis and treatment of pain. Pain 2011;152:S2–15.
51. Yunus MB. Fibromyalgia and overlapping disorders: the unifying concept of central sensitivity syndromes. Semin Arthritis Rheum 2007;36(6):339–56.
52. Bonavita V, De Simone R. Towards a definition of comorbidity in the light of clinical complexity. Neurol Sci 2008;29:S99–102.
53. Plesh O, Adams SH, Gansky SA. Temporomandibular joint and muscle disorder-type pain and comorbid pains in a national US sample. J Orofac Pain 2011;25: 190–8.
54. Marcus DA. Interrelationship of neurochemicals, estrogen, and recurring headache. Pain 1995;62:129–39.
55. Gupta S, McCarson KE, Welch KM, et al. Mechanisms of pain modulation by sex hormones in migraine. Headache 2011;51(6):905–22.
56. Hoffmann RG, Kotchen JM, Kotchen TA, et al. Temporomandibular disorders and associated clinical comorbidities. Clin J Pain 2011;27:268–74.
57. King CD, Wong F, Currie T, et al. Deficiency in endogenous modulation of prolonged heat pain in patients with irritable bowel syndrome and temporomandibular disorder. Pain 2009;143(3):172–8.
58. Galdon MJ, Dura E, Andreu Y, et al. Multidimensional approach to the differences between muscular and articular temporomandibular patients: coping, distress, and pain characteristics [Proceedings Paper]. Oral Surg Oral Med Oral Pathol Oral Radiol Endod 2006;102(1):40–6.
59. Keith D, Shaefer J. Diagnosis and management of temporomandibular joint disorders. In: Mehta N, Maloney G, Bana D, et al, editors. Head, face, and neck pain: science, evaluation, and management. John Wiley; 2009. p. 381–444.
60. Mense S, Simons D, Russel IJ, editors. Muscle pain: understanding its nature, diagnosis and treatment. Philadelphia: Lippincott Williams & Wilkins; 2001.
61. Rammelsberg P, LeResche L, Dworkin S, et al. Longitudinal outcome of temporomandibular disorders: a 5-year epidemiologic study of muscle disorders defined by research diagnostic criteria for temporomandibular disorders. J Orofac Pain 2003;17:9–20.
62. Yap AU, Tan KB, Chua EK, et al. Depression and somatization in patients with temporomandibular disorders. J Prosthet Dent 2002;88(5):479–84.
63. Riley JL, Robinson ME, Wise EA, et al. Sex differences in the perception of noxious experimental stimuli: a meta-analysis. Pain 1998;74:181–7.

64. Cairns BE, Hu JW, Arendt-Nielsen L, et al. Sex-related differences in human pain and rat afferent discharge evoked by injection of glutamate into the masseter muscle. J Neurophysiol 2001;86:782–91.
65. LeResche L. Gender disparities in pain. Clin Orthop Relat Res 2011;469(7): 1770–876.
66. Kehlet H, Troels SJ, Clifford JW. Persistent postsurgical pain: risk factors. Lancet 2006;367:1618–25.
67. Diatchenko L, Slade GD, Nackley AG, et al. Genetic basis for individual variations in pain perception and the development of a chronic pain condition. Hum Mol Genet 2005;14:135–43.
68. Cairns BE. The influence of gender and sex steroids on craniofacial nociception. Headache 2007;47(2):319–24.
69. Pinto PR, McIntyre T, Nogueria-Silva C, et al. Risk factors for persistent postsurgical pain in women undergoing hysterectomy due to benign causes: a prospective predictive study. J Pain 2012;13(11):1045–57.
70. Nie H, Arendt-Nielsen L, Andersen H, et al. Temporal summation of pain evoked by mechanical stimulation in deep and superficial tissue. J Pain 2005;6:348–55.
71. Sarlani E, Grace EG, Reynolds MA, et al. Evidence for up-regulated central nociceptive processing in patients with masticatory myofascial pain. J Orofac Pain 2004;86:41–55.
72. Carlson CR, Bertrand P. Physical self-regulation training for the management of temporomandibular disorders. J Orofac Pain 2001;1:47–55.
73. Yoshihara T. Neuroendocrine responses to psychological stress in patients with myofascial pain. J Orofac Pain 2005;19(3):202–8.
74. Karszun A. Basal circadian cortisol secretion in women with TMD. J Dent Res 2002;81(4):279–83.
75. Zubieta JK, Heitag MM, Smith YR, et al. COMT val168met genotype affects mu-opioid neurotransmitter responses to a stressor. Science 2009;299:1240–3.
76. Martenson ME, Cetas JS, Heinricher MM. Neural basis for stress-induced hyperalgesia. Pain 2009;143(3):236–44.
77. Svensson P, Cairns BE, Wang K, et al. Injection of nerve growth factor into human masseter muscle evokes long-lasting mechanical allodynia and hyperalgesia. Pain 2003;104:241–7.
78. Lobbezoo F, Drangsholt M, Peck C, et al. Topical review: new insights into the pathology and diagnosis of disorders of the temporomandibular joint. J Orofac Pain 2004;18(3):181–90.
79. Raper J. Detrimental effects of chronic hypothalamic-pituitary-adrenal axis activation. From obesity to memory deficits. Mol Neurobiol 1998;18:1–22.
80. Maixner W. Sensitivity of patients with painful temporomandibular disorders to experimentally evoked pain. Pain 1995;63(3):341–51.
81. Palmer SN, Gieseche NM, Body SC, et al. Pharmacogenetics of anesthetic and analgesic agents. Anesthesiology 2005;102(3):663–71.
82. Diatchenko L, Anderson AD, Slade GD, et al. Three major haplotypes of the B_2 adrenergic receptor define psychological profile, blood pressure, and the risk for the development of a common musculoskeletal pain disorder. Am J Med Genet 2006;141:449–62.
83. Meloto CB, Serrano PO, Ribeiro-DaSilva MC, et al. Genomics and the new perspectives for temporomandibular disorders. Arch Oral Biol 2011;56: 1181–91.
84. Slade GD, Daitchenko L, Ohrbach R, et al. Orthodontic treatment, genetics, and risk of temporomandibular disorder. Semin Orthod 2008;14(2):146–56.

85. Rogers RR. Individual differences in endogenous pain modulation as a risk factor for chronic pain. Neurology 2005;65(3):437–43.

86. Woolf CJ. Dissecting out mechanisms responsible for peripheral neuropathic pain: implications for diagnosis and therapy. Life Sci 2004;74(21):2605–10.

87. Sessle BJ. The neural basis of temporomandibular joint and masticatory muscle pain. J Orofac Pain 1999;13:238–45.

88. Litt M, Shafer P, Kreutzer D. Cognitive behavioral treatment for TMD: long term outcomes and moderators of treatment. Pain 2010;151:110–6.

89. Rhudy JL, Bartley EJ, Williams AE, et al. Are there sex differences in affective modulation of spinal nociception and pain? J Pain 2010;11(12):1429–41.

90. Davis MC, Okun MA, Kruszewski D, et al. Sex differences in the relations of positive and negative daily events and fatigue in adults with rheumatoid arthritis. J Pain 2010;11(12):1338–47.

91. Bjørkedal E, Flaten MA. Expectations of increased and decreased pain explain the effect of conditioned pain modulation in females. J Pain Res 2012;5:289–300.

92. Kavaliers M, Choleris E. Sex differences in N-methyl-D-aspartate involvement in kappa opioid and non-opioid predator-induced analgesia in mice. Brain Res 1997;768(1–2):30–6.

93. Gear RW, Miaskowski C, Gordon NC, et al. Kappa-opioids produce significantly greater analgesia in women than in men. Nat Med 1996;2(11):1248–50.

94. Niesters M, Dahan A, Kest B, et al. Do sex differences exist in opioid analgesia? A systematic review and meta-analysis of human experimental and clinical studies. Pain 2010;151:61–8.

95. Dahan A, Sarton E, Teppema L, et al. Sex-related differences in the influence of morphine on ventilatory control in humans. Anesthesiology 1998;88:903–13.

96. Romberg R, Olofsen E, Sarton E, et al. Pharmacokinetic–pharmacodynamic modeling of morphine-6-glucuronide-induced analgesia in healthy volunteers. Anesthesiology 2004;100:120–33.

97. Gear RW, Miaskowski C, Gordon NC, et al. The kappa opioid nalbuphine produces gender- and dose-dependent analgesia and antianalgesia in patients with postoperative pain. Pain 1999;83:339–45.

98. McCartney CJ. A qualitative systematic review of NMDA receptor antagonists in preventive analgesia. Anesth Analg 2004;98:1385–400.

99. Snijdelaar DG, Koren G, Katz J. Effects of perioperative oral amantadine on postoperative pain and morphine consumption in patients after radical prostatectomy: results of a preliminary study. Anesthesiology 2004;100(1):134–41.

100. Tanaka E. Gender-related differences in pharmacokinetics and their clinical significance. J Clin Pharm Ther 1999;24:339–46.

101. Harris RZ, Benet LZ, Schwartz JB. Gender effects in pharmacokinetics and pharmacodynamics. Drugs 1995;50:222–39.

102. Xie CX, Piecoro LT, Wermeling DP. Gender-related considerations in clinical pharmacology and drug therapeutics. Crit Care Nurs Clin North Am 1997;9:459–68.

103. Meyer UA. Overview of enzymes of drug metabolism. J Pharmacokinet Biopharm 1996;24:449–59.

104. Oakley M, Vieira AR. The many faces of genetics contribution to temporomandibular joint disorder. Orthod Craniofac Res 2008;11:125–35.

105. Young EE, Lariviere WR, Belfer I. Genetic basis of pain variability: recent advances [review]. J Med Genet 2012;49:1–9.

106. Tchivileya IE, Lim PF, Smith SB, et al. Effect of catechol-*O*-methyltranferase polymorphism on response to propranolol therapy in chronic musculoskeletal pain: a randomized, double-blind, placebo controlled, crossover pilot study. Pharmacogenet Genomics 2010;20(4):239–48.

107. Kornstein SG, Schatzberg AF, Thase ME, et al. Gender differences in treatment response to sertraline versus imipramine in chronic depression. Am J Psychiatry 2000;157:1445–52.

108. Thase ME, Entsuah R, Cantillon M, et al. Relative antidepressant efficacy of venlafaxine and SSRIs: sex-age interactions. J Womens Health 2005;14: 609–16.

109. Mitchell AA, Gilboa SM, Werler MM, et al, the National Birth Defects Prevention Study. Medication use during pregnancy, with particular focus on prescription drugs: 1976–2008. Am J Obstet Gynecol 2011;205(1):51.e1–8.

110. TERIS. Teratogen information system. University of Washington. Available at: http://depts.washington.edu/terisweb/teris/. Accessed October 23, 2012.

111. Reprotox. Reproductive Toxicology Center. Available at: www.reprotox.org. Accessed October 30, 2012.

112. Daily Med. US National Library of Medicine, National Institutes of Health, Health and Human Services. Available at: http://dailymed.nlm.nih.gov/dailymed/about.cfm. Accessed October 30, 2012.

113. Lact Med. US National Library of Medicine, National Institutes of Health, Health and Human Services. Available at: http://toxnet.nlm.nih.gov/cgi-bin/sis/htmlgen?LACT. Accessed October 30, 2012.

114. Davis AR, Westhoff CL, Stanczyk FZ. Carbamazepine coadministration with an oral contraceptive: effects on steroid pharmacokinetics, ovulation, and bleeding. Epilepsia 2011;52(2):243–7.

115. Wegner I, Edelbroek P, de Haan GJ, et al. Drug monitoring of lamotrigine and oxcarbazepine combination during pregnancy. Epilepsia 2010;51(12): 2500–2.

116. Backman JT, Schröder MT, Neuvonen PJ. Effects of gender and moderate smoking on the pharmacokinetics and effects of the CYP1A2 substrate tizanidine. Eur J Clin Pharmacol 2008;64(1):17–24.

117. Granfors MT, Backman JT, Laitila J, et al. Oral contraceptives containing ethinyl estradiol and gestodene markedly increase plasma concentrations and effects of tizanidine by inhibiting cytochrome P450 1A2. Clin Pharmacol Ther 2005; 78(4):400–11.

118. Tsatsaris V, Cabrol D, Carbonne B. Pharmacokinetics of tocolytic agents. Clin Pharmacokinet 2004;43(13):833–44.

119. Bendixen KH, Baad-Hansen L, Cairns BE, et al. Effects of low-dose intramuscular ketorolac on experimental pain in the masseter muscle of healthy women. J Orofac Pain 2010;24(4):398–407.

120. Nanau RM, Neuman MG. Ibuprofen-induced hypersensitivity syndrome. Transl Res 2010;155(6):275–93.

121. Wolff K, Boys A, Rostami-Hodjegan A, et al. Changes to methadone clearance during pregnancy. Eur J Clin Pharmacol 2005;61(10):763–8.

122. Ardakani YH, Rouini MR. Pharmacokinetics of tramadol and its three main metabolites in healthy male and female volunteers. Biopharm Drug Dispos 2007;28(9):527–34.

123. Greenblatt DJ, Harmatz JS, von Moltke LL, et al. Age and gender effects on the pharmacokinetics and pharmacodynamics of triazolam, a cytochrome P450 3A substrate. Clin Pharmacol Ther 2004;76(5):467–79.

124. Ferrari A, Tiraferri I, Neri L, et al. Why pharmacokinetic differences among oral triptans have little clinical importance: a comment. J Headache Pain 2011;12(1): 5–12.
125. Ferrari A, Pinetti D, Bertolini A, et al. Interindividual variability of oral sumatriptan pharmacokinetics and of clinical response in migraine patients. Eur J Clin Pharmacol 2008;64(5):489–95.
126. Wade A, Pawsey S, Whale H, et al. Pharmacokinetics of two 6-day frovatriptan dosing regimens used for the short-term prevention of menstrual migraine: a phase I, randomized, double-blind, placebo-controlled, two-period crossover, single-centre study in healthy female volunteers. Clin Drug Investig 2009;29(5): 325–37.
127. Lobo ED, Bergstrom RF, Reddy S, et al. In vitro and in vivo evaluations of cytochrome P450 1A2 interactions with duloxetine. Clin Pharmacokinet 2008;47(3): 191–202.
128. McCormack PL, Keating GM. Duloxetine: in stress urinary incontinence. Drugs 2004;64(22):2567–73 [discussion: 2574–5].

Gender Differences in the Growing, Abnormal, and Aging Jaw

Julie Glowacki, PhD[a,b,c],*, Kristina Christoph, DMD[a,d]

KEYWORDS

- Facial bones • Sex characteristics • Maxillofacial development • Aging • Jaw

KEY POINTS

- Craniofacial anomalies are among the most common congenital defects, and the prevalences often show gender differences.
- Gender dimorphism is demonstrated in many of the craniofacial bones along with the gender-specific growth trajectories of the craniofacial bones that are especially notable for the maxilla and mandible.
- Consideration of jaw growth influences by tooth eruption at different ages for girls and boys as well as other gender differences, such as variations in the number of teeth, the presence of palatal tori, and other factors contributing to patterns of malocclusion, are aids to clinicians in diagnosis and treatment planning.
- Facial aging in dentate patients is characterized by retrusion of the midface in relation to the lower face. With edentulism, there is a gender-specific age-related loss of height in both jaws, a greater loss of ridge height and mandibular bone mineral content in women, and an increase in cortical bone mineral content in men that may reflect a gender-specific functional adaptation.
- Systemic osteoporosis, which is more prevalent in women than men, is correlated with some measurements in the jaws, but radiographs are not approved for the diagnosis of osteoporosis.

INTRODUCTION

Despite wide variations in the size and shape of the human face, head, and body, there is remarkable consistency for gender-specific facial traits, quantifiable by cephalometric and surface methods. Orthodontists, reconstructive surgeons, forensic

Neither author has any disclosures.
[a] Department of Orthopedic Surgery, Brigham and Women's Hospital, 75 Francis Street, Boston, MA 02115, USA; [b] Department of Orthopedic Surgery, Harvard Medical School, 250 Longwood Avenue, Boston, MA 02115, USA; [c] Department of Oral and Maxillofacial Surgery, Harvard School of Dental Medicine, 188 Longwood Avenue, Boston, MA 02115, USA; [d] Harvard School of Dental Medicine, 188 Longwood Avenue, Boston, MA 02115, USA
* Corresponding author. Orthopedic Research, Brigham and Women's Hospital, 75 Francis Street, Boston, MA 02115.
E-mail address: jglowacki@rics.bwh.harvard.edu

Dent Clin N Am 57 (2013) 263–280
http://dx.doi.org/10.1016/j.cden.2013.01.005
0011-8532/13/$ – see front matter © 2013 Elsevier Inc. All rights reserved.

scientists, and archeologists require normal reference landmarks and have recon-firmed gender dimorphism for several craniofacial traits in populations around the globe. Technological advances introduced greater precision in surface and skeletal parameters of size and shape in normal individuals. The relationships between the growing jaws and tooth eruption are complex, but they also show gender-specific trajectories in children and adolescents. Disturbances in genetic, endocrine, and nutri-tional regulatory controls result in gender-specific and nonspecific disorders. Gender differences are evident in jaw abnormalities, including craniofacial deformities and malocclusions, as well as incidental findings of variation in the number of teeth and the presence of palatal tori. There are also gender-specific differences in the aging jaw, with acceleration of jaw bone atrophy on loss of teeth, especially in women. Aging, systemic osteoporosis, local periodontal disease, and tooth loss contribute to jaw bone loss.

GENDER DIFFERENCES IN THE GROWING JAW
Morphometrics of the Adult Orofacial Skeleton

Despite wide variations in the size and shape of the human face, head, and body, there is remarkable consistency for gender-specific facial traits, quantifiable by cephalo-metric and surface methods. It is generally thought that those traits have important implications for the role of sexual selection in the evolution of anthropoid faces and for theories of human facial attractiveness.[1] This information is of great importance in forensic, archeological, and anthropologic sciences, as well as for cosmetic and reconstructive surgery. Second to the pelvis, cranial remains are the most useful part of the skeleton for determining gender. There are many studies that show gender differences in facial traits (**Fig. 1**) and in growth rates for specific bones. Cohorts have been characterized, in some cases, to establish norms for surgical planning for chil-dren with craniofacial deformities. A striking observation in one such investigation revealed minimal heterogeneity in gender-specific traits and striking individual varia-tions in nonspecific traits[2]; this suggests a potent mechanism(s) for maintaining the dimorphic traits. Most measures of the craniofacial complex are 5% to 9% larger in men than in women.[3] A study of dental students showed that most cephalometric measures were larger for men than women, with several exceptions including the nasal bone, foramen magnum, and inner orbital distance.[4] A detailed study of serial

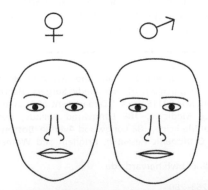

Fig. 1. Gender dimorphic facial characteristics, with the female image having a narrower forehead, cheek, nose, jaw, and chin and a higher browridge than the male image.

lateral cephalograms showed that gender dimorphism of cephalometric measures of the craniofacial skeleton, especially the lengths of the anterior cranial base, maxilla, and mandible, was apparent by 14 years of age.[5] The adolescent growth spurt in boys was accompanied by the most substantial increases in facial growth. There was also a trend for a more horizontal direction of facial growth in the girls. The neurocranium is often used as a control region where growth seems to decelerate at 4 to 6 years of age, perhaps because of the cessation of brain growth. A recent analysis showed gender-specific growth trajectories for the face and that girls' average growth ceased between 12 to 14 years of age, whereas boys' facial development continued thereafter.[6] Another notable finding was the absence of correlation between individual forms as newborns and adults, whereas there was a strong correlation with adult form at 3 years of age. Thus, 3-year-old children possess a high correlation with their adult morphology. Furthermore, individual trajectories vary before 3 years of age; group patterns of growth become homogeneous and reproducible thereafter. Because of the limitations of radiographic methods for studying shape differences, 3-dimensional topographic tools have been developed for quantitative descriptors. Validation studies with surface laser scans described significant gender and racial differences for browridge and chin morphologies.[7] Gender had a large discriminatory effect on browridge and chin shapes, the latter being more pointed in women; but the studies also revealed the importance of ancestry on specific parameters of both regions.

Data from a longitudinal anthropometric analysis of craniofacial variables during the transition from deciduous and mixed to permanent dentition support the view that tooth eruption influences postnatal growth of the craniofacial skeleton.[8] Boys had larger values than girls for all facial variables examined, but the percent of annual changes in many parameters were often significantly greater for girls than boys. In the transition from deciduous to mixed dentition, there were decreases in head breadth and length. In the period of mixed dentition, there were increases in those dimensions. There was dichotomy in periods of maximum growth: between 9.8 and 10.7 years for boys and between 8.5 and 10.7 years for girls.

Chromosomal aberrations, nutritional insufficiencies, and metabolic disorders influence craniofacial growth. The evaluation of children with idiopathic growth hormone (GH) deficiency shows the importance of GH for development of the craniofacial skeleton, particularly for advancement of the maxilla and elongation of the mandible.[9] Short-term and long-term GH therapies resulted in catch-up growth, especially in the maxilla and mandibular ramus.

It is thought that dimorphic facial traits are related to endocrinological development, but the timing and mechanisms are unclear. An example is the association of testosterone levels with parameters of facial shape that was demonstrated in a study of healthy adolescent subjects. Broader forehead, chin, jaw, and nose, as quantified by magnetic resonance imaging (MRI)–based parameters, were found for the boys compared with girls and were correlated with plasma testosterone levels.[10] Further, those facial cues were associated with accurate sex identification from MRI-reconstructed facial images and the facial parameters that were most accurate predictors of male identification were correlated with plasma testosterone levels of the subject. One large study indicated maximal orofacial shape change during the adolescent growth spurt for boys but not for girls.[2] Complications about the effect of hormones, however, arise from concerns about certain studies' reliance on a single measurement, variations within groups, cross-cultural group differences, and the complicated multivariate statistical tools used for data analysis.

To address the hypothesis that prenatal hormone status may have a major and enduring influence on face shape, Fink and colleagues[11] used a surrogate marker for early exposure to testosterone and estrogen. They showed significant correlations for facial shape landmarks with the 2D/4D ratio (lengths of 2D to 4D). There is a body of indirect evidence suggesting that testosterone stimulates prenatal growth of the fourth finger and that estrogen promotes growth of the second finger; the interpretation is that a low 2D/4D ratio (with the fourth finger longer than the second) is a marker for a uterine environment relatively high in testosterone.[12] It is notable that new experimental evidence that the digit ratio is a lifelong signature of prenatal hormonal exposure comes from studies with mice; the dimorphic presence and activity of androgen and estrogen receptors in digits in early embryos (E17) underlie the dimorphic 2D/4D length ratios.[13] This evidence that the 2D/4D ratio is determined in the mouse embryo provides a plausible biologic basis for the correlative human data.

Thus, it is clear that there are differences between male and female craniofacial parameters and their rates of change during growth. Large, powered studies support the view that certain parameters of craniofacial growth accelerate during pubescence, at least for boys. Other studies indicate that facial shape may be determined by in utero exposure to sex hormones. Finally, there is a great impact of tooth eruption on changes in jaw size and shape. These principles are gleaned from association studies, but future work with appropriate animal models may provide significant information about the mechanisms of these gender-specific outcomes.

Mandible

Evidence shows separate gender dimorphisms for the shape and for the size of the mandible. A landmark investigation of the variation in contour of the mentum osseum in 180 mandibles equally representing adults from 9 geographic regions provided quantitative evidence of gender dimorphism, with a broad chin characterizing men in diverse cultural groups.[14] Gender dimorphism for the shape of mandible was shown to exist at birth, especially in the ramus and mental regions.[15] Those shape differences, however, decrease with age as the female mandible becomes more similar to the shape of the male mandible. Size dimorphism predominates thereafter, but other shape differences become apparent after 13 years of age, chiefly at the ramus and symphysis. Many longitudinal studies confirm that dramatic changes in craniofacial growth occur during the first 5 years, especially in the mandible. Mandibular length showed the greatest changes in growth, followed by ramus height and corpus length.[16] Analysis of longitudinal data for patients at defined intervals revealed that the most rapid increase in length was between 6 and 12 months of age, with significantly greater rates for the boys than the girls. By 5 years of age, boys had significantly larger mandibles than girls; boys, however, had achieved a smaller percent of adult size than the girls. Fossil evidence suggests that the degree of chin size dimorphism may have diminished over time.[17]

Maxilla

Cephalometric analysis of annual lateral cranial radiographs of 38 individuals showed that from 8 to 18 years of age, sagittal growth of the maxilla was significantly greater in girls (0.29 mm/y) than in boys (0.13 mm/y) and that the anterior and posterior downward movement of the maxilla was greater in boys (1.21 mm/y) than in girls (0.71 mm/y).[18] Dental arch dimensions (width, length, and vault depth) showed significant changes during the mixed dentition stage and with the continuous eruption of teeth, but only the maxillary vault depth was gender dimorphic.[19] MRI data available from 55 healthy children aged 1.0 month to 15.3 years were used to model changes in maxillary volume for boys and girls.[20] Boys had larger maxillary volumes at all ages. There were 3 periods of growth for both boys and girls: steady growth during the first 5 years of life, followed by a more rapid rate between 5 and 11 years of age (coincident with the norms for eruption of permanent teeth) and slowing to a plateau between 11 and 15 years of age. Moorrees and colleagues[21] had emphasized the importance of eruption of the permanent teeth on the period of accelerated maxillary growth. Other studies indicate an adolescent growth spurt in the development of the maxilla occurring later in 52 boys[22] than in 50 girls.[23] An experimental study showing impaired nasomaxillary growth in gonadectomized newborn mice suggests that sex hormones are indispensible for postnatal development,[24] but the relevance to humans is unknown.

There is also dimorphism for the dimensions of the incisive canal and of the bone anterior to it. Men have longer and wider canals and dramatically thicker anterior bone than do women.[25] Those findings are important when planning surgery in the anterior maxilla.

Dentition

There is controversy about whether the emergence pattern of primary teeth is earlier in girls[26] or in boys.[27–29] It has been suggested that the discrepancies may be caused by the fact that counts of emerged teeth may not be normally distributed and that teeth emerge as pairs and, thus, require advanced nonparametric statistical tools.[30]

The generally accepted belief of precocious dental emergence pattern of permanent teeth in girls[31] has been confirmed in several recent analyses, although there can be important influences of socioeconomic factors, craniofacial morphology, and systemic diseases.[32] Tooth emergence in girls was 4.5 months earlier in the maxilla and 5.3 months earlier in the mandible than for boys.[33] Other analyses confirm earlier emergence pattern in girls.[34,35] Compared with Hurme's[31] tables from 1951, the emergence of maxillary dentition was at least 3 months later or earlier in a 2003 report, depending on the tooth, whereas mandibular patterns were the same.[36]

It has been suggested that there is greater gender dimorphism in dimensions of permanent than deciduous teeth.[37] A study of dental casts indicated that the tooth crowns of males were significantly broader than those of females, especially in the permanent dentition.[38] Serial casts showed that subjects with small or broad primary incisors and canines developed the same size differences in permanent teeth. A study with material from Herculaneum samples (79 AD, Naples) validated the permanent canine as the tooth with greatest power for gender determination of adolescents.[39]

GENDER DIFFERENCES IN JAW ABNORMALITIES
Craniofacial Anomalies

Craniofacial anomalies are among the most common congenital defects, and prevalences often show gender differences. Orofacial clefts are of the most common craniofacial defects, affecting 1 in every 500 to 1000 births worldwide.[40] Their causes are complex, involving many genetic and environmental factors. Approximately 70% of cases of cleft lip and/or palate occur as isolated entities termed *nonsyndromic*. The *syndromic* cases are associated with a wide range of malformations, including those arising from mendelian or single gene disorders, chromosomal abnormalities, or teratogenic effects. Well-known syndromes associated with orofacial clefting include DiGeorge syndrome, Treacher Collins syndrome, Pierre Robin sequence, and Van der Woude syndrome. Females are more likely than males to have an additional malformation associated with an orofacial cleft, which may include malformations of the abdominal cavity (umbilical and inguinal hernia) or deformities of the extremities or ears.[41,42]

Isolated cleft lip occurs in 1 per 1000 births and is seen more frequently in boys (80%) than in girls.[43] At 6 weeks *in utero*, the developing upper lip consists of 2 medial nasal prominences located toward the center of the face. Immediately adjacent to them are 2 maxillary prominences located at either side of the face. Normally, by the seventh week *in utero*, the bilateral maxillary prominences have fused with the medial prominence, forming the upper lip as well as the most anterior portion of the palate, called the primary palate. The primary palate, also known as the premaxilla, will support the 4 maxillary incisor teeth. Failure of fusion will result in either a unilateral or bilateral cleft lip. It may vary in severity from a slight defect in the vermillion border to a cleft extending into the nose and/or through the alveolar process to the incisive foramen. The cause of the male gender predilection is not known.

In contrast, there is a greater occurrence of cleft palate in females (67%) than in males.[43] A proposed explanation for the gender predilection is a difference in the timing of secondary palate development. The development of the mature hard palate involves the integration of 3 joining structures (**Fig. 2**). The primary palate forms separately from the posterior secondary palate. The incisive foramen is located at the center of the junction between the primary and secondary palates and serves as the passageway between the anterior maxilla and floor of the nasal cavity for the nasopalatine nerve as well as a branch of the sphenopalatine artery. The incisive foramen is

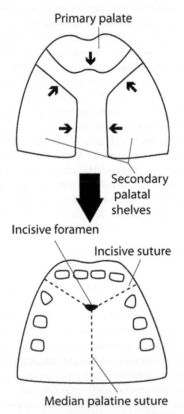

Fig. 2. Development of the hard palate. Bilateral palatal shelves ascend and fuse (*small arrows*) to form the secondary palate while fusing anteriorly with the primary palate. The incisive foramen marks the center of the 3 coalescing structures.

also considered a dividing landmark between anterior and posterior cleft deformities. The secondary palate begins to form in the sixth week in utero as 2 shelflike outgrowths of the maxillary prominences, called the palatine shelves, which initially grow in a downward direction. In the seventh week *in utero*, the bilateral palatal shelves ascend and coalesce to form the secondary palate. In the anterior direction, both shelves fuse with the primary palate, with the incisive foramen marking the midline. If the palatal shelves fail to fuse with one another, a cleft palate occurs, through which the oral and nasal cavities communicate. The frequency of an isolated cleft palate is 1 per 2500 births. The palatal shelves fuse approximately 1 week later in girls; this extended period may contribute to a greater occurrence of cleft palate in females than males.[43]

Cleft lip and cleft palate frequently occur together. Approximately 45% of cases involve both cleft lip and palate, whereas 30% are cleft palate alone and 25% are cleft lip alone.[44] Combined cleft lip and palate occurs more often in males, as does cleft lip alone. Cases of combined cleft lip and palate and cleft lip alone are thought to be etiologically related, but cleft palate alone is thought to be a separate entity. This finding is consistent with the different developmental origins of the lip and primary palate compared with the secondary palate.[45]

Other craniofacial defects also display gender predilections. Hemifacial microsomia is a condition that affects 1 per 5600 births.[46] It encompasses several craniofacial abnormalities, including the oculoauriculovertebral spectrum and Goldenhar syndrome, all of which usually involve hypoplasia of the maxillary, temporal, and zygomatic bones. In one study, patients with hemifacial microsomia were 40% more likely to be male,[47] and other studies agree with a male predilection.[46,48] Similarly, males are more likely to be affected by craniosynostosis, characterized by premature closure of one or more sutures of the skull, which affects 1 per 2500 births. Craniosynostosis is a feature of more than 100 genetic syndromes, the most common ones being Crouzon, Apert, Pfeiffer, Carpenter, and Saethre-Chotzen.[43,49]

Malocclusion

Studies using serial cephalometrics show gender differences in malocclusions. In a study conducted by Siriwat and Jarabak,[50] gender dimorphism was found to be the lowest among class I malocclusions and progressively increased with class II division I, class II division II, and class III malocclusions. There was a greater pattern of hypodivergence in males, which occurs when the mandible grows further forward in a horizontal direction as opposed to a hyperdivergent or more vertical direction. Males demonstrated a tendency toward prognathism, whereas females demonstrated a tendency toward orthognathism and retrognathism.

A cephalometric study performed by Baccetti and colleagues[51] demonstrated significant gender dimorphism in the development of class III malocclusions, particularly starting from 13 years of age. Beginning at the pubertal and postpubertal ages, the major gender differences include shorter anterior cranial base, shorter midfacial and mandibular lengths, and shorter upper and lower anterior facial heights in females compared with males. Beginning as early as 6 years of age, however, class III females consistently displayed shorter cranial bases compared with class III males; this is a characteristic of class III females that can be distinguished in early development. Male patients with class III malocclusion presented with significantly larger linear dimensions of the maxilla, mandible, and anterior facial heights when compared with female patients during circumpubertal and postpubertal periods. Understanding gender differences in growth patterns of malocclusions can aid clinicians in proper diagnosis and treatment planning.

Tooth Agenesis, Supernumerary Teeth, and Palatal Tori

Gender prevalence discrepancies are also seen in tooth agenesis, supernumerary teeth, and palatal tori. A lack of induction of embryologic tissues in tooth development can result in tooth agenesis (missing 1 or more teeth), whereas abnormal induction can result in the development of supernumerary teeth (1 or more additional teeth). Their causes are multifactorial, that is, influenced by both genetic and environmental factors. Tooth agenesis is the most common congenital anomaly in humans. The teeth most often affected are third molars, followed by second premolars and permanent maxillary lateral incisors.[44] Prevalence rates of tooth agenesis are reported higher in females compared with males.[52,53] One study found gender differences in the type of missing tooth, with male/female ratios of 2:1 in upper lateral incisor agenesis and 0.5:1.0 in premolar agenesis.[54]

In contrast to tooth agenesis, supernumerary teeth exhibit an overall male predominance.[43,52,55] Supernumerary teeth most commonly occur between the maxillary central incisors (mesiodens), followed by distal to the maxillary third molars (distomolars), the premolar region (perimolar), and the canine and lateral incisor regions.[44,56] Although supernumerary teeth in the midline occur more often in males, those in the incisor region are more common in females.[55]

The torus palatinus is a common exostosis located in the midline vault of the hard palate. The bilateral palatine processes of the maxilla meet at the intermaxillary suture, and this suture provides a site for excess bone formation.[57] Although most palatal tori are small (less than 2 cm in diameter), they can continue to grow throughout life.[44] Although the cause of palatal tori is not known, there is a pronounced female/male ratio of 2:1.[44,58,59]

GENDER DIFFERENCES IN THE AGING JAW
Skeletal Aging and Osteoporosis

Skeletal status is commonly described by bone mineral content ([BMC] in grams) and bone mineral density ([BMD] in grams per square centimeter) and assessed by dual-energy x-ray absorptiometry at the spine and femoral neck. By those measures, peak bone mass is achieved by 30 years of age; the BMD of men is significantly higher than that of women. Osteoporosis is defined as having a value of BMD more than 2.5 standard deviations below normal gender-specific reference values for BMD. With age, there is a decline in BMD, resulting in an increased risk of fractures that occur spontaneously or as the result of mild trauma. These fractures are termed *fragility fractures* and most commonly occur in the distal radius, vertebrae, and hip. At the onset of menopause, there is an acceleration of bone loss. For men, age-related bone loss is more gradual and to a lesser extent. A study of 1715 elders aged 67 to 93 years showed gender dimorphism in rates of bone loss in that age span; the percent change in BMD at the femoral neck was -7.7% per decade for women and -2.3% for men ($P = .002$).[60] This loss of bone mass was reflected in changes in calculated compressive strength of the femoral neck at -14.8% for women and -3.0% for men ($P<.0001$). There are clear osteoprotective effects of estrogen, testosterone, and adrenal dehydroepiandrosterone and their age-related declines contribute to skeletal aging.[61]

Osteoporosis and the Jaws

The relationship between systemic osteoporosis and oral/maxillofacial bone health is complex. The literature is controversial about the generalizability of the impact of systemic osteoporosis on the oral/maxillofacial bones.[62]

Dental radiographs and cephalograms provide convenient measures that may be useful for monitoring bone changes in individuals. Commonly used measures are changes in alveolar crestal height, residual ridge height in edentulous regions, gonion index, mental index, antegonial index, panoramic mandibular index, and density score relative to phantoms. All studies indicate larger values for males than for females throughout the lifespan. Evidence from longitudinal studies indicates that increases in those parameters, particularly in lower facial height and forward growth of the mandible, continue into the fourth decade for both men and women.[63]

Some studies suggest that there is potential for dental radiographic measures to identify patients with osteoporosis, but the magnitude of the correlation may not be large. Various radiomorphometric indices of the mandible were shown to be significantly correlated with BMD in lumbar spine or femoral neck,[64,65] but the relationships are often weak[66] or show unacceptable false positives and negatives.[67] Radiomorphometric measurements of cortical width at the mental foramen showed significant interactions between gender and age and between gender and dental status.[68] Inconsistencies may reflect heterogeneity of the studied population. Careful selection of subjects may provide more useful data. An analysis of men with chronic kidney disease requiring hemodialysis showed similar quantifiable changes caused by severe secondary hyperparathyroidism in hand and jaw bones, reflecting cortical erosion and trabecular diminution in both.[69] Qualitative assessment of porosity of the inferior mandibular cortex is another parameter used as an index of bone loss.[70] There is a stronger relationship for features of trabecular architecture on periapical radiographs between patients with osteoporosis (with documented hip fracture) and controls; the anterior maxilla and posterior mandible showed the greatest differences between groups.[71] A similar method was applied to a cohort of women with serial radiographs and showed that for each 0.01-mm/y loss of trabeculae (node-to-terminus length) there was an increase in hip fracture rate by 2.9-fold.[72] In sum, although differences can be shown for jaw parameters between osteoporotic and control subjects, there is no quantitative definition of oral/maxillofacial osteoporosis as there is for the axial and appendicular skeleton. The mandible may not be considered a common site for osteoporotic fragility fractures, but some studies indicate a significant correlation between the frequency of mandible fractures and systemic osteoporosis.[73] Although radiographs are not approved for the diagnosis of osteoporosis, it has been suggested that dentists have an important opportunity to identify patients at risk of osteoporosis and to recommend referral for evaluation and management by osteoporosis specialists.[74]

Effects of Age on the Dentate Jaws

Although all bones undergo skeletal aging, the maxillofacial complex undergoes unique patterns of resorption that result in functional and aesthetic changes. These changes are accounted for by changes in supporting alveolar bone and muscles of mastication. Although many of the facial stigmata of aging are related to soft tissue changes, some are secondary to age-related hollowing of supporting skeletal structures. Computer-assisted tomographic studies with dentate patients show that the midfacial becomes retrusive with age in relation to the upper face for both men and women.[75] Recession of the pyriform and maxillary angles results in posterior positioning of the nasolabial fold and upper lip.[76] The mandible shows resorption in some measured regions and expansion in other measurements.[77]

Effects of Age on the Edentulous Jaws

Without teeth, there is little functional load on the jaws. The bone of the residual alveolar ridge is continuously reduced, and there is a decrease in the height of the lower face. The classic longitudinal study by Tallgren[78] showed the greatest loss of height on extraction, followed by continuous reduction of height in both jaws, with resorption in the maxilla occurring in a centripetal direction and in the mandible it is centrifugal. This rotation results in a reduction in facial height and secondary prognathism. The extent of residual ridge resorption ([RRR] **Fig. 3**A) is greatest in the anterior regions of both jaws[79] and greater for women than for men.[80,81] The maxilla demonstrates more rapid and severe alveolar bone atrophy after tooth loss than the mandible. Initially, maxillary height is retained with progressive loss of width, resulting in a knife-edged ridge. This shape is difficult for denture use and for implant placement. Subsequent progressive loss of height can result in pneumatization of the maxillary sinuses. The accompanying loss of soft tissue and maxillary migration in the superior and posterior directions result in decreased fullness of the upper lip and decreased lower facial height; those changes are more extreme in women than in men.[82]

As assessed from dental panoramic radiographs, mandibular cortical width is significantly lower for women than men at all ages, with an acceleration in thinning for women after 42.5 years of age.[83] Serial mandibular BMC measurements showed significantly greater loss over 3 years for women than for men (**Fig. 3**B), with the calculated average annual loss significantly greater in women (1.5%) than in men (0.9%).[84] That study involved patients less than 81 years of age. A study with edentulous mandibles from cadaveric subjects between 69 and 90 years of age showed gender

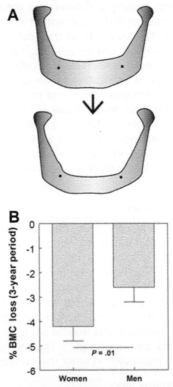

Fig. 3. (*A*) Age-related loss of height in edentulous mandible. (*B*) Comparison of the rate of loss of BMC in the edentulous mandible for women and men between 70 and 81 years of age. (*Data from* von Wowern N. Bone mineral content of mandibles: normal reference values–rate of age-related bone loss. Calcif Tissue Int 1988;43:193–8.)

dimorphism with an age-related increase in BMC for men older than 80 years (**Fig. 4**).[85] The speculation was that functional adaptation to the loss of height was achieved in elderly men but not in women. Additional studies with BMC information with more patients older than 80 years and including the duration of edentulism would be helpful to test for gender differences, differences between the maxilla and mandible, and relative effects on trabecular and cortical bone.

Effects of Age and Gender on Salivary Glands

There is emerging evidence that advances in oral health care have resulted in improved retention of teeth in the elderly.[86] Nevertheless, elders are vulnerable to oral diseases caused by poor hygiene; disabilities and dependency; medications; history of radiation or nerve damage; and other diseases, including Sjögren syndrome, Alzheimer disease, diabetes, anemia, rheumatoid arthritis, hypertension, Parkinson disease, and stroke. Xerostomia is defined as the subjective perception of oral dryness. Xerostomia, in addition to discomfort and difficulty wearing dentures, increases a person's risk of gingivitis, tooth decay, and mouth infections. It is accepted that chronic dry mouth can contribute to tooth decay[87] and that salivary flow rate, pH, and buffering capacity have an impact on caries susceptibility. Many studies have shown that chewing sugar-free gum after meals results in a significant decrease in the incidence of dental caries and that the benefit is caused by stimulating salivary flow rather than any chewing gum ingredient.[88] Nevertheless, it has not been shown that there are differences in any specific salivary component or property between caries-free and caries-positive groups.[89] This finding is likely caused by the complexity of factors that contribute to caries. Another complicating factor is that saliva from the different glands has different composition and likely different activities, but they are not well mixed in the oral cavity; thus, different regions of the mouth are exposed to different components.

The normal for unstimulated whole saliva flow rate is taken as greater than 0.2 mL/min. The prevalence of very low unstimulated salivary flow in young and middle-aged adults is 11% to 18%.[90] There is reproducible evidence that unstimulated salivary flow rates in healthy young adults are much lower in women than men[90-92] and that salivary gland size can explain the gender difference.[93]

There are age-related increases in xerostomia and in aspects of salivary gland function. Unstimulated flow rates of whole and submandibular saliva as well as stimulated parotid and submandibular saliva decline with advancing age.[89] A detailed analysis of a small number of women and men showed significantly lower secretion rates and

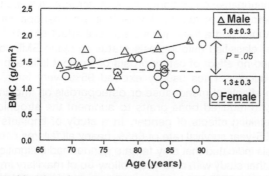

Fig. 4. BMC of cortical border of 25 atrophic cadaveric mandibles. Data from Ref.[85] suggest functional adaptation in males in response to RRR.

lower pH in unstimulated saliva in women; even when corrected for numbers of medications, there were significant age-related declines in secretion rate and in pH.[94] Because of the impact of common age-related diseases and medications on salivary flow, large population-based studies are useful to unravel the effect of age. Multiple regression analysis of 1006 patients between 35 and 75 years of age showed significant effects of age and caloric intake on flow rates.[95] A study with 1427 individuals between 20 and 69 years of age determined that advanced age, female gender, and lower number of teeth were associated with low salivary flow rates, but the age of risk was 50 years for women and 60 years for men.[90] The use of xerogenic medications was also associated with low flow rates but was significant only in the older patients. There is a wide variation in the effect of age on salivary flow rate. Autoantibody data were available for a group of 178 female patients in a rheumatology practice.[91] Patients with any of the sicca-associated antibodies (anticentromere, anti-Ro, and/or anti-La) showed the age-related decrease in the salivary production rate. There was no relationship between the salivary production rate and age for the autoantibody-negative patients. At least for women, those autoantibodies are associated with an increased odds ratio of dry mouth by as much as 180 to 480.

Oral discomfort, related to dry mouth and decreased salivary flow, is among the subjective symptoms of menopause. Recent information suggests that estrogen receptors in salivary glands and oral mucosal epithelial cells mediate the protective antiapoptotic effects of estrogen on those tissues.[96] A study of 64 menopausal women showed that the mean unstimulated saliva flow rate and concentration of 17β-estradiol were significantly lower for those with xerostomia.[97] There was an inverse correlation between xerostomia severity and saliva 17β-estradiol. These mechanisms can help to explain the gender dimorphism of Sjögren syndrome (male/female ratio of 1:9). There is abundant evidence that estrogen replacement therapy (ERT) relieves many women of these problems.[98] One study indicated that responsiveness to ERT was associated with the immunocytochemical presence of estrogen receptors in oral tissue.[99] In a study with objective outcome measures, saliva flow was increased after 3, 6, and 12 months of hormone treatment; this was accompanied by subjective relief of dry mouth sensation.[100]

Effects of Gender on Success of Endosseous Implants

Endosseous implants placed into jaws transmit functional load to the bone and reduce atrophy of alveolar bone. Jaffin and Berman[101] identified the implant failure rate to be elevated in sites with poor-quality bone (ie, with thin cortical bone and poor trabecular architecture), suggestive of osteopenia. A limited number of studies examined the effects of age or menopause on implant failure. A retrospective study showed significantly higher maxillary failure rate for implants in postmenopausal women than in premenopausal women and a trend for a beneficial effect of ERT.[102] Another retrospective study that classified osteoporosis status by spine BMD found an effect of current smoking and no effect of osteoporosis on implant failure in the mandible.[103] Because implant success rates usually exceed 95%, very large studies may be needed to test the effects of menopause or osteoporosis on implant success. Analyses of patients who required bone grafts to augment the atrophic jaw for implant placement show striking effects of gender. In a study of implants in grafted jaws, with a poor overall 5-year survival rate of 68%, nearly all failures occurred in women; multivariate analysis indicated that only female gender had a significant effect on the failure rate.[104] Another study with a 10-year follow-up of maxillary implants with onlay bone grafting showed a 10% failure in women compared with 3% in men ($P<.05$).[105] The difference was not explained by smoking habits or marginal bone loss. The latter team of investigators reported no effect of gender or smoking on implant failure in a series with interpositional bone grafting to restore maxillary volume.[106] These studies show the importance of careful selection of patients for surgical options for maxillary reconstruction.

SUMMARY

Despite wide variations in the size and shape of the human face, head, and body, there is remarkable consistency for quantifiable gender-specific facial traits. Gender-specific growth trajectories of the craniofacial bones are especially notable for the mandible and maxilla. Craniofacial anomalies are among the most common congenital defects, and prevalences often show gender differences. Eruption of the deciduous and permanent teeth influence jaw growth at different ages for girls and boys. In addition, there are gender differences in clinical findings of variations in tooth number and presence of palatal tori. An understanding of these differences in patterns of malocclusions can aid clinicians in diagnosis and treatment planning.

Facial aging in dentate patients is characterized by retrusion of the midface in relation to the lower face. With edentulism, there is a gender-specific age-related loss of height in both jaws, a greater loss of ridge height and mandibular bone mineral content in women, and an increase in cortical bone mineral content in men that may reflect a gender-specific functional adaptation. Systemic osteoporosis, which is more prevalent in women than men, is correlated with some measurements in the jaws, but radiographs are not approved for diagnosis of osteoporosis. Salivary gland size and unstimulated flow rate are lower in women than in men. With aging, there is loss of salivary gland secretion and function, especially at menopause and in women positive for sicca-associated antibodies. These disturbances in genetic, endocrine, and nutritional regulatory controls result in gender-specific and nonspecific disorders.

ACKNOWLEDGMENTS

The authors appreciate Karen Aneshansley for the Figs.

REFERENCES

1. Weston EM, Friday AE, Liò P. Biometric evidence that sexual selection has shaped the hominin face. PLoS One 2007;2:e710.
2. Dean D, Hans MG, Bookstein FL, et al. Three-dimensional Bolton-Brush Growth Study landmark data: ontogeny and sexual dimorphism of the Bolton standards cohort. Cleft Palate Craniofac J 2000;37:145–56.
3. Forsberg CM. Facial morphology and ageing: a longitudinal investigation in young adults. Eur J Orthod 1979;1:15–23.
4. Ingerslev CH, Solow B. Sex differences in craniofacial morphology. Acta Odontol Scand 1975;33:85–94.
5. Ursi WJ, Trotman CA, McNamara JA Jr, et al. Sexual dimorphism in normal craniofacial growth. Angle Orthod 1993;63:47–56.
6. Bulygina E, Mitteroecker P, Aiello L. Ontogeny of facial dimorphism and patterns of individual development within one human population. Am J Phys Anthropol 2006;131:432–43.
7. Garvin HM, Ruff CB. Sexual dimorphism in skeletal browridge and chin morphologies determined using a new quantitative method. Am J Phys Anthropol 2012; 147:661–70.

8. Gazi-Coklica V, Muretić Z, Brcić R, et al. Craniofacial parameters during growth from the deciduous to permanent dentition–a longitudinal study. Eur J Orthod 1997;19:681–9.

9. Funatsu M, Sato K, Mitani H. Effects of growth hormone on craniofacial growth. Angle Orthod 2006;76:970–7.

10. Marečková K, Weinbrand Z, Chakravarty MM, et al. Testosterone-mediated sex differences in the face shape during adolescence: subjective impressions and objective features. Horm Behav 2011;60:681–90.

11. Fink B, Grammer K, Mitteroecker P, et al. Second to fourth digit ratio and face shape. Proc Biol Sci 2005;272:1995–2001.

12. Manning JT, Scutt D, Wilson J, et al. The ratio of 2nd to 4th digit length: a predictor of sperm numbers and concentrations of testosterone, luteinizing hormone and oestrogen. Hum Reprod 1998;13:3000–4.

13. Zheng Z, Cohn MJ. Developmental basis of sexually dimorphic digit ratios. Proc Natl Acad Sci U S A 2011;108:16289–94.

14. Thayer ZM, Dobson SD. Sexual dimorphism in chin shape: implications for adaptive hypotheses. Am J Phys Anthropol 2010;143:417–25.

15. Coquerelle M, Bookstein FL, Braga J, et al. Sexual dimorphism of the human mandible and its association with dental development. Am J Phys Anthropol 2011;145:192–202.

16. Liu YP, Behrents RG, Buschang PH. Mandibular growth, remodeling, and maturation during infancy and early childhood. Angle Orthod 2010;80:97–105.

17. Plavcan JM. Sexual dimorphism in primate evolution. Am J Phys Anthropol 2001;116:25–53.

18. Alió-Sanz J, Iglesias-Conde C, Pernía JL, et al. Retrospective study of maxilla growth in a Spanish population sample. Med Oral Patol Oral Cir Bucal 2011; 16:e271–7.

19. Louly F, Nouer PR, Janson G, et al. Dental arch dimensions in the mixed dentition: a study of Brazilian children from 9 to 12 years of age. J Appl Oral Sci 2011; 19:169–74.

20. Langford RJ, Sgouros S, Natarajan K, et al. Maxillary volume growth in childhood. Plast Reconstr Surg 2003;111:1591–7.

21. Moorrees CF, Gron AM, Lebret LM, et al. Growth studies of the dentition: a review. Am J Orthod 1969;55:600–16.

22. Savara BS, Singh IJ. Norms of size and annual increments of seven anatomical measures of maxillae in boys from three to sixteen years of age. Angle Orthod 1968;38:104–20.

23. Singh IJ, Savara BS. Norms of size and annual increments of seven anatomical measures of maxillae in girls from three to sixteen years of age. Angle Orthod 1966;36:312–24.

24. Fujita T, Ohtani J, Shigekawa M, et al. Effects of sex hormone disturbances on craniofacial growth in newborn mice. J Dent Res 2004;83:250–4.

25. Güncü GN, Yıldırım YD, Yılmaz HG, et al. Is there a gender difference in anatomic features of incisive canal and maxillary environmental bone? Clin Oral Implants Res 2012. [Epub ahead of print].

26. Kaul SS, Pathak RK, Santosh BS. Emergence of deciduous teeth in Punjabi children, north India. Z Morphol Anthropol 1992;79:25–34.

27. Ramirez O, Planells P, Barberia E. Age and order of eruption of primary teeth in Spanish children. Community Dent Oral Epidemiol 1994;22:56–9.

28. Choi NK, Yang KH. A study on the eruption timing of primary teeth in Korean children. ASDC J Dent Child 2001;68:244–9.

29. Soliman NL, El-Zainy MA, Hassan RM, et al. Relationship of deciduous teeth emergence with physical growth. Indian J Dent Res 2012;23:236–40.
30. Bastos JL, Peres MA, Peres KG, et al. Infant growth, development and tooth emergence patterns: a longitudinal study from birth to 6 years of age. Arch Oral Biol 2007;52:598–606.
31. Hurme VO. Standards of variation in the eruption of the first six permanent teeth. Child Devel 1948;19:213–31.
32. Almonaitiene R, Balciuniene I, Tutkuviene J. Factors influencing permanent teeth eruption. Part one–general factors. Stomatologija 2010;12:67–72.
33. Diamanti J, Townsend GC. New standards for permanent tooth emergence in Australian children. Aust Dent J 2003;48:39–42.
34. Leroy R, Bogaerts K, Lesaffre E, et al. The emergence of permanent teeth in Flemish children. Community Dent Oral Epidemiol 2003;31:30–9.
35. Wedl JS, Schoder V, Blake FA, et al. Eruption times of permanent teeth in teenage boys and girls in Izmir (Turkey). J Clin Forensic Med 2004;11:299–302.
36. Rousset MM, Boualam N, Delfosse C, et al. Emergence of permanent teeth: secular trends and variance in a modern sample. J Dent Child (Chic) 2003; 70:208–14.
37. Moorrees CF, Thomsen SO, Jensen E, et al. Mesiodistal crown diameters of the deciduous and permanent teeth in individuals. J Dent Res 1957;36:39–47.
38. Thilander B. Dentoalveolar development in subjects with normal occlusion. A longitudinal study between the ages of 5 and 31 years. Eur J Orthod 2009;31: 109–20.
39. Viciano J, Aleman I, D'Anastasio R, et al. Odontometric sex discrimination in the Herculaneum sample (79 AD, Naples, Italy), with application to juveniles. Am J Phys Anthropol 2011;145:97–106.
40. Marazita ML. Genetic etiologies of facial clefting. In: Mooney MP, Siegel MI, editors. Understanding craniofacial anomalies: the etiopathogenesis of cranio-synostoses and facial clefting. New York: Wiley-Liss; 2002. p. 147–61.
41. Meskin LH, Pruzansky S. A malformation profile of facial cleft patients and their siblings. Cleft Palate J 1969;6:309–15.
42. Ingalls TH, Taube IE, Klingberg MA. Cleft lip and cleft palate: epidemiologic considerations. Plast Reconstr Surg 1964;34:1–10.
43. Sadler TW. Langman's medical embryology. 9th edition. Philadelphia: Lippincott Williams & Wilkins; 2004.
44. Neville BD, Damm DD, Allen CM, et al. Oral and maxillofacial pathology. 3rd edition. St Louis: Saunders; 2009. p. 79–81.
45. Dixon MJ, Marazita ML, Beaty TH, et al. Cleft lip and palate: understanding genetic and environmental influences. Nat Rev Genet 2011;12(3):167–78.
46. Poon CC, Meara JG, Heggie AA. Hemifacial microsomia: use of the OMENS-Plus classification at the Royal Children's Hospital of Melbourne. Plast Reconstr Surg 2003;111:1011–8.
47. Werler MM, Sheehan JE, Hayes C, et al. Demographic and reproductive factors associated with hemifacial microsomia. Cleft Palate Craniofac J 2004;41: 494–500.
48. Rollnick BR, Kaye CL, Nagatoshi K, et al. Oculoauriculovertebral dysplasia and variants: phenotypic characteristics of 294 patients. Am J Med Genet 1987;26: 361–75.
49. Reardon W, Wilkes D, Rutland P, et al. Craniosynostosis associated with FGFR3 pro250arg mutation results in a range of clinical presentations including unisu-tural sporadic craniosynostosis. J Med Genet 1997;34:632–6.

50. Siriwat PP, Jarabak JR. Malocclusion and facial morphology is there a relationship? An epidemiologic study. Angle Orthod 1985;55:127–38.
51. Baccetti T, Reyes BC, McNamara JA Jr. Gender differences in class III malocclusion. Angle Orthod 2005;75:510–20.
52. Brook AH. A unifying aetiological explanation for anomalies of human tooth number and size. Arch Oral Biol 1984;29:373–8.
53. Larmour CJ, Mossey PA, Thind BS, et al. Hypodontia—a retrospective review of prevalence and etiology. Part I. Quintessence Int 2005;36:263–70.
54. Küchler EC, Risso PA, Costa Mde C, et al. Studies of dental anomalies in a large group of school children. Arch Oral Biol 2008;53:941–6.
55. Küchler EC, Costa AG, Costa Mde C, et al. Supernumerary teeth vary depending on gender. Braz Oral Res 2011;25:76–9.
56. Bath-Balogh M, Fehrenbach MJ. Illustrated dental embryology, histology, and anatomy. 2nd edition. St Louis: Elsevier Saunders; 2006. p. 65–9.
57. Williams PL, Warwick R, Dyson M, et al. Osteology. In: Gray's anatomy. 37th edition. Edinburgh, Scotland: Churchill Livingstone; 1989. p. 354.
58. Reichart PA, Neuhaus F, Sookasem M. Prevalence of torus palatinus and torus mandibularis in Germans and Thai. Community Dent Oral Epidemiol 1988;16:61–4.
59. Haugen LK. Palatine and mandibular tori. A morphologic study in the current Norwegian population. Acta Odontol Scand 1992;50:65–77.
60. Sigurdsson G, Aspelund T, Chang M, et al. Increasing sex difference in bone strength in old age: the Age, Gene/Environment Susceptibility-Reykjavik study (AGES-REYKJAVIK). Bone 2006;39:644–51.
61. LeBoff MS, Glowacki J. Sex steroids, aging, and bone. In: Rosen C, Glowacki J, Bilzekian JP, editors. The aging skeleton. San Diego (CA): Academic Press; 1999. p. 159–74.
62. Jeffcoat MK. Osteoporosis: a possible modifying factor in oral bone loss. Ann Periodontol 1998;3:312–21.
63. Bondevik O. Dentofacial changes in adults. J Orofac Orthop 2012;73:277–88.
64. Law AN, Bollen AM, Chen SK. Detecting osteoporosis using dental radiographs: a comparison between four methods. J Am Dent Assoc 1996;127:1734–42.
65. Devlin H, Horner K. Mandibular radiomorphometric indices in the diagnosis of reduced skeletal bone mineral density. Osteoporos Int 2002;13:373–8.
66. Drozdzowska B, Pluskiewicz W, Tarnawska B. Panoramic-based mandibular indices in relation to mandibular bone mineral density and skeletal status assessed by dual energy x-ray absorptiometry and quantitative ultrasound. Dentomaxillofac Radiol 2002;31:361–7.
67. Passos JS, Gomes Filho IS, Sarmento VA, et al. Women with low bone mineral density and dental panoramic radiography. Menopause 2012;19:704–9.
68. Dutra V, Yang J, Devlin H, et al. Radiomorphometric indices and their relation to gender, age, and dental status. Oral Surg Oral Med Oral Pathol Oral Radiol Endod 2005;99:479–84.
69. Henriques JC, Castilho JC, Jacobs R, et al. Correlation between hand/wrist and panoramic radiographs in severe secondary hyperparathyroidism. Clin Oral Investig 2012. [Epub ahead of print].
70. Devlin H, Karayianni K, Mitsea A, et al. Diagnosing osteoporosis by using dental panoramic radiographs: the OSTEODENT project. Oral Surg Oral Med Oral Pathol Oral Radiol Endod 2007;104:821–8.
71. White SC, Rudolph DJ. Alterations of the trabecular pattern of the jaws in patients with osteoporosis. Oral Surg Oral Med Oral Pathol Oral Radiol Endod 1999;88:628–35.

72. White SC, Atchison KA, Gornbein JA, et al. Change in mandibular trabecular pattern and hip fracture rate in elderly women. Dentomaxillofac Radiol 2005; 34:168–74.
73. Werning JW, Downey NM, Brinker RA, et al. The impact of osteoporosis on patients with maxillofacial trauma. Arch Otolaryngol Head Neck Surg 2004; 130:353–6.
74. Ganguly R, Ramesh A. Screening for osteoporosis with panoramic radiographs. J Mass Dent Soc 2012;61:44–5.
75. Pessa JE, Zadoo VP, Mutimer KL, et al. Relative maxillary retrusion as a natural consequence of aging: combining skeletal and soft-tissue changes into an integrated model of midfacial aging. Plast Reconstr Surg 1998;102:205–12.
76. Shaw RB Jr, Kahn DM. Aging of the midface bony elements: a three-dimensional computed tomographic study. Plast Reconstr Surg 2007;119:675–81.
77. Shaw RB Jr, Katzel EB, Koltz PF, et al. Aging of the mandible and its aesthetic implications. Plast Reconstr Surg 2010;125:332–42.
78. Tallgren A. The continuing reduction of the residual alveolar ridges in complete denture wearers: a mixed-longitudinal study covering 25 years. J Prosthet Dent 1972;27:120–32 Reproduced in J Prosthet Dent 2003;89:427–35.
79. Kovačić I, Knezović Zlatarić D, Celebić A. Residual ridge atrophy in complete denture wearers and relationship with densitometric values of a cervical spine: a hierarchical regression analysis. Gerodontology 2012;29:e935–47.
80. Nishimura I, Hosokawa R, Atwood DA. The knife-edge tendency in mandibular residual ridges in women. J Prosthet Dent 1992;67:820–6.
81. Hirai T, Ishijima T, Hashikawa Y, et al. Osteoporosis and reduction of residual ridge in edentulous patients. J Prosthet Dent 1993;69:49–56.
82. Richard MJ, Morris C, Deen BF, et al. Analysis of the anatomic changes of the aging facial skeleton using computer-assisted tomography. Ophthal Plast Reconstr Surg 2009;25:382–6.
83. Roberts M, Yuan J, Graham J, et al. Changes in mandibular cortical width measurements with age in men and women. Osteoporos Int 2011;22:1915–25.
84. von Wowern N. Bone mineral content of mandibles: normal reference values–rate of age-related bone loss. Calcif Tissue Int 1988;43:193–8.
85. Ulm CW, Solar P, Ulm MR, et al. Sex-related changes in the bone mineral content of atrophic mandibles. Calcif Tissue Int 1994;54:203–7.
86. Müller F, Naharro M, Carlsson GE. What are the prevalence and incidence of tooth loss in the adult and elderly population in Europe? Clin Oral Implants Res 2007;18:2S–14S.
87. Available at: http://www.ada.org/sections/newsAndEvents/pdfs/ltr_dry_mouth_110427.pdf. Accessed January 8, 2013.
88. Stookey GK. The effect of saliva on dental caries. J Am Dent Assoc 2008;139: 11S–7S.
89. Dodds MW, Johnson DA, Yeh CK. Health benefits of saliva: a review. J Dent 2005;33:223–33.
90. Flink H, Bergdahl M, Tegelberg A, et al. Prevalence of hyposalivation in relation to general health, body mass index and remaining teeth in different age groups of adults. Community Dent Oral Epidemiol 2008;36:523–31.
91. Takada K, Suzuki K, Okada M, et al. Salivary production rates fall with age in subjects having anti-centromere, anti-Ro, and/or anti-La antibodies. Scand J Rheumatol 2006;35:23–8.
92. Yamamoto K, Kurihara M, Matsusue Y, et al. Whole saliva flow rate and body profile in healthy young adults. Arch Oral Biol 2009;54:464–9.

93. Inoue H, Ono K, Masuda W, et al. Gender difference in unstimulated whole saliva flow rate and salivary gland sizes. Arch Oral Biol 2006;51:1055–60.
94. van der Putten GJ, Brand HS, De Visschere LM, et al. Saliva secretion rate and acidity in a group of physically disabled older care home residents. Odontology 2013;101:108–15.
95. Yeh CK, Johnson DA, Dodds MW. Impact of aging on human salivary gland function: a community-based study. Aging (Milano) 1998;10:421–8.
96. Välimaa H, Savolainen S, Soukka T, et al. Estrogen receptor-beta is the predominant estrogen receptor subtype in human oral epithelium and salivary glands. J Endocrinol 2004;180:55–62.
97. Agha-Hosseini F, Mirzaii-Dizgah I. Unstimulated saliva 17β-estradiol and xerostomia in menopause. Gynecol Endocrinol 2012;28:199–202.
98. Wardrop RW, Hailes J, Burger H, et al. Oral discomfort at menopause. Oral Surg Oral Med Oral Pathol 1989;67:535–40.
99. Forabosco A, Criscuolo M, Coukos G, et al. Efficacy of hormone replacement therapy in postmenopausal women with oral discomfort. Oral Surg Oral Med Oral Pathol 1992;73:570–4.
100. Eliasson L, Carlén A, Laine M, et al. Minor gland and whole saliva in postmenopausal women using a low potency oestrogen (oestriol). Arch Oral Biol 2003; 48:511–7.
101. Jaffin RA, Berman CL. The excessive loss of Branemark fixtures in type IV bone: a 5-year analysis. J Periodontol 1991;62:2–4.
102. August M, Chung K, Chang Y, et al. Influence of estrogen status on implant osseointegration. J Oral Maxillofac Surg 2001;59:1285–9.
103. Holahan CM, Koka S, Kennel KA, et al. Effect of osteoporotic status on the survival of titanium dental implants. Int J Oral Maxillofac Implants 2008;23: 905–10.
104. Schliephake H, Neukam FW, Wichmann M. Survival analysis of endosseous implants in bone grafts used for the treatment of severe alveolar ridge atrophy. J Oral Maxillofac Surg 1997;55:1227–33.
105. Nyström E, Nilson H, Gunne J, et al. A 9-14 year follow-up of onlay bone grafting in the atrophic maxilla. Int J Oral Maxillofac Surg 2009;38:111–6.
106. Nyström E, Nilson H, Gunne J, et al. Reconstruction of the atrophic maxilla with interpositional bone grafting/Le Fort I osteotomy and endosteal implants: a 11-16 year follow-up. Int J Oral Maxillofac Surg 2009;38:1–6.

Violence and Abuse
Core Competencies for Identification and Access to Care

Lisa A. Thompson, DMD[a],*, Mary Tavares, DMD, MPH[a],
Daphne Ferguson-Young, DDS, MSPH[b], Orrett Ogle, DDS[c],
Leslie R. Halpern, MD, DDD, PhD, MPH[d]

KEYWORDS

- Violence/abuse • Chronic illness • Curricula • Core competencies • Access
- Interdisciplinary

KEY POINTS

- Apply violence/abuse/neglect in the differential diagnosis of all female patients with orofacial injuries.
- Apply a well-documented record that includes mechanism of injury to orofacial region/associated injuries, and history, if any, of prior assault.
- Record other health disparities/chronic illnesses and how violence/abuse/neglect affect the life span of the victim.
- Apply core competencies at the individual, health center, and community levels that will enable the skills to identify, intervene, and prevent future injuries.
- Interdisciplinary education on violence/abuse needs to be standardized and incorporated into dental school and continuing education curricula.

INTRODUCTION

"Interpersonal violence (violence and abuse) is the intentional use of physical force or power, threatened or actual, against oneself, against another person or against a group or community, which results in a high likelihood of injury, death, psychological harm, maldevelopment, or deprivation" (WHO, 2011).[1] It occurs in the context of a broad range of human relationships including violence within the family: child abuse and neglect, intimate partner violence (IPV), and elder abuse.[2–4] It is estimated that

---

All authors have nothing to disclose.
[a] Oral Health Policy and Epidemiology, Harvard School of Dental Medicine, 188 Longwood Avenue, Boston, MA 02115, USA; [b] General Practice Residency, School of Dentistry, Meharry Medical College, 1005 DB Todd Jr. Boulevard, Nashville, TN 37208, USA; [c] 28 Roger Street, Hempstead, NY 11550, USA; [d] Oral and Maxillofacial Surgery, Meharry Medical College, 1005 DB Todd Jr. Boulevard, Nashville, TN 37208, USA
* Corresponding author.
E-mail address: lisa_thompson@hsdm.harvard.edu

more than 2.5 million women are abused annually, and 30% to 50% of all female homicides are perpetrated by former or current intimate partners.[5,6] Within the past 2 to 3 decades, violence and abuse (V/A) has been recognized as a significant public health problem among female patients.[5-9] Beyond the physical and psychological repercussions, a significant number of female victims have lower health-related quality of life and more frequent use of health services.[5-7]

A growing awareness of the scope and effects of V/A have led various health care bodies, including the American Medical Association (AMA), the American College of Obstetricians and Gynecologists (ACOGS), and, most recently, the Institute of Medicine (IOM), to recommend that all patients be asked routinely about abuse, regardless of their presenting injury or symptoms.[5-9] The American Dental Association (ADA) developed an educational policy for identifying all victims of abuse. Dental providers were advised to look for symptoms such as conflicting histories of injury, behavioral changes, and multiple injuries at various stages of healing, as well as recoil behavior during dental examinations. In 1999, the American Academy of Pediatrics and the American Academy of Pediatric Dentistry concurred that "in all 50 states, physicians and dentists are required to report suspected cases of child abuse to social service or law-enforcement agencies and to collaborate in order to increase the prevention, detection, and treatment of these conditions."[9,10]

In a viewpoint article of the ADA News (2006), Colangelo[11] summarized the importance of increasing the dental community's understanding of and response to domestic violence, because of the common involvement of the head, neck, and oral cavity. An estimated 75% of physical abuse cases result in injuries to the head, neck, and/or mouth, areas that are clearly visible to the dental team during examination. With more than 50% of adults and children visiting the dentist at least once per year, oral health care providers are in routine contact with affected patients. However, studies show that these providers are not always aware of the pivotal role they can play even though the dentist and his or her team are in an ideal position to identify a significant number of patients who have experienced V/A. In a survey of dentists, only 6% of respondents reported that they commonly suspected spousal abuse among their female patients.[9] Concerns reported among these dentists that may affect their likelihood to inquire about IPV include inadequate professional training in detecting an abuse victim and ambiguity in orofacial signs of abuse. Likewise, there may be various reasons for why female patients do not report IPV, including reluctance to admit the true cause of an injury, shame, denial, fear, poor communication between the provider and patient, or desire to protect the assailant.[12,13]

This article provides compelling evidence that supports the unique position occupied by dental professionals within the arena of the detection, intervention, and prevention of V/A. The authors review the epidemiology of orofacial risk factors for V/A, and diagnostic tools and surveys for identifying victims of all ages, and suggest interdisciplinary educational curricula and specific algorithms to provide the necessary core competencies for identifying victims in the oral health care environment. In addition, evidence is presented to characterize the disproportionate number of female patients who are victims. By doing so, the oral health care provider will successfully identify and prevent future injuries to their patients within the community setting.

EPIDEMIOLOGY
Overview in Adults

Tilden and colleagues[14] demonstrated that "dentists and dental hygienists are least likely to suspect abuse in children, elders, or young adults." Other research found that only a small percentage of providers screen for V/A, even when there are visible signs of head and neck injuries.[15] In addition, reports of child abuse by dental staff comprise less than 1% of all reports made.[15,16] The perpetrator(s) and their victims often return to the same dental office for care, thinking it unlikely that the dentist will screen for possible abuse.[17,18] Dental therapeutics can be particularly uncomfortable for victims of abuse, owing to feelings of loss of control.[16–18] Walker and colleagues[19] evaluated women with a history of trauma and reported greater dental fear, while women with high dental fear scores were nearly twice as likely to have been victims of multiple assaults. In a study of female patients with temporomandibular disorder, those with a history of physical abuse reported significantly more pain, anxiety, and depressive symptoms than patients with a history of sexual abuse or no history of abuse. In a study of female patients with orofacial pain, nearly 69% had a history of abuse, significantly related to greater levels of depression and psychological distress, increased anxiety, decreased capacity to cope with stressful events, and increased pain severity.[19–21] These results suggest that victims of abuse may have difficulty finding adequate coping strategies for facial pain, and their psychological distress may exacerbate their facial pain disorders.[19–21]

Child Abuse

All 50 US states and the US territories have mandatory child abuse and neglect-reporting laws that require certain professionals and institutions to report suspected maltreatment to child-protective services (CPS).[22,23] Dental neglect, as defined by the American Academy of Pediatric Dentistry, is the "willful failure of parent or guardian to seek and follow through with treatment necessary to ensure a level of oral health essential for adequate function and freedom from pain and infection."[24] Numerous studies have characterized craniofacial, head, face, and neck injuries to occur in more than half of cases of child abuse, regardless of gender.[23,25,26] For 2010, three-fifths of reports of alleged child abuse and neglect were made by professionals: teachers (16.4%), law-enforcement and legal personnel (16.7%), and social services staff (11.5%). The number of reported child fatalities resulting from child abuse and neglect, however, has fluctuated during the past 5 years. In addition, studies have supported the mandate of laws for abuse and neglect by mandating not only signs of oral trauma but also caries, gingivitis, and other oral health problems.[22,23,25,26]

Some authorities believe that the oral cavity may be a central focus for physical abuse and neglect because of its significance in communication and nutrition. In the area of cognitive, behavioral, and emotional well-being, witnessing V/A can have significant effects on children and adolescents.[23,25,26] Children who live in violent household(s) were at risk for physical injury either directly or indirectly, the most common mechanism of injury being a direct hit.[27,28] Children younger than 5 years were more likely than older children to sustain head or facial injury. Some 60% of children younger than 2 years were injured while being held by a parent. A high proportion of adolescents were injured during an attempt to intervene in the altercation between the adults.[27,28] As such, children and adolescents seen by the oral health care provider for a facial or dental injury should include V/A as a possible cause, regardless of gender (see later sections on identification/educational strategies).[22,23,25,26,28]

Elder Abuse

While dental professional groups are lending more attention to the area of domestic violence and child abuse, there is a paucity of data examining elder abuse and neglect (EAN).[29–31] EAN is defined as intentional actions that cause harm or create a serious risk of harm (whether or not it is intended) to an adult older than 65 years by a caregiver or other person who stands in a trusted relationship with the elder.[29] Because women live longer than their male cohorts, significant data have suggested that abuse and neglect of older women is a serious public health problem.[29,30] A total of 91,000 women between the ages of 50 and 79 years in the Women's Health Initiative provided prevalence data on abuse and neglect. Eleven percent reported abuse at baseline, and after prospective follow-up 5% still reported abuse.[30]

Elder abuse, whether in women or men, is often left in the shadows.[30,31] A 2010 survey conducted by predoctoral students at the University of California, Los Angeles (UCLA) School of Dentistry highlights some of the discrepancies in dental school education addressing elder abuse. Overall, dental students felt inadequately prepared to both detect and report elder abuse, and need more education on the psychosocial aspects of older adults.[31] As stated by Gironda and colleagues,[31] "little attention is given to elder abuse by professional organizations and may further contribute to the dental community's lack of reporting." This situation is evident, even among practicing dentists, in the low rates of detecting and reporting of EAN. In one survey of 407 dentists, 7% reported having suspected abuse and 1% had filed a report.[31] There was no separation between reporting by male or female practitioners. With current prevalence estimates of elder mistreatment ranging between 3.2% and 27.5% in general population studies, it is estimated that for every case of elder abuse, neglect, exploitation, or self-neglect reported to authorities, about 5 more cases go unreported (Fact Sheet: National Center on Elder Abuse).[32] This evidence pleads the case to assure that the dental workforce is properly training its staff on reporting elder mistreatment.

Several factors contribute to the complexity in screening for elder abuse. To identify victims of abuse and neglect, one must distinguish among characteristics of normal aging, physical manifestations of disease, and physical signs of abuse. "Not all mucosal or skin lesions or bruises or discolorations of the orofacial structures are indicators of abuse. Bruises and abrasions may be the unintentional result of medications administered intravenously or intramuscularly or caused accidentally by caregivers."[10] In addition to a thorough head, neck, and oral examination, a comprehensive and valid history that includes questions of a patient's activities of daily living, independent activities of daily living, living situation, and who helps take care of the patient are essential to forming a differential diagnosis and screening for elder abuse. Elder abuse victims may be victims of physical, emotional, psychological, or financial abuse, or neglect from individuals with whom they live, partners, adult children, caregivers, other family members, or employees of a nursing facility or institution.[10] As such, the diminished physical and cognitive capabilities, and social isolation superimposed with the differing definitions and terminology of abuse make it more difficult to diagnose EAN.[33,34] The recent laws on the mandatory reporting of EAN have prompted health care specialties to revisit ways for identification and intervention (see sections on education/competencies).

Orofacial Injuries as Diagnostic Tools

Interpersonal violence is a frequent cause of orofacial injuries in females, with most injuries occurring in individuals between the ages of 15 and 45 years.[8,35–39] The prevalence of IPV-related orofacial injuries, however, is underestimated. There has been a paucity of well-designed epidemiologic studies that measure more precisely the frequency of IPV-related orofacial injuries (**Table 1**). Injury sustained during interpersonal assaults is reported to account for 5% to 59% of all facial injuries.[8,35–39,43] Reports from emergency department visits indicate that more than 75% of the time,

Table 1
Frequency estimates of maxillofacial injuries in victims of IPV

Authors,[Ref.] Year	Design[a]	Data Set[b]	Age Range (y)	n (%)[c]	Sex	Injury
Zacharides et al,[75] 1990	Retrospective	Chart review	16–62	51 (9)	F	HNF
Fisher et al,[76] 1990	Cross-sectional	Chart review	10–78	23 (20)	F	HNF
Berrios and Grady,[35] 1991	Retrospective	Chart review	16–66	149 (68)	F	HNF
Ochs et al,[77] 1996	Cross-sectional	Cohort	18–51	15 (94)	F	HNF
Muelleman et al,[12] 1996	Cross-sectional	Cohort	19–65	121 (51)	F	HNF
Hartzell,[78] 1996	Retrospective	Chart review	15–63	7 (30)	F	Ocular
Huang et al,[40] 1998	Retrospective	Chart review	15–45	109 (36)	F	HNF
Perciaccante et al,[41] 1999	Cross-sectional	Cohort	24–56	34 (31)	F	HNF
Greene et al,[79] 1999	Retrospective	Chart review	32 (Mean)	29 (22)	F	HNF
Le et al,[80] 2002	Retrospective	Chart review	15–71	85 (30)	F	HNF
Crandall et al,[38] 2004	Cross-sectional	Chart review	16–65	145 (72)	F	HNF
Halpern and Dodson,[42] 2006	RCT	Cohort	27–64	63 (31)	F	HNF

Abbreviations: HNF, head, neck, and face; IPV, intimate partner violence; RCT, randomized controlled trial.
[a] Study design.
[b] Origin of data set.
[c] n, frequency (%) of IPV injuries.
Adapted from Wilson S, Dodson TB, Halpern LR. Maxillofacial injuries in intimate partner violence. In: Mitchell C, Anglin D, editors. Intimate partner violence: a health-based perspective based. New York: Oxford University Press; 2009. p. 201–16.

women who presented with facial trauma had concomitant injuries within the oral cavity, especially in young adults.[8,35–37]

Motor vehicle collisions and interpersonal assaults have been recognized as 2 of the primary mechanisms by which orofacial injuries occur, although the etiology depends on the population studied.[8,35–39] An Australian study of 2581 patients with radiographic evidence of facial fractures found that 1135 were secondary to interpersonal violence, 286 were secondary to a motor vehicle accident, and the remainder resulted from a variety of mechanisms. Most victims of the motor vehicle type were male and the most frequently sustained injury was mandible fracture(s). Alcohol use was involved in 87% of these assault-related injuries.[43]

A retrospective study of facial trauma in women by Huang and colleagues[40] in 1998 showed that there was often inadequate documentation regarding the circumstances of the facial injury. The investigators concluded that IPV may be severely underreported in women presenting with orofacial injuries. Among further studies,[40,43,44] Dutton and Strachen[44] examined the motives of men who committed IPV and interpersonal violence assaults against women seen in the emergency department. Possible motives were, it was concluded, the need for power and the maintenance of gender roles in the assailant's relationships. The investigators suggested that assaults to the face and head reinforce the assailant's dominance and control by leaving visible wounds as reminders of their power.[44] The residual effect of injury, that is, scars, facial asymmetries, damage to dentition, loss of masticatory function, and psychological wounds, persist as painful reminders of the abuse.[40,43,44]

Diagnostic protocols have been implemented to evaluate orofacial injuries as markers for IPV in the emergency setting.[41,45,46] Perciaccante and colleagues[41] evaluated head, neck, and facial injuries as markers of IPV in women. Of the 100 injured women, 58 had head, neck, and facial injuries, 31 of whom were victims of IPV. A woman who had head, neck, and facial injuries was 7.5 times more likely than a woman who had other injuries to be a victim of IPV. Halpern and colleagues[46] repeated this approach and tested the external validity of the protocol using the 2 variables (1) head, neck, facial injury location and (2) a verbal questionnaire associated with IPV-related injuries from the preliminary studies by Perciaccante and colleagues[41,45,46] By comparing 2 hospitals that differed by geographic location, socioeconomic status, and health care cost, their results suggested that clinicians can use injury location in conjunction with the Partner Violence Screen (PVS) score to stratify (ie, as high or low) the risk of self-report of IPV-related injuries.[46] Additional studies have determined that, in terms of detecting women with IPV-related injuries, diagnostic protocol proposed by the investigators is 40 times more likely to report an IPV-related injury, compared with 11 times more likely with the standard operating procedure of the emergency department (odds ratio 40; $P<.01$). The sensitivity of the diagnostic protocol was superior to standard operating procedures, but specificities were equivalent.[47] A predictive model using location of head, neck, and facial injury and responses to a verbal questionnaire stratifies the risk of self-report of causes of IPV-related injury.[42] This risk was modified by other variables of age and race and was tested in a predictive model for goodness of fit using an independent set of patients with which to compare the model. Injury location, positive responses to the questionnaire, and age can significantly facilitate early diagnosis of IPV.[42]

Although the aforementioned tools appear valid, there is still controversy on whether routine screenings for IPV should be performed in health care settings. In 2004 the US Preventive Services Task Force found insufficient evidence to recommend for or against routine screening of women for IPV.[27,48] A systematic review was published in the Cochrane Database of Systematic Reviews in 2004 regarding screening for domestic violence and intervention programs for females who had dental or facial injuries.[48] The investigators found no eligible randomized controlled trials on this topic, and concluded that "there is no evidence to support or refute the effectiveness of screening and intervention programs detecting and supporting victims of domestic violence with dental or facial injuries".[48] Nevertheless, there are individual studies suggesting the value of screening for V/A. Taliaferro[49] has written a review article on the topic of screening and identification of V/A in females. She emphasized the need to assess risk versus benefit in such screening of individual patients. Although anecdotal evidence suggests the benefits of screening, there are potential risks to such questionnaires, including selection bias, misclassification, reproducibility, and generalizability.[42,46–50] Further research is needed to determine whether diagnostic protocols can help to significantly increase the identification of victims of V/A and reduce future injuries.

Educational Strategies for the Practitioner

In 2006, the ADA News ran a commentary summarizing the importance of increasing the dental community's education, understanding, and obligation to recognize the signs and symptoms of family violence.[51,52] In 2008, the American Association of Oral and Maxillofacial Surgeons issued a consensus statement: "Oral and maxillofacial surgeons are dedicated to the health and well-being of all our patients, including those affected by V/A, post-traumatic stress disorders, or traumatic brain injury."[53] Education about V/A in the training of oromaxillofacial surgeons and dentists, however, has been insufficient even when the signs of abuse are present. Reasons for lack of identification may be divided into 2 types: (1) inadequate education on the approach to identify victims and (2) barriers to questioning that include patients accompanied by their partners and/or family members, cultural norms, and personal embarrassment by the doctor. Some dental professionals fear that there will be litigation if they are mistaken.[15,22,47]

Educators in oral health at the public health level have taken a variety of major steps to provide the knowledge base needed by dentists to identify victims of domestic violence more effectively. The Prevent Abuse and Neglect through Dental Awareness (PANDA) was initiated in the early 1990s by Dr Lynn Mouden-Douglas and coordinated through Delta Dental. PANDA provides information on the history of family violence in our society, clinical examples of confirmed cases of child abuse and neglect, and discussions of legal and liability issues involved in reporting child maltreatment. More than 46 states and several international coalitions have replicated this model.[34] In 2008, PANDA expanded training in abuse/neglect detection to the entire family: children, adults, and the elderly. Oral manifestations of sexually transmitted diseases, fearfulness of the dental examination, difficulty sitting or walking, and fear of the reclined position of the chair should alert the health care practitioner to signs and symptoms suggestive of physical or sexual abuse.[34]

Within the past 10 years, educational curricula for identifying victims have been introduced into the predoctoral and postdoctoral residency training curricula of a significant number of dental and medical schools around the United States.[54] Through the observation of what works and does not work within dental schools, a few strategies and approaches for future curricular pursuits have been outlined. Topics about abuse, if they were in the curricula, included the responsibilities of the oral health provider, as well as physical and behavioral indicators and referral protocols (see later discussion). The topics least emphasized, however, were about the education of the abused as an intervention, and the impact of V/A on society.[10] Research has indicated that dental students with IPV training before attending dental school had significantly higher rates of actual knowledge than the dental students without any prior IPV training.[54,55] Furthermore, it was noted that dental students who received IPV training in dental school had significantly higher actual knowledge than the dental students without access to IPV training in dental school.[54,55] The study also found that 10% of all dental students reported being a victim of IPV whether it was through sexual, physical, or threats of violence. Although a personal encounter may be useful as dental students relate to patients of IPV, it will not necessarily increase the actual knowledge or perceived knowledge of IPV.[55]

Nelms and colleagues[56] conducted a study through domestic shelters, which revealed that victims often experienced injury to more than 1 location in the head and neck region. The study further indicated that many of the victims who needed dental work as a consequence of the abusive episode did not seek care because of lack of finances. For the individuals who did seek out dental services, a large percentage of the respondents did not ask about their injuries. The study findings indicated regarding IPV, it would be prudent for dental professionals to recognize the signs of abuse, ask questions, and make the appropriate referrals for assistance. The dental profession faces barriers in relation to domestic violence. Education is critical in both dental schools and professional organizations, to train the dental team in how to conduct an interview and provide support to the victim.[56]

Gibson-Howell and colleagues[54] published data from surveys conducted among United States dental schools. By 2007 to 2008, 96% of dental schools included some curricula on child abuse. (For IPV and elder abuse, the percentage was unknown.) In dental hygiene schools, 70% had curricula in child abuse, 54.9% included elder abuse, and 46% included IPV. The topics relevant to the domestic violence part of the dental curricula included (1) responsibility of the health care professional, (2) physical and behavioral indicators, and (3) prevalence. In addition, 96% of dental schools included some curricula on child abuse; for IPV and elder abuse, however, the percentage was unknown. In dental hygiene schools, 70% had curricula on child abuse, 54.9% included elder abuse, and 46% included IPV.[53]

Several predoctoral education models are currently in place that can serve as case exemplars for intervention models, one of which is based at the Minnesota School of Dentistry. The Program Against Sexual Violence designed *Family Violence: An Intervention Model for Dental Professionals* for dental school and continuing education curricula. This model educates dental professionals about the signs of abuse and neglect, and teaches proactive and appropriate intervention. There is a series of DVDs available, and continuing education is encouraged by the state of Minnesota.[57] Another program has been developed in Boston at Tufts School of Dental Medicine (Gul G, personal communication, 2004). **Fig. 1** depicts this schema, which defines a flow of patients from the community who become de-identified for safety and examined thoroughly for both oral and overall health and well-being, so that further referrals can be sought to prevent future injuries to all victims. **Fig. 2** supports an interdisciplinary approach for combining oral health and the overall health and well-being of victims. Further data, as yet unpublished, are being collected by the authors of this article.

At the University of California, San Francisco, Hsieh and colleagues[52] published results of a survey indicating that dentists encounter major barriers to screening for domestic violence, including having the partner at the office visit, a lack of training, and the dentist's own embarrassment. In response, the team developed the AVDR tutorial, an acronym for Ask, Validate, Document, and Refer. The AVDR intervention was designed to help patients without imposing the unreasonable expectation that dentists solve the problem of family violence (**Box 1**). "After taking the tutorial," the investigators noted, "dentists reported that they would be more likely to inquire about a patient's safety after recognizing injuries to the head or neck."[52]

Because of the complex nature of EAN, it would be of use to have an educational schema to help put persons' oral health status in the context of their physical and

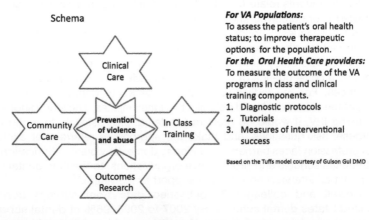

Fig. 1. Program structure.

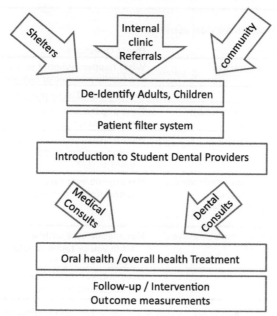

Fig. 2. Model in the dental center.

cognitive capabilities as well as a time frame in which their oral health care needs should be met.[31] One study attempts to define oral neglect in long-term care facilities, to create a framework by which to both define oral neglect and execute a plan to address the oral health of the residents. It was determined by this study that for acute and chronic stages of oral disease the total time for oral neglect was equal to 8 and 35 days, respectively.[33,34] **Table 2** defines the specific questions that were used in

---

Box 1
The AVDR model for identification of victims of V/A

Asking

Practitioners should ask about abuse privately and confidentially. Family members should not be used to interpret. Be nonjudgmental in tone and wording.

Validating

Dentists should provide validating messages showing compassion and providing comfort.

Documenting

Findings should be carefully and completely documented. Use direct quotations, accurate charting, radiographs, and photographs when indicated.

Referring

Victims should be referred to community advocates. Although victims may refuse referral, repeated offering assures them that help is available when they are ready.

Adapted from Gerbert B, Caspers N, Bronstone A, et al. A qualitative analysis of how physicians with expertise in domestic violence approach the identification of victims. Arch Intern Med 1999;131:578–4.

Table 2
Questions to use to screen for elder abuse

General Questions	Direct Questions
Do you feel safe where you live?	What happens when/if you disagree with a family member or caregiver?
Are you alone a lot?	Are you yelled at or punished in any way?
Do you know someone you can turn to when problems arise?	Does anyone at home threaten to hurt you or make you uncomfortable or afraid?
Do you make your own decisions about your life?	Have you ever been forced to stay in your home or room or do something you didn't want to do?
Do you need help with your medications, checkbook, meal preparation, transportation, bathing, toileting, or dressing?	Has anyone ever taken anything of yours without your permission?
Does any family member drink excessive alcohol or take drugs?	Has anyone ever withheld food or medications from you or failed to take care of you when you needed help?
	Have you ever signed or been forced to sign a document that you didn't understand?

Adapted from Johnson TE, Boccia AD, Strayer MS. Elder abuse and neglect: detection, reporting, and intervention. Spec Care Dentist 2001;21(4):141–6.

this study to screen for elder abuse.[34] This work helps the dental community to help define EAN, set a framework for a treatment plan, educate institutions about EAN, and set expectations for the treatment of oral disease.[33,34] Dental educators and researchers are beginning to insert the topic of EAN into the curriculum of dental health professionals in specific geographic areas, dictated primarily by state reporting laws.[10,31–34] Arising from the research conducted by the UCLA School of Dentistry, new curriculum units are in place within predoctoral dental education that focus on the ethical and legal aspects of reporting suspected abuse and neglect, and the health and cultural aspects unique to the older population.[10,31–34]

ORAL HEALTH AND VIOLENCE AND ABUSE ACROSS THE LIFE SPAN OF THE INDIVIDUAL

The aforementioned evidence-based data support the premise that V/A is a significant public health problem.[49,52–58] Specifically it is a major, if not leading contributor to premature death, disability, and illness among women.[49,52–58] Studies support the premise that lifetime occurrence of abuse in women is associated with an increased prevalence of age-related chronic diseases and health disparities affecting their life span.[56,57] Victims with current or past exposure to V/A have significantly increased susceptibility to numerous health disparities such as behavioral health problems, cardiovascular disease, immune and reproductive health disorders, depression, alcohol, tobacco and drug abuse, and other chronic illnesses.[56,58] However, little is known about the mechanistic pathways of harsh life events that lead to physical health problems.[2,56–58] Studies do suggest that childhood maltreatment and adult IPV are associated with persistent stimulation of neuroendocrine and inflammatory cascades.[2,56–58] Specifically, pediatric cohort studies correlate exposure to physical violence with higher levels of systemic inflammation.[59,60] In addition, stress-related mental health exposure during child and adolescent development potentiates hormonal cascades; that is, cortisol release that initiates and exacerbates physical health problems.[2,59,60] Violence and abuse have serious long-term medical consequences that last long after the initial trauma, as shown by the work of Felitti and colleagues.[61,62] Koss and Heslet[63] reported that those who had experienced abuse accessed the health care system 2 to 2.5 times as often as those not exposed to abuse. The increased risk of negative health outcomes manifest themselves in more physical health problems, more frequent use of medical and mental health care services, higher levels of depression, more frequent suicide attempts, and increased substance abuse.[64–66] Other research has found associations between exposure to V/A and increased frequency of surgical procedures and mental health services, and visits to general practitioners, emergency departments, and hospitals.[64–68] **Fig. 3** illustrates the conditions and health risk behaviors that are known or suspected to have a correlation with lifetime exposure to abuse. It is quite evident from this detailed schema that health care services are significantly burdened by the population of those who have experienced abuse.[67]

Along with the immense human costs associated with incidents of domestic violence, there are also steep fiscal costs. Nationwide, every year hundreds of thousands of women are the victims of domestic violence and the cost to the local communities is exceedingly high. Between January 1, 2012 and September 30, 2012 the New York City's Domestic Violence Hotline advocates answered 85,020 calls (an average of 311 calls per day). In 2011 the New York Police Department responded to 257,813 domestic violence incidents, which averages more than 700 incidents per day. All of this resulted in immense fiscal cost to the city. It was reported that in 2005 the city spent at least $227 million (not including state or federal funds) on emergency, police, and other services related to domestic violence. Nearly $180 million, or almost 80% of the total cost, was for emergency social services such as providing shelter for victims and counseling. In the same year, nearly 4000 women in New York City were treated in emergency departments for injuries that they acknowledged were due to IPV, resulting in nearly $3 million in direct health care costs. In a 2000 report from New York City's Bellevue Hospital it was estimated that 21% of all injuries in women admitted through Bellevue Hospital Shock Trauma Unit requiring urgent surgery were the result of partner abuse. This cost was never reported. However, in a 2003 study by the National Center for Injury Prevention and Control, it was estimated that the direct health care costs of IPV against women in the United States was $4.1 billion.

The financial impact of health care resources is illustrated by physician and hospital visits. Women with a history of V/A had up to 20% higher total health care costs (approximately $439 annually), and the elevation in costs continued long after the violence ended.[64,65] Rivara and colleagues[66] found evidence among a randomly selected sample of women that health care costs were 36% higher for women who reported experiences with childhood physical and sexual abuse. As a result, the health care system spends many billions of dollars each year treating the consequences of this exposure—too often without addressing the underlying causes.[64–66] Health care could be improved if physicians were to identify the underlying cause of the patient's symptoms while referring to violence victimization.[64–66]

Oral Health/Human Saliva as a Biomarker for Violence and Abuse

Technology has afforded the opportunity to use biological fluids (ie, blood, urine, lymph) to monitor disease pathways. As such, there is a growing interest in using human biomarkers to determine disease presence and progression.[67] Human saliva has been applied as a "diagnostic alphabet" for numerous clinical applications such as oral cancer, cardiovascular disease (CVD), autoimmune diseases, and diabetes.[67,68]

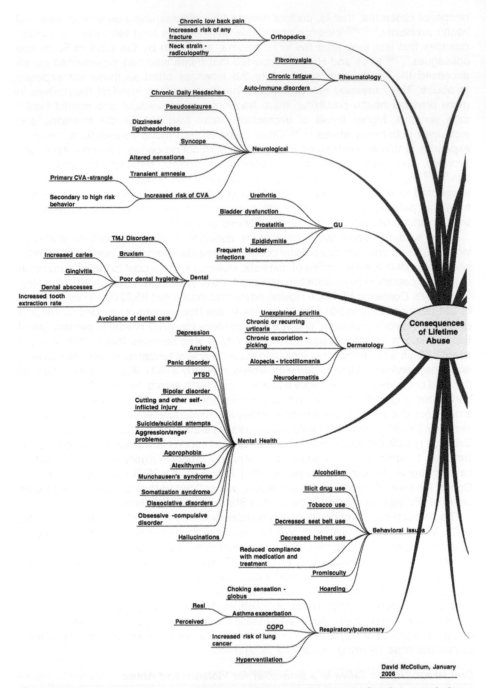

Fig. 3. Known and suspected consequences of lifetime experiences of violence and abuse (COLEVA). ACTH, corticotropin; C-section, cesarean section; COPD, chronic obstructive pulmonary disease; CVA, cerebrovascular accident; ENT, ear/nose/throat; GERD, gastroesophageal reflux disease; GU, genitourinary; HIV, human immunodeficiency virus; Ob-Gyn, obstetric/gynecologic; PTSD, posttraumatic stress disorder; STIs, sexually transmitted infections; TMJ, temporomandibular joint.

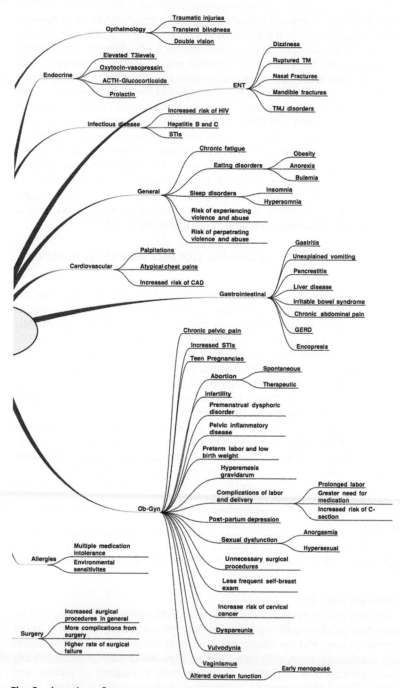

Fig. 3. (*continued*)

The advantages of salivary sampling include noninvasive approaches to collection, cost effectiveness in application, and painlessness to patients.[69–71] It provides an ideal vehicle by which to evaluate biomarkers of clinical relevance.[69–72] Several inflammatory mediators assessed in oral fluids include C-reactive protein (CRP), interleukin (IL)-6, IL-8, IL-1β, tumor necrosis factor α, and secretory immunoglobulins.[69–72] The growing interest in biomarkers of clinical relevance has extended to the use of saliva as a tool to investigate IPV.[69,71] Out and colleagues[72] evaluated differences in CRP in saliva in relation to systemic inflammation and CVD. In a cross-sectional prospective study of women in a shelter for victims of domestic violence, using plasma and salivary sampling, there were significant differences in CRP between victims of domestic violence with CVD in comparison with women who were not victims. The salivary marker for CRP was reliable in distinguishing between high-risk patients with CVD who were victims of IPV, and controls, who had significantly lower levels of CRP. Although these results should be viewed with caution, saliva may have the potential as a diagnostic tool in monitoring several health disparities associated with exposure to V/A.[69–72]

CORE COMPETENCIES NEEDED FOR ADDRESSING VIOLENCE AND ABUSE IN PATIENT CARE

From a practical perspective, dentists may the most pivotal point of contact for the identification of victims of domestic violence in a health care setting (see earlier discussion). Although some progress has been made using the evidence presented in this article, it is still only the tip of the iceberg. Training and education about the effect of V/A on the overall health and well-being of all victims still need to be honed. The recognition and identification of victims must occur along more than one tier of responsibility; that is, among different disciplines of health care. There is a new calling for core competencies at the local, community, and national levels that can be applied to identify and intervene in the traumatic life events of V/A.[1,2,73,74]

In 2005, the Academy on Violence and Abuse (AVA) was chartered to address the issues set forth by the IOM, AMA, and ADA with respect to victims' health and well-being.[73] Within the last 5 years, the AVA has built a model of public health surveillance by collaborating with educators/clinicians among the health specialties of medicine, dentistry, public health, dental hygiene, and psychology. The groundwork for a model of core competencies has thus been undertaken.[73,74]

Core Competencies

These competencies are composed of 3 tiers of responsibility: (1) individual provider, (2) the educational/research institution, and (3) the health care center of the community.[74]

Individual health care provider

The basis for competency at the individual level is understanding what V/A is; that is, definitions, epidemiology, distinguishing between the myth and reality of victims, acute and chronic presentations, and the relationship between harsh life events and health problems most significantly seen in female victims. The health care provider should then apply these principles to population-based models in respect of culture and community norms. Clinical criteria need to be reinforced by the provider to assess, intervene, and keep the victims safe (the reader is referred to Ref.[74] for further specifics).

Academic institution/training programs

Core competencies at this level include developing curricula from an interdisciplinary framework, with learner-centered training focusing not only on identification but, more importantly, on prevention. Educators should learn about how V/A is hidden by developing clinical competencies with case scenarios. Faculty support and mentoring allows for accessible nondiscriminatory counseling for both trainee and trainer. The promotion of learner safety, self-care, and partnering in community education intervention and prevention will assure an institutional environment free of V/A.

Health system requirements

Accreditation of institutions should be predicated on policies for core competencies. There should be competencies specific to each specialty based on the needs of the population that it treats. Best practice in care and management of victims, as well as the requirement for continuing education credit for yearly recertification of licensure, should be implemented. Research within and between health care institutions should be encouraged so as to develop more cost-effective approaches to intervention, because harsh life events precipitate health disparities that affect the life span of the victim of V/A.

These proposed standards are just a springboard from which all health care/behavioral health specialties can develop profession-specific competencies that will enable the skills to identify, intervene in, and prevent future injuries and health disparities resulting from V/A (for further discussion, the reader is referred to Refs.[73,74]). **Box 2** lists several approaches to help set the foundation for educational approaches to identification and intervention, and the enforcement of core competencies throughout the community setting.[53,74]

SUMMARY AND FUTURE DIRECTIONS

The oral health care provider and his or her staff are in the most pivotal position as first responders to expediently identify victims of V/A and refer them for further interventional care, especially with their female patient population. Women are at a disproportionately greater risk for injury and subsequent health disparities that significantly affect their life span. Seventy-five percent of all injuries from V/A present in the head, neck, and face. Interdisciplinary collaborations with medical colleagues are encouraged because physicians receive minimal training in oral health and dental injury and disease, and thus may not detect dental aspects of abuse or neglect as readily as they do child abuse and neglect involving other areas of the body.

Changes at the national, educational, public health, and private practice levels of dentistry and medicine are still needed to make identification of V/A and intervention a priority. The core competencies are a beginning, but more work needs to be done.

Box 2
Future directions for identification/intervention/prevention of violence/abuse

1. Applying violence/abuse/neglect as a differential diagnosis in all patients with orofacial injuries

2. Educating patients with head and facial injuries on the increased risk(s) associated with recurrent injuries; that is, co-occurring traumatic brain injury

3. Encouraging referrals for V/A counseling, including bedside danger assessment and safety planning before discharge

4. Research using prospective clinical studies to further examine orofacial and other injury types as clinical markers for violence and abuse

5. The use of interdisciplinary teams to determine how other health disparities of victims affect their health-related quality of life/life span

The opportunity for dental professionals to help victims gain access to support and referral services and, consequently, make a positive difference in the lives of patients must not be overlooked.

REFERENCES

1. World Health Organization. Violence. Geneva (Switzerland): WHO; 2011. Available at: http://www.who.int/topics/violence/en/. Accessed March 3, 2011. (Adapted from World Health Organization (1996). Violence: a public health priority. WHO Global Consultation on Violence and Health. Geneva (Switzerland): document WHO/EHA/SPI.POA.2).
2. Krug EG, Dahlberg LL, Mercy JA, et al, editors. World report on violence and health. Geneva (Switzerland): World Health Organization; 2002.
3. Tjaden PG, Thoennes N. Full report of the prevalence, incidence, and consequences of violence against women: findings from the national violence against women survey. Washington, DC: U.S. Dept. of Justice, Office of Justice Programs, National Institute of Justice; 2000.
4. Krug EG, Dahlberg LL, Mercy JA, et al. Violence by intimate partners. In: Krug E, Dahlberg LL, Mercy JA, editors. World report on violence and health. Geneva (Switzerland): World Health Organization; 2002. p. 89–121.
5. Melnick DM, Maio RF, Blow E, et al. Prevalence of domestic violence and associated factors among Women on a trauma service. J Trauma 2002;53(1):33–7.
6. American College of Obstetricians and Gynecologists. Screening tools-domestic violence. Available at: www.acog.org/departments/dept_notice.cfmrecno=17&bulletin=585. Accessed March 31, 2010.
7. Cantril SV. Trauma system injuries - face. In: Marx JA, Hockberger RS, Walls RM, editors. Rosen's emergency medicine concepts and clinical practice. St Louis (MO): Mosby Publishing; 2002. p. 2766.
8. Centers for Disease Control and Prevention. Prevalence of intimate partner violence and injuries: Washington, 1998. MMWR Morb Mortal Wkly Rep 2000; 49:589–92.
9. Chiodo GT, Tilden VP, Limandri BJ, et al. Addressing family violence among dental subjects: assessment and intervention. J Am Dent Assoc 1994;125:69–75.
10. Senn DR, McDowell JD, Alder ME. Dentistry's role in the recognition and reporting of domestic violence, abuse and neglect. Dent Clin North Am 2001;45(2):343–63.
11. Colangelo G. Responding to family violence. ADA News 2006;37(8):4.
12. Muelleman RL, Lenaghan PA, Pakieser RA. Battered women: injury locations and types. Ann Emerg Med 1996;28(5):486–92.
13. McCauley J, Yurk RA, Jenckes MW, et al. Inside "Pandora's box:" abused women's experiences with clinicians and health services. J Gen Intern Med 1998;13:549–55.
14. Tilden VP, Schmidt TA, Limandri BJ, et al. Factors that influence clinician's assessment and management of family violence. Am J Public Health 1994;84:628–33.
15. Love C, Gerbert B, Caspers N, et al. Dentists' attitudes and behaviors regarding domestic violence. The need for an effective response. J Am Dent Assoc 2001; 132(1):85–93.
16. Mouden LD, Smedstad B. Reporting child abuse and neglect: the dental hygienist's role, Dental hygienist news. Available at: www.dentalcare.com/soap/journals/dh_news/dhn0804/dn01n05 htm. Accessed June 8, 2002.
17. McDowell J. Diagnosing and treating victims of domestic violence. N Y State Dent J 1996;62(4):36–42.

18. Hutchison I, Magennis P, Shepherd J, et al. The BAOMS United Kingdom survey of facial injuries part 1: aetiology and the association with alcohol. Br J Oral Maxillofac Surg 1998;36:4–14.
19. Walker EA, Milgrom PM, Weinstein P, et al. Assessing abuse and neglect and dental fear in women. J Am Dent Assoc 1996;127(4):485–90.
20. Curran SL, Sherman JJ, Cunningham LL, et al. Physical and sexual abuse among orofacial pain patients: linkages with pain and psychologic distress. J Orofac Pain 1995;9(4):340–6.
21. Hender TJ, Sutherland SE. Domestic violence and its relation to dentistry: a call for change in Canadian dental practice. J Can Dent Assoc 2007;73(7):617a–617f.
22. Mouden LD, Bross DC. Legal issues affecting dentistry's role in preventing child abuse and neglect. J Am Dent Assoc 1995;126:1173–80.
23. Katner DR, Brown CE. Mandatory reporting of oral injuries indicating possible child abuse. J Am Dent Assoc 2012;143(10):1087–92.
24. American Academy of Pediatric Dentistry. Definition of dental neglect. Pediatr Dent 2003;25(Suppl):7.
25. Available at: www.aapd.org/media/Policies_Guidelines/G_Childabuse.pdf. Accessed 2010.
26. Needleman HL. Orofacial trauma in child abuse: types, prevalence, management, and the dental profession's involvement. Pediatr Dent 1986;8(1):71–80.
27. Zeitler DL. The abused female oral and maxillofacial surgery patient: treatment approaches for identification and management. Oral Maxillofac Surg Clin North Am 2007;19(2):259–65.
28. Wahl R, Sisk D, Ball T. Clinic-based screening for domestic violence: use of a child safety questionnaire. BMC Med 2004;2:25.
29. Bonnie R, Wallace R, editors. Elder mistreatment: abuse, neglect, and exploitation in an aging America. Washington, DC: National Academies Press; 2003.
30. Liebschutz J, Savetsky JB, Saitz R, et al. The relationship between sexual and physical abuse and substance abuse consequence. J Subst Abuse Treat 2002;22(3):121–8.
31. Gironda MW, Lefever KH, Anderson EA. Dental students' knowledge about elder abuse and neglect and the reporting responsibilities of dentists. J Dent Educ 2010;74(8):824–9.
32. Fulmer T, Strauss S, Russell SL, et al. Screening for elder mistreatment in dental and medical clinics. Gerodontology 2012;29:96–105.
33. Katz RV, Smith BJ, Berkey DB, et al. Defining oral neglect in institutionalized elderly: a consensus definition for the protection of vulnerable elderly people. J Am Dent Assoc 2010;141(4):433–40.
34. Johnson TE, Boccia AD, Strayer MS. Elder abuse and neglect: detection, reporting, and intervention. Spec Care Dentist 2001;21(4):141–6.
35. Berrios DC, Grady D. Domestic violence: risk factors and outcomes. West J Med 1991;155:133–5.
36. McDowell JD. Forensic dentistry: recognizing the signs and symptoms of domestic violence: a guide for dentists. J Okla Dent Assoc 1997;88(2):21–8.
37. Lee KH, Snape L, Steenberg LJ, et al. Comparison between interpersonal violence and motor vehicle accidents in the aetiology of maxillofacial fractures. ANZ J Surg 2007;77:695–8.
38. Crandall ML, Nathens AB, Rivava FP. Injury pattern among female trauma patients: recognizing intentional injury. J Trauma 2004;57:42–5.
39. Haug RH, Prather J, Indresano AT. An epidemiologic survey of facial fractures and concomitant injuries. J Oral Maxillofac Surg 1990;48:926.

40. Huang V, Moore C, Bohrer P, et al. Maxillofacial injuries in women. Ann Plast Surg 1998;41:482–4.
41. Perciaccante VJ, Ochs HA, Dodson TB. Head, neck and facial injuries as markers of domestic violence in women. J Oral Maxillofac Surg 1999;57(7):760–2.
42. Halpern LR, Dodson TB. A predictive model for diagnosing victims of intimate partner violence. J Am Dent Assoc 2006;137:604–9.
43. Leathers R, Shetty V, Black E, et al. Orofacial injury profiles and patterns of care in an inner-city hospital. Int J Oral Biol 1998;23(1):53–8.
44. Dutton DG, Strachan CE. Motivational needs for power and spouse-specific assertiveness in assaultive and non-assaultive men. Violence Vict 1987;2: 145–56.
45. Feldhaus KM, McLain J, Amsbury HL. Accuracy of three3 brief screening questions for detecting partner violence in the emergency department. JAMA 1997; 277(17):439–41.
46. Halpern LR, Perciaccante VJ, Hayes C, et al. A protocol to diagnose intimate partner violence in the emergency room setting. J Trauma 2006;60(5):1101–5.
47. Halpern LR, Parry B, Hayward G, et al. A comparison of 2 protocols to detect intimate partner violence. J Oral Maxillofac Surg 2009;67:1453–9.
48. Coulthard P, Yong S, Adamson L, et al. Domestic violence screening and intervention programs for adults with dental or facial injury. Cochrane Database Syst Rev 2004;(2):CD004486.
49. Taliaferro E. Screening and identification of intimate partner violence. Clin Fam Pract 2003;5(1):89–100.
50. Lipsky S, Caetano R, Field CA, et al. Violence-related injury and intimate partner violence in an urban emergency department. J Trauma 2004;57(2):352–9.
51. Kenney J. Domestic violence: a complex healthcare issue for dentistry today. Forensic Sci Int 2006;159:S121–5.
52. Hsieh N, Herzig K, Gansky S, et al. Changing dentists' knowledge, attitudes and behavior regarding domestic violence through an interactive multimedia tutorial. J Am Dent Assoc 2006;137(5):596–603.
53. Halpern LR. Orofacial injuries as markers for intimate partner violence. Oral Maxillofac Surg Clin North Am 2010;22(2):239–46.
54. Gibson-Howell JC, Gladwin MA, Hicks MJ, et al. Instruction in dental curricula to identify and assist domestic violence victims. J Dent Educ 2008;72(1):1277–89.
55. Connor P, Nouer S, Mackey SA. Dental students and intimate partner violence: measuring knowledge and experience to institute curricular change. J Dent Educ 2011;75(8):1010–9.
56. Nelms A, Gutmann M, Solomon E, et al. What victims of domestic violence need from the dental profession. J Dent Educ 2009;73(4):490–6.
57. Short S, Tiedemann J, Rose T. Family violence: an intervention model for dental professionals. Northwest Dent 1997;76(5):32–5.
58. Campbell J. Health consequences of intimate partner violence. Lancet 2002;359: 1331–6.
59. Brown DW, Anda RF, Tiemeier H, et al. Adverse childhood experiences and the risk of premature mortality. Am J Prev Med 2009;37(5):389–96.
60. Danese A, Pariante CM, Caspi A, et al. Childhood maltreatment predicts adult inflammation in a life-course study. Proc Natl Acad Sci U S A 2007;104:1319–24.
61. Felitti VJ, Anda RF, Nordenberg D, et al. The relationship of adult health status to childhood abuse and household dysfunction. Am J Prev Med 1998;14:245–58.
62. Middlebrooks JS, Audage NC. The effects of childhood stress on health across the lifespan. Atlanta (GA): Centers for disease control and prevention, National

center for injury prevention control; 2008. Available at: www.cdc.gov/ncipc/pub-res/effects_of_childhood_stress.htm. Accessed June 17, 2012.

63. Koss MP, Heslet L. Somatic consequences of violence against women. Arch Fam Med 1992;1(1):53–9.

64. Davis J, Combs-Lane A, Smith D. Victimization and health risk behaviors: implications for prevention programs. In: Kendall-Tackett KA, editor. Health consequences of abuse in the family: a clinical guide for evidence-based practice. Washington, DC: American Psychological Association; 2003. p. 179–95.

65. Max W, Rice DP, Finkelstein E, et al. The economic toll of intimate partner violence against women in the United States. Violence Vict 2004;19(3):259–72.

66. Rivara FP, Anderson ML, Fishman P, et al. Healthcare utilization and costs for women with a history of intimate partner violence. Am J Prev Med 2007;32(2): 89–96.

67. Dolezal T, McCollum D. Hidden costs in healthcare. In: Dolezal T, McCollum D, Callahan M, et al, editors. The economic impact of violence and abuse. Academy on Violence and Abuse; 2009. p. 1–12.

68. Bonomi AE, Anderson ML, Rivara FP, et al. Health care utilization and costs associated with childhood abuse. J Gen Intern Med 2008;23(3):294–9.

69. Pfaffe T, Cooper-hite J, Beyerlein P, et al. Diagnostic potential of saliva: current state and future applications. Clin Chem 2011;57(5):675–87.

70. Rao PV, Reddy AP, Lu X, et al. Proteonomic identification of salivary biomarkers of type-2 diabetes. J Proteome Res 2009;8(1):239–45.

71. Fernandez-Botran R, Miller JJ, Burns V, et al. Correlations among inflammatory markers in plasma, saliva, and oral mucosal transudate in postmenopausal women with past intimate partner violence. Brain Behav Immun 2011;25:314–21.

72. Out D, Hall RJ, Granger DA, et al. Assessing salivary C-reactive protein: longitudinal associations with systemic inflammation and cardiovascular disease risk in women exposed to intimate partner violence. Brain Behav Immun 2012;26(4): 543–51.

73. Academy on Violence and Abuse, Highlights of Proceedings form the 2009 Conference: Sowing Seeds of Academic Change-Nurturing New Paradigms. Trauma, Violence and Abuse 2010. Available at: http://tva.sagepub.com/content/ 11/2/83. Accessed April, 2010.

74. Competencies needed by health professionals for addressing exposure to violence and abuse in patient care. Academy on Violence and Abuse. In: Family Violence Prevention Fund pre-conference institute hosted by the AVA and the Family Violence Prevention Fund, October 8, 2009 entitled "Creating Core Competencies for Health Education on Violence and Abuse." 2010. p. 1–20.

75. Zachariades N, Koumoura F, Konsolaki-Agouridaki F. Facial Trauma in women resulting from violence by men. J Oral Maxillofac Surg 1990;48(12):1250–3.

76. Fisher E, Kraus H, Lewis VL. Assaulted women: Maxillofacial injuries in rape and domestic violence. Plast Reconstr Surg 1990;86(1):161–2.

77. Ochs H, Neuenschwande MC, Dodson TB. Are head, neck and facial injuries markers of domestic violence? J Am Dent Assoc 1996;127(6):757–61.

78. Hartzell K, Botek AA, Goldberg KH. Orbital fractures in women due to sexual assault and domestic violence. Ophthalmology 1996;103(6):953–7.

79. Greene D, Maas CS, Carvalo G, et al. Epidemiology of facial injury in female blunt assault trauma cases. Arch Facial Plast Surg 1999;(4):288–91.

80. Le B, Dierks SJ, Veeck BA, et al. Maxillofacial injuries associated with domestic violence. J Oral Maxillofac Surg 2001;59:1279–83.

The Impact of Gender on Caries Prevalence and Risk Assessment

Esperanza Angeles Martinez-Mier, DDS, MSD, PhD[a,b,]*,
Andrea Ferreira Zandona, DDS, MSD, PhD[c,d,e]

KEYWORDS

- Dental caries • Risk assessment • Risk management • Gender disparities

KEY POINTS

- A gender gap created by biologic and cultural influences, including behavioral and dietary variations, places women at a disadvantage in oral health.
- Cultural and social differences between men and women influence their oral health status by affecting their exposure to risk factors and shaping their access to protective factors and care.
- The large biologic differences between men and women and their relationship to oral health have not been sufficiently studied.
- There is a definite lack of evidence in regard to gender differences and dental caries. Therefore, there is a need to develop the evidence necessary to meet the oral health needs of both women and men.

INTRODUCTION
Disease Description

See **Box 1** for a description of dental caries.

Risk Factors for Dental Caries

The World Health Organization (WHO) defines risk as the probability of an adverse event or a factor that can raise this probability.[10] Thus, identifying the risk factors

Funding sources: Dr Martinez-Mier: Delta Dental, Glaxo Smith Klein, HRSA, IUPUI CSL. Dr Ferreira Zandona: IUPUI CSL, NIDCR, Glaxo Smith Klein, NIEHS.
Conflict of interest: None.
[a] Fluoride Research Program, Indiana University School of Dentistry, 415 Lansing Street, Indianapolis, IN 46202, USA; [b] Department of Preventive and Community Dentistry, Binational/Cross-Cultural Health Enhancement Center, Oral Health Research Institute, Indiana University School of Dentistry, 415 Lansing Street, Indianapolis, IN 46202, USA; [c] Graduate MSD/MS Preventive Dentistry Program, Indiana University School of Dentistry, 415 Lansing Street, Indianapolis, IN 46202, USA; [d] Early Caries Research Program, Indiana University School of Dentistry, 415 Lansing Street, Indianapolis, IN 46202, USA; [e] Department of Preventive and Community Dentistry, Oral Health Research Institute, Indiana University School of Dentistry, 415 Lansing Street, Indianapolis, IN 46202, USA
* Corresponding author. Department of Preventive and Community Dentistry, Oral Health Research Institute, Indiana University School of Dentistry, 415 Lansing Street, Indianapolis, IN.
E-mail address: esmartin@iu.edu

Dent Clin N Am 57 (2013) 301–315
http://dx.doi.org/10.1016/j.cden.2013.01.001
0011-8532/13/$ – see front matter © 2013 Elsevier Inc. All rights reserved.

dental.theclinics.com

Box 1
Description of dental caries

Dental caries remains the most common childhood disease worldwide,[1,2] disproportionally affecting women in many populations.[3–6] Dental caries is a site-specific, multifactorial disease that results from individual biofilm composition and metabolism,[7] which is influenced by several biologic factors. These biologic determinants include saliva, diet, and possibly genetic factors. At the individual or population level, multiple cultural, behavioral, and socioeconomic factors also influence caries development. Well-documented gender differences in these factors have also been reported to influence oral health status.

Although dental caries is multifactorial and complex, it is preventable. Fluoride and sealants have proven to prevent dental caries.[8] However, prevention of this disease is largely influenced by patient behaviors and attitudes as well as access to preventive dental services.[9]

---

that correlate to the individual burden of the disease[11] has been a long-standing goal. Caries management at the public health level[12–14] or individual level[15,16] relies on the identification of risk factors for correct categorization of a community or an individual and appropriate policy or management plan implementation. Unfortunately, the most reliable indicator of future risk is previous caries experience,[15,17] which is an antithesis when the aim is prevention of the disease. There is a multitude of variables that are included in risk prediction models[18]; the issue is very complex because the predictive values are influenced by many factors, and it is unlikely that any individual risk factor will provide a strong predictive value.[16]

There is evidence indicating that many caries risk factors provide a gender bias, placing women at a higher caries risk than men.[3] These factors may include different salivary composition and flow rate, hormonal fluctuations, dietary habits, genetic variations, and particular social roles among their family.[19] Additionally, there are systemic diseases that have been found to be associated with caries and to have an association with the female gender.[20]

Risk factors can be regarded as those that are risk indicators and those that are risk modifiers. There are risk factors related to the host (past caries experience, teeth, saliva, patient age, sociodemographic factors, behavioral factor, genetic factors), those related to the diet (type, quantity, frequency), those related to the dental biofilm (bacterial counts, genera and species, bacterial metabolism, and metagenomics), and those that are protective factors (adequate fluoride exposure, good oral hygiene, and positive dietary behaviors).

Risk Factors Related to the Host

Past caries experience

This predictor is the single most reliable predictor of future risk and evidence supports its inclusion in considerations of risk assessment to increase sensitivity.[21,22] Epidemiologic studies have shown a positive strong correlation between past caries experience and future caries development.[23,24] The presence of caries in the mother and siblings increases the risk for a young child.[25] Caries prevalence in primary teeth can help predict future caries in permanent teeth.[26] If young girls are found to have a higher caries prevalence,[27–29] it can place them at a higher future risk.[30] In adults, there is a moderate association between existing caries and the risk of developing root caries.[31]

Teeth

Caries risk differs among different morphologic tooth types and between primary and permanent teeth. In permanent teeth, molars are more susceptible, followed by premolars, incisors, and canines.[32,33] Lesion progression on individual teeth also differs according to tooth type, with lesions on molars progressing faster than lesions in premolars and anterior teeth.[34] In the primary dentition, in early childhood caries (ECC), anterior teeth are more susceptible.[35] Occlusal surfaces are the most susceptible surfaces to caries,[36-44] followed by approximal surfaces.[42] Higher caries prevalence among girls may be explained by earlier eruption of teeth,[19] hence, longer exposure of teeth to the cariogenic oral environment, although to date there is no evidence.[20]

Saliva

In individuals with markedly reduced salivary function, caries activity is significantly increased.[45] Unstimulated flow rates are usually more predictable of caries risk and, when significantly low, can be isolated as a dominant risk factor.[46] However, the equation can be balanced and the risk altered by protecting agents, such as fluoride,[46] because of the prolonged retention time of fluoride in the mouth and the absence of diluting and clearance functions of saliva. There is an indication that fluctuating hormone levels in women and the associated physiologic changes during events, such as puberty, menstruation, and pregnancy, alter the biochemical composition of saliva and overall saliva flow rate.[19,47] These changes would make the oral environment significantly more cariogenic for women than for men and provide a possible explanation of the gender differences in caries rates.[19]

Age

Epidemiologic surveys of caries show an increase in caries prevalence with age. Newly erupted teeth (nonmature) are more susceptible to caries, particularly at pit and fissure sites.[48,49] The susceptibility also seems increased by the difficulty of cleaning the teeth until they have reached the occlusal plane.[50] Accordingly, children are at greatest risk at those ages when teeth have just erupted.[51] The earlier eruption pattern in girls could place them at a higher risk during teeth eruption years.[19] As children reach young adulthood, there is some indication that the caries incidence slows down.[52] The elderly are particularly at a greater risk for root caries; however, elderly women are not at a particularly higher risk.[53,54]

Sociodemographic factors: race, culture, ethnicity, income, and education level

Sociodemographic factors are seen as potential contributors to risk.[22] The data are controversial; some studies have found a clear relationship[55-57] between sociodemographic factors, whereas others failed to identify this relationship as significant.[22] It is clear that the impact depends on several variables or a combination of variables being studied, for instance, tooth surface, age, gender, and country. There are indications that race contributes to caries risk,[27,58-61] usually associated with income and education level; but few studies look at ethnicity as a variable.[62] Recent data have examined genetic variations observed in different populations and their association to dental caries.[63] Those in the lower-income brackets are likely to be at a higher risk for caries[56,57] as well as those in rural areas.[57] In children, the impact of sociodemographic factors on ECC differs among countries.[60,64,65] There is some indication that sociodemographic factors are a risk factor for caries in primary teeth[66,67] but not on permanent teeth.[68]

The issue of gender is controversial. In children, girls were found to have a higher risk for caries,[27-29] whereas others have found it to be a modifier,[69] and yet others found boys to have a higher or similar risk.[4] In adults, white men have been found to be at a higher risk for root caries,[53,54] whereas studies on other tooth surfaces have either found no effect of gender on caries risk[70] or found women to be at a higher risk.[3,4,19] It is likely that the culture-based division of labor and gender-based dietary preferences play a role in the gender bias on caries risk.[3] Genome-wide association studies have found caries susceptible and caries protective loci, some of which are X-linked, that influence variation in taste, saliva, and enamel proteins, affecting the oral environment and the microstructure of enamel, which may partly explain gender differences in caries.[3] Because of the complexity of the data related to sociodemographic factors in caries risk assessment and management, they should be considered as a modifier or potential contributor to risk.[22,71]

Behavior

Positive oral health attitudes and behaviors have been associated with decreased caries prevalence.[72–74] Positive oral health behaviors are regular tooth brushing, regular use of fluorides, and consumption of little or no sugar.[75] However, there are concerns about the reliability of measuring behavior, and mostly behavioral variables are not found to be good predictors of caries risk.[75,76] There is a tendency by anthropologists to favor explanations of the increased caries risk in women to factors involving behavior, including sexual division of labor and women's domestic role in food production.[19] There are suggestions that higher caries prevalence among women could be caused by easier access to food supplies and frequent snacking during food preparation[19] and by behaviors related to access to dental care.[74] In certain countries, the gender difference in oral health seems to involve social and religious causes, such as son preference, ritual fasting, and dietary restrictions during pregnancy.[3,4]

Risk Factors Related to the Diet

Diet

Diet plays an important role in dental caries. There is a large body of evidence linking frequent consumption of fermentable carbohydrates and caries prevalence. Historical studies have linked the shift from lower to higher sugar consumption to an increase in dental caries prevalence.[77,78] The classic Vipeholm study demonstrated the relationship between an increase in sugar consumption and the different types of sugars to an increment in dental caries.[79] More recent data compiled from 90 countries examining sugar consumption and dental caries in 12-year-old children related an increase in decay/missing/filled (DMFT) scores with sugar consumption.[80] Sucrose is considered the most cariogenic sugar because it can form glucan,[81] which enables bacterial adhesion to the teeth and restricts diffusion acid and buffers in the plaque.[82] However, in industrialized nations, the sugar-caries relationship is not always found, suggesting that other factors, for instance, other aspects of diet, exposure to fluoride, and genetic effects, need to be considered as explanatory.[80,83,84] Some foods, such as milk and milk products, provide a protective effect.[85,86] In children, gender differences in food tastes does not corroborate with gender differences in caries rates because boys have been reported to prefer sugary foods,[87] but preferences may be influenced by the mother's preferences[88] and culture.[89,90] In adults, women have been reported to prefer carbohydrates and sugary foods,[91] although no gender difference has been reported in the frequency of consumption of sugary snacks.[92,93]

ECC and baby bottle tooth decay

The distinct clinical presentation of ECC has not been consistently associated with poor feeding practices.[94] Studies have been inconclusive in associating prolonged bottle use, use of the bottle at bedtime,[76] the contents of the bottle,[71] or nursing ad libitum[94] with caries risk.

Risk Factors Related to the Dental Biofilm

Microbiological counts

Despite the univariate associations of *Streptococcus mutans* counts and lactobacilli levels with caries prevalence,[95] the correlation with future risk is weak.[22] There have been many findings indicating an association of microbial counts and caries in children with differing levels of confidence,[95–97] although this association was not found in root caries.[98] The accuracy of salivary tests for mutans streptococci in predicting future caries in the whole population is less than 20% to 50%.[99] In populations with low caries prevalence, the caries predictability of microbiological tests is further decreased.[100] Lactobacilli microbiological tests are even less sensitive at predicting caries than the mutans tests.[101] There have not been reported gender differences in bacterial counts.[102–105]

Protective Factors

Oral hygiene

Although caries might be reduced by the mechanical removal of plaque, the evidence that tooth brushing reduces caries is weak; effectiveness of mechanical cleaning alone is hard to evaluate because tooth brushing is usually done using fluoridated toothpaste.[71] Additionally, most patients do not remove it effectively.[106] There is evidence that any condition that affects the patients' ability to maintain good oral hygiene are positively associated with caries risk.[25] Girls tend to have significantly higher scores than boys for desire to improve oral care and toothbrushing.[107–109]

Fluoride exposure

Fluoride in various forms is significant evidence of being efficacious on the prevention of dental caries.[110–122] Fluoride's main mechanism of action is posteruptive, controlling the initiation and progression of carious lesions by promoting remineralization of early caries lesions and reducing sound enamel demineralization.[123] Differences in fluoride have been reported among racial groups; however, these differences have been described as complex and are in need of further investigation.[124] Gender differences in fluoride exposure have not been correlated with differences in caries prevalence.[109]

Prevalence and Incidence of Dental Caries in the United States

Based on data from the National Health and Nutrition Examination Survey from 1999 to 2002,[125] the mean number of caries in permanent teeth (DMFT) among children and adults in the United States is reported in **Tables 1** and **2**.

Table 1
Mean number of caries in permanent teeth (DMFT) among children in the United States

Age	Mean	95% Confidence Interval	Total Sample	Total Weighted Population
6–11	0.42	(0.35, 0.48)	2149	23 569 639
12–15	1.74	(1.49, 1.99)	2333	15 556 985
16–19	3.20	(2.98, 3.42)	2155	15 006 863
Mean for males (6–19)	1.44	(1.27, 1.62)	3327	27 680 453
Mean for females (6–19)	1.70	(1.55, 1.85)	3310	26 453 034

Data from NIDCR/CDC. NIDCR/CDC Dental, Oral, and Craniofacial Data Resource Center. 2012. Available at: http://drc.hhs.gov/index.htm. Accessed October 2012.

Table 2
Mean number of caries in permanent teeth (DMFT) among adults in the United States

Age (y)	Mean	95% Confidence Interval	Total Sample	Total Weighted Population
20–39	7.14	(6.77, 7.52)	3149	73 758 539
40–59	13.53	(13.03, 14.03)	2614	70 407 492
60+	20.01	(19.55, 20.46)	2989	41 735 510
Mean for males (6–19)	11.83	(11.35, 12.31)	4159	89 342 776
Mean for females (6–19)	13.02	(12.56, 13.49)	4593	96 558 766

Data from NIDCR/CDC. NIDCR/CDC Dental, Oral, and Craniofacial Data Resource Center. 2012. Available at: http://drc.hhs.gov/index.htm. Accessed October 2012.

Dental caries in the United States is no longer a population-wide problem but it is endemic to specific population subsets. In general, dental caries disproportionally affects the poor and racial and ethnic minorities, with women suffering more from the disease than men.[12] However, gender differences in caries prevalence or access to treatment have been reported to be decreasing or no longer exist for some age and racial groups. For example, among 2 to 5 year olds, boys were reported to have 20.0% untreated caries from 2001 to 2004, whereas girls had 20.1%.[126]

Worldwide Prevalence and Incidence of Dental Caries

Worldwide, dental caries continues to be the most prevalent disease of childhood, particularly in the Americas, the Eastern Mediterranean, and Southeast Asian regions. In 2003, it was estimated that 5 billion people worldwide suffered from dental caries.[126] Based on the reported data, it is not always possible to discern if gender differences present global patterns. Other distinct trends in dental caries prevalence have emerged worldwide, with certain regions observing a decline in the prevalence of disease and others, mostly low-income countries, reporting a continuous increase.

However, even in countries where dental caries continues to increase, the distribution of disease also affects certain segments of the population disproportionately.[1] In general, in countries with a high-income economy, dental caries disproportionally affect the poor and racial and ethnic minorities, with women suffering more from the disease than men. In countries with middle- and low-income economies, dental caries is a highly prevalent disease often characterized by marked differences within the same country.[1] In the United States and Europe, 20% of children suffer 60% to 80% of the disease. A similarly skewed distribution is found throughout the world, with some children having none or very few caries and others having a high number.

Many epidemiologic studies conducted around the world have recorded oral health data of 12-year-old children. In many countries, this is the last age at which data can be easily obtained through the school systems. For this reason, prevalence data for children is often more accurate than that of adults, which is often based on estimates in many countries. The most commonly used index for assessing caries prevalence and treatment needs among populations has been the DMFT index.[127] This index is based on subjective visual examination. Because the DMFT index does not include radiographs, it has been shown to underestimate the prevalence and treatment needs.[127]

In the current article, prevalence estimates were extracted from the WHO Oral Health Country/Area Profile Project for 12-year-old children using the DMFT index.[128] This database is updated and expanded continuously, with monthly updates. Data ranges are presented by region; however, meaningful comparisons worldwide are not feasible mostly because of temporal differences for data collection.

- For the Americas region, data are derived from surveys conducted in 12-year-old children from 1987 (Argentina) to 2008 (El Salvador). The region is home to countries from low, middle, and high incomes; as such, the contrasts in caries prevalence are stark, ranging from a DMFT of 0.2 for Bermuda to 6.7 for Martinica.
- For Europe, data are derived from surveys conducted in 12-year-old children from 1985 to 1990 (Armenia, Georgia, and Kazakhstan) to 2009 to 2010 (Belgium and Croatia). The region is home to countries with middle and high incomes, with DMFTs ranging from of 0.65 for Cyprus to 4.8 for Croatia.
- For Africa, data are derived from surveys conducted in 12-year-old children from 1981 (Angola) to 2003 to 2004 (Nigeria), with multiple countries having never reported or collected DMFT data nationally. The region is home to countries with low and middle incomes, with DMFTs ranging from of 0.3 for Togo and Tanzania to 4.9 for Mauritius.
- For the Eastern Mediterranean region, data are derived from surveys conducted in 12-year-old children from 1990 (Djibouti) to 2007 to 2008 (Sudan and Libya). The region is home to countries from low, middle, and high incomes, with DMFTs ranging from of 0.4 for Egypt to 5.9 for Saudi Arabia.
- For the Southeast Asia region, data are derived from surveys conducted in 12-year-old children from 1984 (Maldives) to 2009 (Indonesia). The region is home to countries from low and middle incomes, with DMFTs ranging from of 0.5 for Nepal to 3.9 for India.
- Finally, for the Western Pacific region, data are derived from surveys conducted in 12-year-old children from 1984 (Micronesia) to 2007 (Malaysia), with several countries having never reported or collected DMFT data nationally. The region is home to countries from low, middle, and high incomes, with DMFTs ranging from of 0.8 for Hong Kong to 4.8 for Brunei and Tokelau.

Dental caries has been reported to disproportionally affect women in many populations around the world. The magnitude of this disparity by gender increases from childhood to adolescence and into adulthood. This difference was observed as early as 4000 BP. Surveys conducted in Bangladesh, Hungary, India, Nepal, Spain, Sri Lanka, and in isolated traditional Brazilian villages have reported higher caries rates in women than men.[1–6,129] Following a similar pattern as that observed for caries, tooth loss in women is greater than in men and has been linked to caries and parity. However, in a patter similar to that observed for the United States, gender inequalities have recently been reported to be decreasing or no longer exist beyond adolescence through the reproductive years.[130]

Clinical Correlation

The treatment of dental diseases is expensive, accounting for between 5% and 10% of total health care expenditures in industrialized countries. In the United States, the Centers for Disease Control and Prevention reported that in 2009 to 2010, 14% of children aged 3 to 5 years had untreated dental caries. For children aged 6 to 9 years, 17% had untreated dental caries; and 11% of adolescents aged 13 to 15 years had untreated dental caries.[131] Differences in untreated caries also reflect disparities among racial and ethnic populations and the poor. On the other hand, in most low-income countries, more than 90% of caries is untreated.

There is extensive data from high-income countries reporting medical and dental services use differences among genders, with women being reported to use services more frequently than men.[132,133] Differences in untreated decay among genders have also been reported for certain communities in low-income countries. For example, women in small, rural, isolated communities in Guatemala were most likely to have their teeth extracted and replaced by dentures, reflecting their concern with appearance as well as their of fear pain and their desire to ensure the best possible marriage.[130]

SUMMARY AND DISCUSSION

A gender bias placing women at a disadvantage in oral health has been reported in many regions in the world and has been associated with genetic, hormonal, and cultural influences, including behavioral and dietary variation. Although there are some reports that have indicated that definite biologic (sex) and social (gender) differences exist, much is not known.

Cultural and social differences between men and women can influence their oral health status in several different ways. Marked differences in daily lives can affect their exposure to risk factors and also shape their access to protective factors and care.

The large biologic differences between men and women and their relationship to oral health have not received sufficient attention. This point is especially relevant because it is well known that biologic factors are partly responsible for differences in disease incidence and prevalence. Other than hormonal variation during reproductive cycles and their relationship to periodontal health, little has been studied in the context of oral health.

The current article indicates the lack of evidence in regard to gender differences and dental caries. There is a definite need to develop the evidence base necessary to meet the oral health needs of both women and men. This evidence would support the development of tools that would aid clinicians in determining the caries activity and risk status of patients in real time. This information would then be used to tailor appropriate preventive intervention strategies to improve the oral health of both genders.

REFERENCES

1. Van PalensteinHelderman W. Priorities in oral health care in non-EME countries. Int Dent J 2002;52(1):30–4.
2. Beltran-Aguilar ED, Barker LK, Canto MT, et al. Surveillance for dental caries, dental sealants, tooth retention, edentulism, and enamel fluorosis–United States, 1988-1994 and 1999-2002. MMWR Surveill Summ 2005;54(3):1–43.
3. Lukacs JR. Sex differences in dental caries experience: clinical evidence, complex etiology. Clin Oral Investig 2011;15(5):649–56.
4. Lukacs JR. Gender differences in oral health in South Asia: metadata imply multifactorial biological and cultural causes. Am J Hum Biol 2011;23(3): 398–411.
5. Nieto Garcia VM, Nieto Garcia MA, Lacalle Remigio JR, et al. Oral health of school children in Ceuta. Influences of age, sex, ethnic background and socio-economic level. Rev Esp Salud Publica 2001;75(6):541–9 [in Spanish].
6. Temple DH. Variability in dental caries prevalence between male and female foragers from the Late/Final Jomon period: implications for dietary behavior and reproductive ecology. Am J Hum Biol 2011;23(1):107–17.
7. Thylstrup A, Bruun C, Holmen L. In vivo caries models–mechanisms for caries initiation and arrestment. Adv Dent Res 1994;8(2):144–57.
8. Centers for Disease Control and Prevention (CDC). Ten great public health achievements–United States, 1900-1999. MMWR Morb Mortal Wkly Rep 1999; 48(12):241–3.

9. Anderson M. Risk assessment and epidemiology of dental caries: review of the literature. Pediatr Dent 2002;24(5):377–85.
10. Brundtland GH. From the World Health Organization. Reducing risks to health, promoting healthy life. JAMA 2002;288(16):1974.
11. Bader JD, Shugars DA, Bonito AJ. A systematic review of selected caries prevention and management methods. Community Dent Oral Epidemiol 2001; 29(6):399–411.
12. Petersen PE. Sociobehavioural risk factors in dental caries - international perspectives. Community Dent Oral Epidemiol 2005;33(4):274–9.
13. Hausen H, Karkkainen S, Seppa L. Application of the high-risk strategy to control dental caries. Community Dent Oral Epidemiol 2000;28(1):26–34.
14. Watt RG. Strategies and approaches in oral disease prevention and health promotion. Bull World Health Organ 2005;83(9):711–8.
15. Zero D, Fontana M, Lennon AM. Clinical applications and outcomes of using indicators of risk in caries management. J Dent Educ 2001;65(10):1126–32.
16. Fontana M, Zero DT. Assessing patients' caries risk. J Am Dent Assoc 2006; 137(9):1231–9.
17. Fontana M, Santiago E, Eckert GJ, et al. Risk factors of caries progression in a Hispanic school-aged population. J Dent Res 2011;90(10):1189–96.
18. Twetman S, Fontana M. Patient caries risk assessment. Monogr Oral Sci 2009; 21:91–101.
19. Lukacs JR, Largaespada LL. Explaining sex differences in dental caries prevalence: saliva, hormones, and "life-history" etiologies. Am J Hum Biol 2006;18(4): 540–55.
20. Ferraro M, Vieira AR. Explaining gender differences in caries: a multifactorial approach to a multifactorial disease. Int J Dent 2010;2010:649643.
21. Bader JD, Perrin NA, Maupome G, et al. Exploring the contributions of components of caries risk assessment guidelines. Community Dent Oral Epidemiol 2008;36(4):357–62.
22. Disney JA, Graves RC, Stamm JW, et al. The University of North Carolina Caries Risk Assessment study: further developments in caries risk prediction. Community Dent Oral Epidemiol 1992;20(2):64–75.
23. Steiner M, Buhlmann S, Menghini G, et al. Caries risks and appropriate intervals between bitewing x-ray examinations in schoolchildren. Schweiz Monatsschr Zahnmed 2011;121(1):12–24.
24. Sheiham A. Impact of dental treatment on the incidence of dental caries in children and adults. Community Dent Oral Epidemiol 1997;25(1):104–12.
25. NIH Consensus Development Conference on Diagnosis and Management of Dental Caries Throughout Life. Bethesda, MD, March 26-28, 2001. Conference Papers. J Dent Educ 2001;65(10):935–1179.
26. Helm S, Helm T. Correlation between caries experience in primary and permanent dentition in birth-cohorts 1950-70. Scand J Dent Res 1990;98(3): 225–7.
27. Ditmyer M, Dounis G, Mobley C, et al. Inequalities of caries experience in Nevada youth expressed by DMFT index vs. significant caries index (SiC) over time. BMC Oral Health 2011;11:12.
28. Ismail AI, Sohn W, Lim S, et al. Predictors of dental caries progression in primary teeth. J Dent Res 2009;88(3):270–5.
29. Declerck D, Leroy R, Martens L, et al. Factors associated with prevalence and severity of caries experience in preschool children. Community Dent Oral Epidemiol 2008;36(2):168–78.

30. Alm A, Wendt LK, Koch G, et al. Caries in adolescence - influence from early childhood. Community Dent Oral Epidemiol 2012;40(2):125–33.
31. DePaola PF, Soparkar PM, Tavares M, et al. Clinical profiles of individuals with and without root surface caries. Gerodontology 1989;8(1):9–15.
32. Macek MD, Beltran-Aguilar ED, Lockwood SA, et al. Updated comparison of the caries susceptibility of various morphological types of permanent teeth. J Public Health Dent 2003;63(3):174–82.
33. Mejare I, Kallestal C, Stenlund H, et al. Caries development from 11 to 22 years of age: a prospective radiographic study. Prevalence and distribution. Caries Res 1998;32(1):10–6.
34. Ferreira Zandona A, Santiago E, Eckert GJ, et al. The natural history of dental caries lesions: a 4-year observational study. J Dent Res 2012;91(9):841–6.
35. Wyne A, Darwish S, Adenubi J, et al. The prevalence and pattern of nursing caries in Saudi preschool children. Int J Paediatr Dent 2001;11(5):361–4.
36. Hopcraft MS, Morgan MV. Pattern of dental caries experience on tooth surfaces in an adult population. Community Dent Oral Epidemiol 2006;34(3): 174–83.
37. Hannigan A, O'Mullane DM, Barry D, et al. A caries susceptibility classification of tooth surfaces by survival time. Caries Res 2000;34(2):103–8.
38. Richardson PS, McIntyre IG. Susceptibility of tooth surfaces to carious attack in young adults. Community Dent Health 1996;13(3):163–8.
39. Chestnutt IG, Schafer F, Jacobson AP, et al. Incremental susceptibility of individual tooth surfaces to dental caries in Scottish adolescents. Community Dent Oral Epidemiol 1996;24(1):11–6.
40. McDonald SP, Sheiham A. The distribution of caries on different tooth surfaces at varying levels of caries–a compilation of data from 18 previous studies. Community Dent Health 1992;9(1):39–48.
41. Dummer PM, Oliver SJ, Hicks R, et al. Factors influencing the initiation of carious lesions in specific tooth surfaces over a 4-year period in children between the ages of 11-12 years and 15-16 years. J Dent 1990;18(4):190–7.
42. Berman DS, Slack GL. Susceptibility of tooth surfaces to carious attack. A longitudinal study. Br Dent J 1973;134(4):135–9.
43. Carlos JP, Gittelsohn AM. Longitudinal studies of the natural history of caries. II. A life-table study of caries incidence in the permanent teeth. Arch Oral Biol 1965;10(5):739–51.
44. Barr JH, Diodati RR, Stephens RG. Incidence of caries at different locations on the teeth. J Dent Res 1957;36(4):536–45.
45. Powell LV, Mancl LA, Senft GD. Exploration of prediction models for caries risk assessment of the geriatric population. Community Dent Oral Epidemiol 1991; 19(5):291–5.
46. Katz S. The use of fluoride and chlorhexidine for the prevention of radiation caries. J Am Dent Assoc 1982;104(2):164–70.
47. Dodds MW, Johnson DA, Yeh CK. Health benefits of saliva: a review. J Dent 2005;33(3):223–33.
48. Ahmad N, Gelesko S, Shugars D, et al. Caries experience and periodontal pathology in erupting third molars. J Oral Maxillofac Surg 2008;66(5):948–53.
49. Shugars DA, Elter JR, Jacks MT, et al. Incidence of occlusal dental caries in asymptomatic third molars. J Oral Maxillofac Surg 2005;63(3):341–6.
50. Carvalho JC, Ekstrand KR, Thylstrup A. Dental plaque and caries on occlusal surfaces of first permanent molars in relation to stage of eruption. J Dent Res 1989;68(5):773–9.

51. Carvalho JC, Ekstrand KR, Thylstrup A. Results after 1 year of non-operative occlusal caries treatment of erupting permanent first molars. Community Dent Oral Epidemiol 1991;19(1):23–8.
52. Mejare I, Stenlund H, Zelezny-Holmlund C. Caries incidence and lesion progression from adolescence to young adulthood: a prospective 15-year cohort study in Sweden. Caries Res 2004;38(2):130–41.
53. Douglass CW, Jette AM, Fox CH, et al. Oral health status of the elderly in New England. J Gerontol 1993;48(2):M39–46.
54. Joshi A, Douglass CW, Jette A, et al. The distribution of root caries in community-dwelling elders in New England. J Public Health Dent 1994;54(1): 15–23.
55. Bohannan HM, Klein SP, Disney JA, et al. A summary of the results of the National Preventive Dentistry Demonstration Program. J Can Dent Assoc 1985;51(6):435–41.
56. Krustrup U, Petersen PE. Dental caries prevalence among adults in Denmark–the impact of socio-demographic factors and use of oral health services. Community Dent Health 2007;24(4):225–32.
57. Shah N, Sundaram KR. Impact of socio-demographic variables, oral hygiene practices, oral habits and diet on dental caries experience of Indian elderly: a community-based study. Gerodontology 2004;21(1):43–50.
58. Divaris K, Fisher EL, Shugars DA, et al. Risk factors for third molar occlusal caries: a longitudinal clinical investigation. J Oral Maxillofac Surg 2012;70(8): 1771–80.
59. Ritter AV, Preisser JS, Chung Y, et al. Risk indicators for the presence and extent of root caries among caries-active adults enrolled in the xylitol for Adult Caries Trial (X-ACT). Clin Oral Investig 2012;16(6):1647–57.
60. Postma TC, Ayo-Yusuf OA, van Wyk PJ. Socio-demographic correlates of early childhood caries prevalence and severity in a developing country–South Africa. Int Dent J 2008;58(2):91–7.
61. Cruz GD, Chen Y, Salazar CR, et al. Determinants of oral health care utilization among diverse groups of immigrants in New York City. J Am Dent Assoc 2010; 141(7):871–8.
62. Harris R, Nicoll AD, Adair PM, et al. Risk factors for dental caries in young children: a systematic review of the literature. Community Dent Health 2004; 21(Suppl 1):71–85.
63. Tannure PN, Kuchler EC, Lips A, et al. Genetic variation in MMP20 contributes to higher caries experience. J Dent 2012;40(5):381–6.
64. Warren JJ, Weber-Gasparoni K, Marshall TA, et al. A longitudinal study of dental caries risk among very young low SES children. Community Dent Oral Epidemiol 2009;37(2):116–22.
65. Spencer AJ, Wright FA, Brown LM, et al. Changing caries experience and risk factors in five- and six-year-old Melbourne children. Aust Dent J 1989;34(2): 160–5.
66. Ditmyer MM, Dounis G, Howard KM, et al. Validation of a multifactorial risk factor model used for predicting future caries risk with Nevada adolescents. BMC Oral Health 2011;11:18.
67. Sayegh A, Dini EL, Holt RD, et al. Caries in preschool children in Amman, Jordan and the relationship to socio-demographic factors. Int Dent J 2002;52(2):87–93.
68. Vanobbergen J, Martens L, Lesaffre E, et al. The value of a baseline caries risk assessment model in the primary dentition for the prediction of caries incidence in the permanent dentition. Caries Res 2001;35(6):442–50.

69. Campus G, Lumbau A, Lai S, et al. Socio-economic and behavioural factors related to caries in twelve-year-old Sardinian children. Caries Res 2001;35(6): 427–34.
70. Lukacs JR. Gender differences in oral health in South Asia: metadata imply multifactorial biological and cultural causes. Am J Hum Biol 2011;23(3): 398–411.
71. Reisine ST, Psoter W. Socioeconomic status and selected behavioral determinants as risk factors for dental caries. J Dent Educ 2001;65(10):1009–16.
72. Levin L, Shenkman A. The relationship between dental caries status and oral health attitudes and behavior in young Israeli adults. J Dent Educ 2004; 68(11):1185–91.
73. Litt MD, Reisine S, Tinanoff N. Multidimensional causal model of dental caries development in low-income preschool children. Public Health Rep 1995; 110(5):607–17.
74. Vehkalahti MM, Paunio IK. Occurrence of root caries in relation to dental health behavior. J Dent Res 1988;67(6):911–4.
75. Grytten J, Rossow I, Holst D, et al. Longitudinal study of dental health behaviors and other caries predictors in early childhood. Community Dent Oral Epidemiol 1988;16(6):356–9.
76. Douglass JM, Tinanoff N, Tang JM, et al. Dental caries patterns and oral health behaviors in Arizona infants and toddlers. Community Dent Oral Epidemiol 2001;29(1):14–22.
77. Fisher FJ. A field survey of dental caries, periodontal disease and enamel defects in Tristan da Cunha. Br Dent J 1968;125(10):447–53.
78. Toverud G. The influence of war and post-war conditions on the teeth of Norwegian school children. II. Caries in the permanent teeth of children aged 7-8 and 12-13 years. Milbank Mem Fund Q 1957;35(2):127–96.
79. Gustafsson BE, Quensel CE, Lanke LS, et al. The Vipeholm dental caries study; the effect of different levels of carbohydrate intake on caries activity in 436 individuals observed for five years. Acta Odontol Scand 1954;11(3–4): 232–64.
80. Woodward M, Walker AR. Sugar consumption and dental caries: evidence from 90 countries. Br Dent J 1994;176(8):297–302.
81. Mattos-Graner RO, Smith DJ, King WF, et al. Water-insoluble glucan synthesis by mutans streptococcal strains correlates with caries incidence in 12- to 30-month-old children. J Dent Res 2000;79(6):1371–7.
82. Tinanoff N, Palmer CA. Dietary determinants of dental caries and dietary recommendations for preschool children. J Public Health Dent 2000;60(3):197–206 [discussion: 207–9].
83. Harel-Raviv M, Laskaris M, Chu KS. Dental caries and sugar consumption into the 21st century. Am J Dent 1996;9(5):184–90.
84. Downer MC, Drugan CS, Blinkhorn AS. Correlates of dental caries in 12-year-old children in Europe: a cross-sectional analysis. Community Dent Health 2008; 25(2):70–8.
85. Yoshihara A, Watanabe R, Hanada N, et al. A longitudinal study of the relationship between diet intake and dental caries and periodontal disease in elderly Japanese subjects. Gerodontology 2009;26(2):130–6.
86. Adegboye AR, Twetman S, Christensen LB, et al. Intake of dairy calcium and tooth loss among adult Danish men and women. Nutrition 2012;28(7–8):779–84.
87. Cooke LJ, Wardle J. Age and gender differences in children's food preferences. Br J Nutr 2005;93(5):741–6.

88. Maciel SM, Marcenes W, Watt RG, et al. The relationship between sweetness preference and dental caries in mother/child pairs from Maringá-Pr, Brazil. Int Dent J 2001;51(2):83–8.
89. Ostberg AL, Halling A, Lindblad U. Gender differences in knowledge, attitude, behavior and perceived oral health among adolescents. Acta Odontol Scand 1999;57(4):231–6.
90. Joshi N, Rajesh R, Sunitha M. Prevalence of dental caries among school children in Kulasekharam village: a correlated prevalence survey. J Indian Soc Pedod Prev Dent 2005;23(3):138–40.
91. Drewnowski A, Kurth C, Holden-Wiltse J, et al. Food preferences in human obesity: carbohydrates versus fats. Appetite 1992;18(3):207–21.
92. Grogan SC, Bell R, Conner M. Eating sweet snacks: gender differences in attitudes and behaviour. Appetite 1997;28(1):19–31.
93. Maciel SM, Marcenes W, Sheiham A. The relationship between sweetness preference, levels of salivary mutans streptococci and caries experience in Brazilian pre-school children. Int J Paediatr Dent 2001;11(2):123–30.
94. Policy on early childhood caries (ECC): classifications, consequences, and preventive strategies. Pediatr Dent 2008;30(Suppl 7):40–3.
95. Kanasi E, Johansson I, Lu SC, et al. Microbial risk markers for childhood caries in pediatricians' offices. J Dent Res 2010;89(4):378–83.
96. Wan AK, Seow WK, Walsh LJ, et al. Association of Streptococcus mutans infection and oral developmental nodules in pre-dentate infants. J Dent Res 2001; 80(10):1945–8.
97. Milgrom P, Riedy CA, Weinstein P, et al. Dental caries and its relationship to bacterial infection, hypoplasia, diet, and oral hygiene in 6- to 36-month-old children. Community Dent Oral Epidemiol 2000;28(4):295–306.
98. Ellen RP, Banting DW, Fillery ED. Longitudinal microbiological investigation of a hospitalized population of older adults with a high root surface caries risk. J Dent Res 1985;64(12):1377–81.
99. Russell JI, MacFarlane TW, Aitchison TC, et al. Prediction of caries increment in Scottish adolescents. Community Dent Oral Epidemiol 1991;19(2):74–7.
100. Klock B, Emilson CG, Lind SO, et al. Prediction of caries activity in children with today's low caries incidence. Community Dent Oral Epidemiol 1989;17(6):285–8.
101. Wilson RF, Ashley FP. Identification of caries risk in schoolchildren: salivary buffering capacity and bacterial counts, sugar intake and caries experience as predictors of 2-year and 3-year caries increment. Br Dent J 1989;167(3):99–102.
102. Ge Y, Caufield PW, Fisch GS, et al. Streptococcus mutans and Streptococcus sanguinis colonization correlated with caries experience in children. Caries Res 2008;42(6):444–8.
103. Hegde PP, Ashok Kumar BR, Ankola VA. Dental caries experience and salivary levels of Streptococcus mutans and Lactobacilli in 13-15 years old children of Belgaum city, Karnataka. J Indian Soc Pedod Prev Dent 2005;23(1):23–6.
104. Shi S, Deng Q, Hayashi Y, et al. A follow-up study on three caries activity tests. J Clin Pediatr Dent 2003;27(4):359–64.
105. De Soet JJ, van Gemert-Schriks MC, Laine ML, et al. Host and microbiological factors related to dental caries development. Caries Res 2008;42(5):340–7.
106. Ogaard B, Seppa L, Rolla G. Relationship between oral hygiene and approximal caries in 15-year-old Norwegians. Caries Res 1994;28(4):297–300.
107. Kawamura M, Takase N, Sasahara H, et al. Teenagers' oral health attitudes and behavior in Japan: comparison by sex and age group. J Oral Sci 2008;50(2): 167–74.

108. Al-Ansari JM, Honkala S. Gender differences in oral health knowledge and behavior of the health science college students in Kuwait. J Allied Health 2007;36(1):41–6.
109. Haugejorden O. Using the DMF gender difference to assess the "major" role of fluoride toothpastes in the caries decline in industrialized countries: a meta-analysis. Community Dent Oral Epidemiol 1996;24(6):369–75.
110. Marinho V. Fluoride gel inhibits caries in children who have low caries-risk but this may not be clinically relevant. Evid Based Dent 2004;5(4):95.
111. Marinho V. Substantial caries-inhibiting effect of fluoride varnish suggested. Evid Based Dent 2006;7(1):9–10.
112. Marinho VC. Evidence-based effectiveness of topical fluorides. Adv Dent Res 2008;20(1):3–7.
113. Marinho VC. Cochrane reviews of randomized trials of fluoride therapies for preventing dental caries. Eur Arch Paediatr Dent 2009;10(3):183–91.
114. Marinho VC, Higgins JP, Logan S, et al. Fluoride varnishes for preventing dental caries in children and adolescents. Cochrane Database Syst Rev 2002;(3):CD002279.
115. Marinho VC, Higgins JP, Logan S, et al. Fluoride gels for preventing dental caries in children and adolescents. Cochrane Database Syst Rev 2002;(2):CD002280.
116. Marinho VC, Higgins JP, Logan S, et al. Topical fluoride (toothpastes, mouth rinses, gels or varnishes) for preventing dental caries in children and adolescents. Cochrane Database Syst Rev 2003;(4):CD002782.
117. Marinho VC, Higgins JP, Logan S, et al. Fluoride mouth rinses for preventing dental caries in children and adolescents. Cochrane Database Syst Rev 2003;(3):CD002284.
118. Marinho VC, Higgins JP, Logan S, et al. Systematic review of controlled trials on the effectiveness of fluoride gels for the prevention of dental caries in children. J Dent Educ 2003;67(4):448–58.
119. Marinho VC, Higgins JP, Sheiham A, et al. Fluoride toothpastes for preventing dental caries in children and adolescents. Cochrane Database Syst Rev 2003;(1):CD002278.
120. Marinho VC, Higgins JP, Sheiham A, et al. Combinations of topical fluoride (toothpastes, mouth rinses, gels, varnishes) versus single topical fluoride for preventing dental caries in children and adolescents. Cochrane Database Syst Rev 2004;(1):CD002781.
121. Marinho VC, Higgins JP, Sheiham A, et al. One topical fluoride (toothpastes, or mouth rinses, or gels, or varnishes) versus another for preventing dental caries in children and adolescents. Cochrane Database Syst Rev 2004;(1):CD002780.
122. Wong MC, Clarkson J, Glenny AM, et al. Cochrane reviews on the benefits/risks of fluoride toothpastes. J Dent Res 2011;90(5):573–9.
123. Featherstone JD, Ten Cate JM. Physicochemical aspects of fluoride-enamel interactions. In: Ekstrand J, Fejerskov O, Silverstone LM, editors. Fluoride in dentistry. Copenhagen (Denmark): Munksgaard; 1988. p. 125–49.
124. Martinez-Mier EA, Soto-Rojas AE. Differences in exposure and biological markers of fluoride among white and African American children. J Public Health Dent 2010;70(3):234–40.
125. NIDCR/CDC. NIDCR/CDC Dental, Oral and Craniofacial Data Resource Center. 2012. Available at: http://drc.hhs.gov/index.htm. Accessed October 27, 2012.

126. WHO. Dental diseases and oral health. World health organization global strategy on diet, physical activity and health. 2003. Available at: http://www.who.int/oral_health/publications/en/orh_fact_sheet.pdf. Accessed October 27, 2012.
127. Mejia GC. Measuring the oral health of populations. Community Dent Oral Epidemiol 2012;40(Suppl 2):95–101.
128. AMRO. Oral Health Database. 2012. Available at: http://www.mah.se/CAPP/Country-Oral-Health-Profiles/AMRO/. Accessed October 27, 2012.
129. Shah N. Gender issues and oral health in elderly Indians. Int Dent J 2003;53(6):475–84.
130. Hunter JM, Arbona SI. The tooth as a marker of developing world quality of life: a field study in Guatemala. Soc Sci Med 1995;41(9):1217–40.
131. Dye BA, Li X, Thornton-Evans G. Oral health disparities as determined by selected Healthy People 2020 oral health objectives for the United States, 2009–2010. NCHS data brief no 104 2012. Available at: http://www.cdc.gov/nchs/data/databriefs/db104.htm. Accessed October 27, 2012.
132. Payne S, Doyal L. Older women, work and health. Occup Med (Lond) 2010;60(3):172–7.
133. Doyal L, Naidoo S. Why dentists should take a greater interest in sex and gender. Br Dent J 2010;209(7):335–7.

Sex/Gender Differences in Tooth Loss and Edentulism

Historical Perspectives, Biological Factors, and Sociologic Reasons

Stefanie L. Russell, DDS, MPH, PhD[a],*,
Sara Gordon, DDS, MSc, FRCD(C), FDS-RCSEd[b], John R. Lukacs, PhD[c],
Linda M. Kaste, DDS, MS, PhD[d]

KEYWORDS

- Tooth loss • Sex • Gender • Periodontal diseases • Dental caries

KEY POINTS

- Across history and prehistory into the present day, sex and gender have played, and are likely to continue to play, major roles in differences in dental disease rates, and in the prevalence of tooth loss and edentulism.
- An anthropologic perspective on tooth loss is valuable to clinical dentistry because it provides evolutionary, prehistoric, and ethnographic contexts for understanding an important aspect of oral health in modern humans.
- Whereas in many populations across the world women most certainly had, and continue to have, higher rates of tooth loss and edentulism, differences in tooth loss by sex/gender are likely decreasing in North America.
- The relationship between sex/gender, dental disease, and tooth loss is inherently very complex; it seems likely that both biology and social factors associated with being female are important risk factors for tooth loss.

The retention or loss of permanent teeth is of central importance to an individual's oral health status and to quality of life. The loss of some or all teeth from the permanent dentition is closely associated with myriad dental and metabolic diseases and has multiple causes, including both systemic biological and cross-cultural behavioral etiology. Tooth loss as a measure of oral health has several advantages over other

[a] Department of Epidemiology & Health Promotion, NYU College of Dentistry, 250 Park Avenue South, 6th Floor, New York, NY 10003-1402, USA; [b] Department of Oral Medicine and Diagnostic Sciences, University of Illinois at Chicago, 801 South Paulina Street, MC838, Chicago, IL 60612, USA; [c] Department of Anthropology, 1218 University of Oregon, Eugene, OR 97403, USA; [d] Department of Pediatric Dentistry, University of Illinois at Chicago, 801 South Paulina Street, Room 563A, MC 850, Chicago, IL 60612, USA
* Corresponding author.
E-mail address: stefanie.russell@nyu.edu

Dent Clin N Am 57 (2013) 317–337
http://dx.doi.org/10.1016/j.cden.2013.02.006
0011-8532/13/$ – see front matter © 2013 Elsevier Inc. All rights reserved.

oral health and disease indices, including not only its direct associations with oral function and with overall health and well-being but also the ease by which the presence or absence of teeth can be measured. Sex and gender influence oral disease, including caries and periodontal diseases, and result in differences in tooth retention rates, edentulism, and in the incidence of tooth loss.

Tooth loss is influenced by biology and genetics, but is also a key indicator of dental care utilization and access (ie, teeth are "lost" mainly because someone extracts them), and is inherently associated with culture and attitudes, including patients' and dentists' philosophies of dental care. Indeed, it is a grave error to dismiss the importance of "the complex pattern of roles, responsibilities, norms, values, freedoms, and limitations that define what is thought of as 'masculine' and 'feminine' in a given time and place"[1] in influencing health. This article follows the convention of referring to differences by sex and gender as sex/gender differences, but when speaking solely of biological differences between men and women the authors use the word sex, and when speaking only of differences resulting from the cultural construction of male/female roles, the word gender is used. Differences in oral health are a function of differences in biology (sex) but also of differences in cultural context (gender).

The purposes of this article are:

1. To provide relevant anthropologic and historical background on sex/gender differences in tooth loss
2. To discuss the recent epidemiology of tooth retention and loss, focusing on North America, in the context of sex/gender differences and similarities
3. To elucidate ways in which biology (sex) and culture (gender) are likely to influence differences in tooth retention, tooth loss, and edentulism

SEX/GENDER DIFFERENCES IN TOOTH LOSS: AN ANTHROPOLOGIC PERSPECTIVE

An anthropologic perspective on tooth loss is valuable to clinical dentistry because it provides evolutionary, prehistoric, and ethnographic contexts for understanding an important aspect of oral health in modern humans. This discussion of tooth loss focuses on "dental ablation" and adopts a bidirectional uniformitarian approach: the present informs us about the past; however, knowledge of the past provides a broad comparative context for understanding tooth loss and dental ablation in modern humans.

In anthropological terms, antemortem tooth loss (AMTL) is defined as "loss of teeth during life, as evidenced by progressive resorption of the alveolus,"[2] and differs from tooth ablation, which is defined as "... the deliberate removal of anterior teeth during life."[3] Tooth ablation is a form of intentional dental modification that is commonly grouped with other forms of tooth modification, such as chipping, filing, inlays, and bleaching.[4] The etiology of AMTL and ablation is complex and multicausal.

In prehistory, skeletal series present unique challenges in the differential diagnosis of causal factors leading to loss of teeth before death. It should be noted that distinguishing the culturally mediated practice of tooth ablation from numerous other causes of tooth loss can be difficult, but this issue has a long history. It has been suggested that 7 criteria may be used for the recognition of ritual ablation: (1) no evidence of dental disease, (2) symmetry or near symmetry of tooth loss, (3) repetition of similar pattern of tooth loss in the group, (4) fracture of the labial wall of the alveolar bone, (5) indication that the tooth loss occurred in youth, (6) presence of the practice in neighboring or related groups, and (7) mention of the practice in myths and legends.[5] However, some have criticisms for each of these criteria, contending that a highly irregular pattern of loss contrasts sharply with the highly regular practices of tooth removal documented ethnographically in some African groups.[6]

Although a comprehensive discussion of tooth ablation and AMTL in nonhuman primates is beyond the scope of this report, it should be noted that tooth loss is well documented in the fossil record of many ancestral species. A key example is the "old man" from La Chapelle aux Saints, a Neanderthal fossil that figured prominently in early misunderstanding the Neanderthal's significance in human evolution. The nearly edentulous skull of *Homo erectus* (= *ergaster*) from the site of Dmanisi (about 1.77 million years ago) is probably male and retained only one tooth: the left mandibular canine.[7] This find renewed the debate over how far into the past modern human social structure, life history, care, and compassion may have existed.[7] Some believe that in antiquity, individuals with extensive edentulism must have benefitted from altruistic care and assistance to survive in the absence of a functional dentition.[8] Others, citing edentulism in nonhuman primates, assert that survival with severe masticatory impairment can be present in the absence of "human-like" caring and cooperative behavior.[9,10]

TOOTH LOSS IN PREHISTORY

Teeth may be missing from the dental arch for many reasons, a situation that makes accurate diagnosis of the exact cause of tooth loss difficult in any population. However, the prime cause of AMTL in prehistoric skeletal series is dental disease. While periodontal disease and dental caries have been recognized as the major reasons for AMTL in archaeological samples, severe dental wear and dental trauma also contribute significantly to AMTL.[11] Although sex/gender differences in AMTL from oral diseases are often significant (caries and tooth loss being more common in women than in men), differences in tooth ablation are primarily influenced by culturally mediated behavior and exhibit significant variation by sex and gender, both temporally and regionally. Moreover, although ablation may account for a smaller percentage of teeth lost antemortem than disease, this practice is the focus of intense study by anthropologists because of its global distribution, the diverse sociocultural settings, and the wide range of behaviors with which it is associated. Ablation has been practiced on every continent, from Neolithic to modern times, and may reflect social status, rites of passage (puberty/initiation, marriage), or mourning the death of leader, relative, or loved one.

Tooth ablation was, in many cases, more common in one gender than in the other: for example, the observed variation in anterior tooth loss in circum Arctic populations may have resulted from trauma due to a strenuous lifestyle, and gender-specific use of teeth as tools in subsistence and craft activities.[6] Additional salient examples of ablation are shown in **Table 1**. Ablation has been documented in prehistory from sites in circum Mediterranean North Africa,[12] and more extensively in sub-Saharan Africa.[13–17] Ablation was also practiced more than 10,000 years ago by prehistoric people of the Maghreb, North Africa, and has been documented geographically and chronologically to reveal changing patterns of ablation.[12] The investigators interpret the decreasing frequency of ablation over time, the changing pattern of ablation by sex, and differences in the regional and cultural distribution of the practice as indicating the diversification of social meaning. Prehistoric Southeast Asia provides clear evidence of cultural modification of teeth, such as filing and ablation, which are distinct from congenitally missing teeth in prehistoric samples from Thailand. Patterns of ablation changed over time: early burials were missing mainly maxillary lateral incisors, whereas in later-phase burials maxillary central and all mandibular incisors were missing. Sex differences in missing teeth were not significant in early burials, but females were missing more teeth than males in later-phase burials.

Table 1
Examples of gender-related tooth ablation and antemortem missing teeth from prehistory

Continent	Era	Gender Relationship	Ablation Pattern	Proportion of Sample Affected
Africa[12]	Iberomarusian Period (>20,000 BP to at least 10,000 BP)	Both genders affected, but males > females (average of 6.6 teeth vs 6.3 teeth)	Limited to the upper central incisors	Ablation nearly universal
Africa[12]	Transitional Epipaleolithic Period	Genders equally affected	Minimally involving the lower incisors, involving all 8 incisors roughly half the time	Ablation nearly universal
Africa (Eastern Algeria and Tunisia)[12]	Capsian period (9800 BP)	Females > males (88% vs 38%)		Ablation in 62% of the sample
Africa[12]	Neolithic period	No data		Ablation in 27% of the sample, suggesting a reduction in frequency of this practice
Africa (Sudan)[13]	350 BP to AD 1400	Genders equally affected (males 12.2%, females 13.3%), adults only	Mandibular central, lateral incisors removed in symmetric or asymmetric patterns	Ablation in 9.4% of the sample
Africa (South Africa)[15]	Early Iron Age (ca 1500 BP)	Genders equally affected, same mean age at ablation (males = 15.6 y; females = 16.6 y), ablation occurred across a wide range of ages (11–20 y)	Missing teeth were said to symbolize gang initiation or membership and to enhance the pleasure of oral sexual acts	
Asia (southeast Thailand)[18]	4000–3500 BP	Sex differences in missing teeth not significant in early burials, but females were missing more teeth than males in later-phase burials	Various, involving anterior teeth. Patterns changed over time: early burials missing mainly maxillary lateral incisors, later burials missing maxillary central incisors, mandibular incisors	

Location	Period	Sex difference	Comments	Other
Asia (northwestern Cambodia)[19]	2500–1500 BP	No sex differences were found in number of teeth ablated in maxillae or in mandibles, by site or in the composite	The majority of specimens (83.5% maxilla; 61.1% mandible) exhibited a symmetric pattern of ablation. Filing of anterior teeth was also documented at both sites	79% were congenitally missing at least 1 upper or lower lateral incisor
Asia (northeastern Thailand)[20]	ca 200 BP to ca AD 500	Males tended to exhibit missing lateral incisors more often than females, but the difference was not significant	Most frequent pattern involved missing all 4 lateral incisors	
Asia (Japan)[21]	18,000 BP			Evidence of missing lower central incisors and alveolar remodeling a female specimen
Asia (Japan)[21]	Jomon period (14,000 to about 300 BP)	Males	Upper canines were the principal teeth extracted and indicators of skeletal development (epiphyseal fusion) suggest ablation began at 12–13 y	80%–100%
Asia (China)[21]	Dawenkou Neolithic (6500 BP); practice declines suddenly with the onset of the Longshan culture (4000 BP)[a]	No sex difference	Targeted maxillary incisor and canine teeth normally commenced in early adolescence, or ca 13–15 y	60%–90%

[a] Period of prevalence and subsequent decline of ablation 2000 years earlier than Japan.

An extensive literature on ritual tooth ablation in East Asia focuses on the history, patterns, methods, prevalence, and significance of this widespread practice. Presence of broken roots and root fragments in the alveolar bone of Jomon period males from Tsukumo and Yoshigo suggests that a traumatic method of ablation was common.[21] A comparison of the antiquity and temporal transition in ablation customs in China and Japan reveal differences in the earliest evidence, height of prevalence, and decline in the practice of ablation.[22] The period of prevalence and subsequent decline of ablation in China occurred 2000 years earlier than in Japan, although the type and significance of ablation diversified through time in both countries.

In China, removal of maxillary lateral incisors was the earliest form of tooth ablation and was the principal type practiced until recent times. Indicating attainment of adult status, ablation may also have signified eligibility for marriage and in some areas may indicate clan membership, allowing enforcement of interclan marriage rules.[22] In Japan, a significant increase in the types of ablation through time and across the life span implies an increase in diversification of social meaning. For example, removal of upper canines was associated with adult status, extraction of lower incisors and canines occurred at marriage, and removal of first premolars was a sign of mourning.[23] Different types of ablation have also been interpreted to signify different places of origin. In a significant number of burials, the husband, who had 4 canines removed, was buried in association with his wife, who had maxillary canines and 4 lower incisors removed. Thus, rules of postmarital residence (bilocal, uxorilocal) have been inferred from ablation types in Jomon period Japan, although regional variation (eastern, western) is likely.[23] This interpretation is controversial, and recent research using stable-isotope analysis of diet and biodistance estimates from cranial and dental measurements challenge these earlier theories of social meaning. Persons with ablation of 4 canines appear to have been more dependent on terrestrial dietary resources; conversely, persons with ablation of maxillary canines and 4 lower incisors were more reliant on marine resources.[24] Furthermore, ablation type was unrelated to migratory pattern, but may represent kin-based social units whereby achievement, status, or age were criteria for membership.[25]

TOOTH ABLATION IN THE MODERN WORLD

Tooth ablation is still practiced among diverse ethnic groups in Africa, where it has a long history and a wide range of ritual and practical motivating factors, and poses significant challenges among emigrants to other cultures where ablation is unknown and not practiced.[17,26] For example, ablation of anterior teeth continues among ethnic groups of southern Sudan[26] and Ethiopia.[27] Although mandibular incisor and canines are most frequently removed, anywhere from 2 to 6 mandibular or maxillary teeth may be removed in association with achieving adulthood, enhancing aesthetics, emitting special linguistic sounds, indicating tribal membership, or consuming soft or liquid foods.[26] In Africa, and among some children of African parents living in other parts of the world, there has been a tradition of extirpation of deciduous tooth buds by village healers to rid the child of perceived "tooth worms," a practice called infant oral mutilation.[28,29]

In South Africa, tooth ablation is currently practiced among urban groups of the Western Cape.[15] Two novel motivations for ablation were uncovered in this group; missing teeth were said to symbolize gang initiation or membership and to enhance the pleasure of fellatio. Although some Cape Flats groups refer to the interdental space resulting from ablation as a "passion gap," some researchers refute this motivation as an incorrect and insulting myth, but regard the importance of gang activity and membership a more likely explanation for the "Cape Flats smile."[15]

Whereas an edentulous space or interdental gap in these groups has well-established significance and value, among most European and American groups tooth loss is considered unattractive and is associated with poor standards of health, low socioeconomic status, and a lack of education. Immigrants from ethnic groups practicing tooth ablation often quickly appreciate the difference in cultural meaning associated with missing teeth, and seek dental restoration as a means of improving social acceptance, facilitating articulation and pronunciation of certain standard English sounds, and enhancing food-acquisition ability.[17,26,30]

PRENUPTIAL EDENTULISM AND DOWRY DENTURES

There are several references to gender-based tooth extractions in the current medical and dental literature.[17,26,30–32] In some regions of the world there appears to be persistence of an old tradition of removing all of a young woman's teeth when she approaches a marriageable age. This practice, called prenuptial edentulism, seems to be related to a wish for attractive teeth, or so-called dowry dentures.[33]

Prenuptial edentulism was first described in the Guatemala highlands,[34] where dental disease was rampant, dental care was expensive for villagers, and young women were perceived to be less tough than young men, hence family resources were spent on extractions for girls rather than for boys. In this poor rural population, some young women would inherit their grandmother's dentures. This practice has also been documented among rural Acadian and French-Canadian populations,[33] where some young women would have their maxillary teeth, or all of their teeth, removed before marriage in order to be fitted for dentures, regardless of their current dental health. In one area of Maine, adjacent to the Canadian region where the practice was described, a local dentist reported that dowry dentures are a common high-school graduation gift for Acadian girls.

In several areas of England, dentists have reported full-mouth clearance and subsequent dentures as a wedding gift, especially for women. In his 1980 valedictory address, British Dental Association President D.G.E. Roberts described the practice: "I can recall that, in certain parts of the country, one of the most popular gifts to a young woman intending marriage was to enable her to have her teeth extracted and dentures fitted. Thus the dread of toothache was removed and the future partner spared any trouble and expense."[33]

SEX/GENDER DIFFERENCES IN THE DISTRIBUTION AND DETERMINANTS OF TOOTH LOSS IN MODERN TIMES: NORTH AMERICA

As is the case in history and prehistory, tooth loss in modern humans often differs by sex/gender and by etiology. In general, a higher prevalence of both tooth loss and dental caries has been documented among women than among men in many parts of the world.[35,36] Because most teeth are extracted because of caries,[37–43] it would follow that rates of tooth loss would reflect rates of dental caries, hence the predisposition for women to be more affected than men by this disease. However, because sex/gender differences in tooth loss reflect not only sex/gender disparities in levels of dental disease but also differences in socioeconomic factors, personal and cultural attitudes and beliefs regarding teeth and dental care, and the availability, frequency, and use of both episodic and preventive dental care, the relationship between sex/gender and tooth loss is quite complex.

In the United States, there are few data specific to sex/gender differences in the prevalence of tooth loss prior to the National Health Survey of 1960 to 1962. However, in that report, tooth loss in adults was common (overall, 18% of adults were completely edentulous), and that the prevalence of tooth loss increased dramatically in persons older than 45 years.[44,45] Part of this dramatic increase was likely due to a lack of preventive dental care for children and adults in the early part of the century, which would have affected all but the youngest group of adults, as well as the popularity of the concept of diseased teeth as foci of infection responsible for a host of systemic diseases.[46] Extraction of teeth for the sake of systemic health continued into the 1950s[47] and, though it is likely that some of the tooth loss seen in older adults because of this cohort effect could be seen in studies of adult oral health extending into the later part of the twentieth century, the effect of the concept of focal infection on sex/gender disparities in tooth loss is unknown. One might hypothesize that perhaps sex disparities in rates of diseases thought to be caused by infected teeth (ie, rheumatism, depression) were higher in women than in men, or that more frequent use of both general and dental services by women might have accounted for these differences. What is absolutely apparent, however, is that as early as the National Health Survey of 1960 to 1962, women were more likely than men to be edentulous (19.6% vs 16.4%),[44] and this sex/gender disparity was true for each of the 7 age groups represented in the sample.[45] In Canada from 1970 to 1972, women were more likely than men to be edentulous in all age categories; the largest differences were seen after the age of 30, with 22.9% of women versus 6.1% of men age 30 to 39, 26.5% of women versus 18.0% men age 40 to 49, 38.4% of women versus 30.4% of men age 50 to 59, and 55.7% of women versus 49.5% men age 60 years and older being edentulous.[48]

Rates of tooth loss and edentulism decreased in North America during the latter half of the twentieth century,[49] when the preventive dentistry movement began. Disease rates have been affected by water fluoridation, the pervasive use of topical fluoride in dentifrices and mouth rinses, and the change in the culture of dentistry to emphasize retention of teeth.[47] In the United States between 1988 and 1994, when the Third National Health and Nutrition Examination Survey (NHANES) was conducted, and from 1999 to 2004, the most recent NHANES survey in which a dental examination was performed, rates of edentulism among adults have continued to decline, from 6% to 4%.[50] In Canada, in 1970 to 1972, 23.6% of adults aged 19 or older were edentulous; by 2007 to 2009 the proportion had dropped to 6.4% edentulous overall.[48,49]

Table 2 provides a summary of adult and older adult population-based epidemiologic studies performed in the United States and Canada over the past 25 years that have included data broken down by sex/gender. It is clear that disparities in rates of edentulism by gender have virtually disappeared, with some notable exceptions. In Canada, although rates of edentulism are now similar between men (6.3%) and women (6.5%), women are still more likely to have lost at least 1 tooth (46.7% vs 38.1%).[48] In the United States, there are large and persistent racial and ethnic disparities in oral health; data from the Hispanic Health and Nutrition Examination Survey (HHANES, 1987) demonstrated that among Mexican Americans, 5.2% of females versus 3.5% of males were edentulous.[51] It appears that in recent years, sex/gender differences in edentulism among whites have disappeared. However, among blacks and Hispanics, women are still more likely than men to have missing teeth,[52] although it has been shown that women have higher rates of caries and men more frequently have periodontal disease.[53–55] These differences in disease patterns likely involve behavioral factors (including diet, smoking, patterns of health-protecting behaviors such as oral hygiene practices and dental treatment patterns), but certainly biology is an important contributor to disease rates; specifically, women's reproductive function, including demands of menses, pregnancy, and parity.[35,36,56]

HOW SEX/GENDER MAY INFLUENCE RATES OF TOOTH LOSS

Fig. 1 provides a conceptual model of how sex (biology) and gender (sociobehavioral factors) are likely to influence rates of tooth loss. Relationships between the variables in this conceptual model are complex, and this conceptual framework is necessarily simplified for the sake of clarity. This model does, however, recognize the multifactorial nature of both dental disease (caries and periodontitis) and tooth loss, demonstrating that both sex (genetics, physiology) and gender (the constructed social roles of what it is to be male or female) are important contributors to caries and periodontal diseases, and to tooth loss. In this model several variables mediate the relationship between gender and dental disease; gender is related to behavior (eg, oral hygiene behavior and oral health protective and damaging behaviors such as smoking and diet), which is in turn related to caries and periodontitis. Gender is also related to socioeconomic status variables such as income, education, and occupation, which are related to dental care use and dental insurance. These dental-related factors are in turn related to caries and periodontitis; and, conversely, having dental disease alters patterns of dental care use. In addition, there may in some cases be either a synergistic or antagonistic effect of gender-related and sex-related factors that may increase or decrease rates of disease or tooth loss. For example, changing hormone levels throughout life related to women's reproductive function (including demands of menses, pregnancy, and parity)[35,36,56–59] are likely to affect the periodontium, sometimes in irreversible ways. Destruction of the periodontium, in turn, influences whether teeth are retained or extracted. However, women and men have different patterns of dental utilization that are likely to affect whether teeth are extracted or not. Although it is difficult to say with certainty whether biology or society/culture more profoundly influences levels of dental disease (caries, periodontitis) and tooth loss, most would argue that both factors together are important in the pathway toward tooth loss.[35,36] The specific contributions of sex-related and gender-related factors to different levels and rates of disease, and to tooth retention and loss, are further discussed here.

Sex-Related Factors Influencing Tooth Loss

While much of human biology is shared between the sexes, there are important sex-related differences. First, because tooth loss is irreversible and cumulative, tooth loss is necessarily associated with increased age. Indeed, it is clear from many studies that the most important risk indicator for partial and complete edentulism is age. Women experience lower mortality rates from most of the major causes of death, including heart disease, cancer, respiratory disease, accidents, suicide, and homicide, and women in the United States currently live on average about 5 years longer than men, almost to age 81 years,[60] whereas women in Canada live about 4.5 years longer than men, to age 83 years.[61] Although some have proposed that perhaps women experience more tooth loss simply because they live longer, when well-conducted studies adjust for differing age structures between population subgroups, including those by sex/gender, differences tend to be attenuated, but not absent.[52,62]

Given that differing life expectancies do not completely account for differences in rates of tooth retention and loss, other factors are likely involved. What biological differences between women and men could contribute to differences in tooth loss? The most obvious difference between the sexes is hormonal: women have a different

Table 2
North American adult population based studies including data on tooth loss: sex/gender relationships

Authors	Publication Date	Location	Population	Outcomes	> = <	Notes
Wu B[63]	2011	USA	Americans age 60+ in NHANES 1999–2004	Edentulism	=	
Health Canada[48]	2010	Canada (CMHS)	Canadians 2007–2009	Edentulism	=	6.5% of females and 6.3% males
				Tooth loss (% with any loss)	>	46.7% of males vs 38.1% of females
CDC[64]	2009	USA	White, black, and Hispanic Americans NHANES 1988–1994	Any tooth loss	=	
CDC[64]	2009	USA	White, black, and Mexican Americans NHANES 1999–2004	Any tooth loss	>	Males have reached Healthy People 2010 target of 40% of population with no permanent tooth loss from disease
Jiminez M[52]	2009	USA	White, black, and Mexican Americans NHANES III 1988–1994	Number of missing teeth	= > >	Whites Blacks Mexican Americans
Quandt SA[65]	2009	USA	Older rural adults (African American, White, American Indian)	Number of teeth	=	Males and females overall had the same number of remaining teeth (numbers of teeth lost)
Beltran-Aguilar ED[66]	2005	USA	White, black, and Hispanic Americans NHANES 1988–1994	Missing teeth	=	Females had slightly more missing teeth, but difference not significant

				Retention of teeth (tooth loss)	=	
Gooch BF[67]	2003	USA	Older Adults ≥65 y, BRFSS 1995–1997		=	
CDC[68]	2003	USA	BRFSS 2002	Tooth loss	=	
CDC[69]	1999	USA	BRFSS 1995–1997	Edentulism	=	
CDC[69]	1999	USA	Older adults ≥65 y, BRFSS 1995–1997	Edentulism	=	
Marcus SE[70]	1996	USA	Adult Americans NHANES III 1988–1994	Tooth loss Edentulism	=	Sex/gender not related to tooth retention or tooth loss after adjustment for age
Marcus SE[71]	1994	USA	Adult Americans USA employed adults and seniors 1985–1986	Tooth loss	=	
Ismael AI[51]	1987	USA	Mexican Americans HHANES 1982–1983	Edentulism	>	5.2% of females vs 3.5% of males were edentulous
Hunt RJ[72]	1985	Iowa, USA	Elderly, rural Iowans age 65+	Edentulism	=	For those 80+, slightly higher rate for females; for other ages, rate for females slightly lower than males; no sex/ gender differences in multivariate analyses

Abbreviations: BRFSS, Behavioral Risk Factor Surveillance System; CHMS, Canadian Health Measures Survey; HHANES, Hispanic Health and Nutrition Examination Survey; NHANES, National Health and Nutrition Examination Survey.

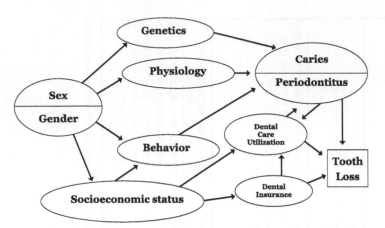

Fig. 1. Conceptual model of the relationship between sex, gender, and tooth loss.

mix of reproduction-related hormones in comparison with men, and most women are likely to experience pregnancy and lactation, often multiple times in their lives. Hormonal variations have been demonstrated to affect oral health. In particular, the intraoral soft-tissue changes that accompany pregnancy, as a result of the complex physiologic alterations, are well documented.[57,73–76] Fluctuations of sex hormones during pregnancy increase oral vasculature permeability, decrease host immunocompetence,[57] and alter levels of oral bacteria,[76,77] thereby increasing susceptibility to oral infection, including periodontal disease.[73] Gingivitis is almost universal during pregnancy,[73,78] and progression of periodontitis during pregnancy has been documented.[79–81] Although the popular belief that pregnancy weakens teeth as a result of calcium depletion is an unsupported hypothesis,[82,83] studies have shown that increased childbearing (parity) is related to tooth loss,[54,56,84–86] possibly through increased hormonal fluctuations that occur because of multiple pregnancies. In addition to hormonal changes that occur during pregnancy, monthly hormonal fluctuations in menses are thought to play a role in gingival inflammation in women,[87] and in fact may exaggerate preexisting inflammation in gingival tissues.[88] There is also evidence that menopause and accompanying osteoporosis are related to periodontitis[89] and tooth loss,[90–93] and conversely that the use of hormone-replacement treatment has been associated with a reduced likelihood of edentulism.[52,94] These results suggest the potential for a protective role of estrogen and progesterone on oral health.

Additional biological differences between the sexes are likely related to dental caries, which persists in most areas of the world as the most common reason for tooth extractions.[37–43,95,96] In most adult populations, including the United States[43,51] and Canada,[48,97] rates of dental caries have been shown to be higher in women. Biological factors that influence the development of caries include salivary flow and sex-linked genetic susceptibility.[98] Saliva protects teeth from dental caries by several mechanisms, including its cleansing effects and its ability to buffer acids produced by dental plaque.[99] Compared with men, women have lower stimulated and unstimulated salivary flow rates[100] and secrete less salivary immunoglobulin A,[101] and menopause is associated with xerostomia.[102] It has been suggested also that hormonally related changes in eating patterns, salivary composition, and salivary flow rates are related to a higher rate of caries in females.[103]

In addition, immune diseases that affect salivary flow disproportionately affect women.[104,105] For example, Sjögren syndrome, which affects about 3% of older women, has an overwhelming preponderance of female patients.[105] Several recent studies have demonstrated that periodontal patients have higher rates of rheumatoid arthritis,[106,107] a disease with a gender bias toward women. It is not clear whether the diseases are simply associated because of shared risk factors and similarities in host response, or whether periodontal pathogens predispose to rheumatoid arthritis in conjunction with other environmental and genetic factors.

Recent studies suggest that a sex-linked gene may explain, to some extent, why rates of dental caries may be higher in women.[108,109] These genes, Amelogenin X (found on the X chromosome) and Amelogenin Y (on the Y chromosome), code for proteins that constitute 90% of the enamel matrix.[109] Although genetic research on caries is yet in its infancy, and genetic and other biological factors that may contribute to gender discrepancies in tooth loss clearly require much more investigation, 2 recent studies in children have supported an association between Amelogenin X and experience of high caries.[110,111] Ultimately, genetic differences may prove to be just as, or more important than, environmental factors in the development of dental caries.[112]

Gender-Related Factors Influencing Tooth Loss

Factors related to tooth loss that are associated with societal gender roles include health-damaging or health-promoting behaviors, such as smoking, diet, and oral hygiene (eg, flossing). Smoking has long been seen as a risk factor for periodontal disease[113,114] and tooth loss,[113,115] and rates of smoking typically vary by gender,[116–118] with higher rates of tobacco use in men, but with large variations of male/female differences in smoking rates by country and culture.[118] Studies that analyze data by sex/gender subgroup, and studies limited to women[119] confirm that smoking is a risk factor for periodontal disease[119,120] and tooth loss among women.[90,113,120,121]

Tooth loss, diet, and nutrition are an important triad, given that mastication of food is a primary function of human dentition. Women and men have been found to have different dietary intakes largely attributed to different energy needs,[122] as well as food preference[123] and belief differences.[123,124] Hence, it would make sense that there might be differences between men and women in the association between tooth loss/edentulism and nutrient intake. Indeed, some researchers have found that nutrient intakes in older persons decreased with impaired dentition status, controlling for age and smoking; in addition, fiber, vitamin, and mineral intake were inversely correlated with masticatory function.[125] Investigators using data from the general United States population (NHANES 1999–2002), however, found similarities in dietary components, although the most reduced components of diets for edentulous persons were fruits for both men and women, and vegetables for women.[126] These data translated as lower α-carotene and β-carotene levels in edentulous males and lower vitamin C levels in females. Edentulous women were also lower on their overall healthy diet scores than their dentate counterparts. Other components of the diet have been found to be related to tooth loss: a recent prospective study found that dietary dairy calcium intake seemed to protect against future tooth loss in both men and women.[127] Another prospective study found that women who had previously changed their diet to one comprising significantly higher intakes of saturated fat, *trans* fat, cholesterol, and vitamin B_{12}, and lower intake of polyunsaturated fat, fiber, carotene, vitamin C, vitamin E, vitamin B_6, folate, potassium, vegetables, and fruits (in other words, a diet predisposing to the development of cardiovascular disease) lost more teeth than women with healthier diets.[128]

In the United States and many other countries, gender is also linked to socioeconomic status, with women, in comparison with men, having less wealth, lower incomes, reduced or underemployment, and, in some cases (but notably not in present-day North America), less education. Socioeconomic status has been inexorably linked to dental disease and tooth loss, with large disparities in dental disease and tooth loss rates evident in both developed[52,129] and developing countries.[130] Income and wealth are closely related to the ability to pay for dental care and to the kind of dental care (ie, preventive vs symptomatic), especially in countries where dental insurance is rare or nonexistent. Therefore, one might assume that men use health care to a greater extent than do women, because of their income and wealth. However, studies on utilization of both medical and dental care show consistently that women are more likely to visit a health care provider than are men,[131] and are more likely to access preventive care, including preventive dental care.[131–133] However, as is true in the general population, disparities among women in rates of dental care use have been reported in relation to socioeconomic status, race/ethnicity, and dental insurance status.[134]

Finally, differences by gender regarding oral health habits, as is the case with healthy general health habits, have been found consistently in favor of females,[135,136] including brushing and flossing. Longitudinal studies have verified the importance of oral hygiene as related to tooth loss[137] and dental disease.[138] Consistently, women appear to brush[139–141] and floss[139,140] more frequently than men. A recent investigation found that gender differences in gingivitis could be explained by oral health behaviors and hygiene status, which were in turn influenced by lifestyle, knowledge, and attitude.[141]

SUMMARY

Across history and prehistory into the present day, sex and gender have played, and are likely to continue to play a major role in differences in rates of dental disease, and in the prevalence of tooth loss and edentulism found between men and women. Whereas in many populations across the world women most certainly have had, and continue to have, higher rates of tooth loss and edentulism, it appears that differences in tooth loss by sex/gender is likely decreasing in North America. However, the relationship between sex/gender, dental disease, and tooth loss is inherently very complex; it seems likely that both biology and social factors associated with being female are important risk factors for tooth loss.

REFERENCES

1. World Health Organization, Department of Gender and Women's Health. Gender, health and aging. 2003. Available at: http://www.who.int/gender/documents/en/Gender_Ageing.pdf. Accessed December 3, 2012.
2. Lukacs JR. Oral health in past populations: context, concepts and controversy. In: Grauer AL, editor. A companion to paleopathology. Chichester (West Sussex), Malden (MA): Wiley-Blackwell; 2012. p. 553–81.
3. Pietrusewsky M, Douglas M. Tooth ablation in old Hawai'i. J Polyn Soc 1993; 102(3):255–72.
4. Alt KW, Pichler SL. Artificial modifications of human teeth. In: Alt KW, Rösing FW, Teschler-Nicola M, editors. Dental anthropology: fundamentals, limits, and prospects. Wein (Austria): Springer; 1998. p. 387–415.
5. Hrdlicka A. Ritual ablation of front teeth in Siberia and America. Smithsonian Misc Collect 1940;99(3).
6. Merbs C. Patterns of activity-induced pathology in a Canadian Inuit population. Archaeol Survey of Canada. 1983. p. 119.

7. Lordkipanidze D, Vejua A, Ferring CR, et al. The earliest toothless hominin skull. Nature 2005;343:717–8.
8. Hublin JJ. The prehistory of compassion. Proc Natl Acad Sci U S A 2009; 106(16):6429–30.
9. De Gusta D. Comparative skeletal pathology and the case for conspecific care in middle Pleistocene hominids. J Archaeol Sci 2002;29:1435–8.
10. De Gusta D. Aubesier 11 is not evidence of Neanderthal conspecific care. J Hum Evol 2003;45:91–4.
11. Milner GR, Larsen CS. Teeth as artifacts of human behavior: intentional mutilation and accidental modification. In: Kelley MA, Larsen CS, editors. Advances in dental anthropology. New York: Wiley-Liss, Inc; 1991. p. 357–78.
12. Humphrey L, Bocaege E. Tooth avulsion in the Maghreb: chronological and geographical patterns. Afr Archaeolo Rev 2008;25(1–2):109–23.
13. Bolhofner KL, Baker BJ. Dental ablation in ancient Nubia: evulsion at the ginefab school site. Am J Phys Anthropol 2012;(Suppl 54):102.
14. Friedlander AH. The physiology, medical management and oral implications of menopause. J Am Dent Assoc 2002;133(1):73–81.
15. Morris AG. Dental mutilation in southern African history and prehistory with special reference to the "Cape Flats Smile". SADJ 1998;53(4):179–83.
16. Willis MS, Swindler DR, Toothaker R. A description of Nuer and Dinka anterior tooth extractions, practices, and a preliminary odontometric analysis of the remaining permanent dentition. In: Zadzińska E, editor. Current trends in dental morphology research. Lódz (Poland): University of Lódz Press; 2005. p. 177–89.
17. Willis MS, Harris LE, Hergenrader PJ. On traditional dental extraction: case reports from Dinka and Nuer en route to restoration. Br Dent J 2008;204(3):121–4.
18. Tayles N. Tooth ablation in prehistoric Southeast Asia. Int J Osteoarch 1996;6(4): 333–45.
19. Domett KM, Newton J, O'Reilly DJ, et al. Cultural modification of the dentition in prehistoric Cambodia. Int J Osteoarch 2011. http://dx.doi.org/10.1002/oa.1245.
20. Nelsen K, Tayles N, Domett K. Missing lateral incisors in Iron Age south-east Asians as possible indicators of dental agenesis. Arch Oral Biol 2001;46(10): 963–71.
21. Takenaka M, Mine K, Tsuchimochi K, et al. Tooth removal during ritual tooth ablation in the Jomon Period. Indo-Pacific Prehist Assoc Bull 2001;21:49–52.
22. Han KX, Nakahashi T. A comparative study of ritual tooth ablation in ancient China and Japan. Anthropol Sci 1996;104(1):43–64.
23. Harunari H. Rules of residence in the Jomon Period, based on the analysis of tooth extraction. In: Pearson RJ, Barnes GL, Hutterer KL, editors. Windows on the Japanese past: studies in archaeology and prehistory. Ann Arbor (MI): Center for Japanese Studies, University of Michigan; 1986. p. 293–310.
24. Kusaka S, Nakano T, Yumoto T, et al. Strontium isotope evidence of migration and diet in relation to ritual tooth ablation: a case study from the Inariyama Jomon site, Japan. J Archaeol Sci 2011;38:166–74.
25. Temple DH, Kusaka S, Sciulli PW. Patterns of social identity in relation to tooth ablation among prehistoric Jomon foragers from the Yoshigo site, Aichi Prefecture, Japan. Int J Osteoarch 2011;21(3):323–35.
26. Willis MS, Schacht RN, Toothaker R. Anterior dental extractions among Dinka and Nuer refugies in the United States: a case series. Spec Care Dentist 2005;25(4): 193–8.
27. Beckwith C, Fisher A. The eloquent surma of Ethiopia. Natl Geogr Mag 1991; 179:77–91.

28. Longhurst R. Infant oral mutilation. Br Dent J 2010;209:591–2.
29. Edwards PC, Levering N, Wetzel E, et al. Extirpation of the primary canine tooth follicles: a form of infant oral mutilation. J Am Dent Assoc 2008;139:442–50.
30. González EL, Pérez BP, Sánchez JA, et al. Dental aesthetics as an expression of culture and ritual. Br Dent J 2010;208:77–80.
31. Friedling LJ, Morris AG. The frequency of culturally derived dental modification practices on the Cape Flats in the Western Cape. SADJ 2005;60(3):97, 99–102.
32. Ikehara-Quebral R, Douglas MT. Cultural alteration of human teeth in the Mariana Islands. Am J Phys Anthropol 1997;104:381–91.
33. Gordon SC, Kaste LM, Barasch A, et al. Prenuptial dental extractions in Acadian women: first report of a cultural tradition. J Womens Health 2011; 20(12):1813–8.
34. Hunter JM, Arbona SI. The tooth as a marker of developing world quality of life: a field study in Guatemala. Soc Sci Med 1995;41(9):1217–40.
35. Lukacs JR. Sex differences in dental caries experience: clinical evidence and complex etiology. Clin Oral Investig 2011;15(5):649–56.
36. Lukacs JR. Gender difference in oral health in South Asia: metadata imply multifactorial biological and cultural causes. Am J Human Biol 2011;23(3):398–411.
37. Caldas AF Jr. Reasons for tooth extraction in a Brazilian population. Int Dent J 2000;50(5):267–73.
38. Chestnutt IG, Binnie VI, Taylor MM. Reasons for tooth extraction in Scotland. J Dent 2000;28(4):295–7.
39. Murray H, Locker D, Kay EJ. Patterns of and reasons for tooth extractions in general dental practice in Ontario, Canada. Community Dent Oral Epidemiol 1996;24(3):196–200.
40. Takala L, Utriainen P, Alanen P. Incidence of edentulousness, reasons for full clearance, and health status of teeth before extractions in rural Finland. Community Dent Oral Epidemiol 1994;22(4):254–7.
41. Morita M, Kimura T, Kanegae M, et al. Reasons for extraction of permanent teeth in Japan. Community Dent Oral Epidemiol 1994;22(5):303–6.
42. Corbet EF, Davies WI. Reasons given for tooth extraction in Hong Kong. Community Dent Health 1991;8(2):121–30.
43. Bailit HL, Braun R, Maryniuk GA, et al. Is periodontal disease the primary cause of tooth extraction in adults? J Am Dent Assoc 1987;114(1):40–5.
44. Kelly JE, Van Kirk LE, Garst CC. Total loss of teeth in adults United States— 1960-1962: data from the National Health Survey. NCHS data brief, Number 1000-Ser. 11-no. 27. Hyattsville (MD): National Center for Health Statistics; 1967.
45. US Department of Health, Education, and Welfare, National Center for Health Statistics. Selected dental findings in adults by age, race, and sex—United States, 1960-1962. Vital Health Stat 11 1965;(7).
46. Dussault G, Sheiham A. Medical theories and professional development: the theory of focal sepsis and dentistry in early twentieth century Britain. Soc Sci Med 1982;16(15):1405–12.
47. Burt BA. Influences for change in the dental health status of populations: an historical perspective. J Public Health Dent 1978;38(4):272–88.
48. Canadian Health Measures Survey (CHMS) 2007-2009: report on the findings of the Oral Health Component. Health Canada Publication; 2009. 100183. Available at: http://www.fptdwg.ca/assets/PDF/CHMS/CHMS-E-tech.pdf. Accessed January 11, 2013.
49. Elani HW, Harper S, Allison PJ, et al. Socio-economic inequalities and oral health in Canada and the United States. J Dent Res 2012;91(9):865–70.

50. Dye BA, Tan S, Smith V, et al. Trends in oral health status: United States, 1988-1994 and 1999-2004. National Center for Health Statistics. Vital Health Stat 11 2007;(248):1–92.

51. Ismail AI, Burt BA, Brunelle JA. Prevalence of total tooth loss, dental caries, and periodontal disease in Mexican-American adults: results from the southwestern HHANES. J Dent Res 1987;66(6):1183–8.

52. Jimenez M, Dietrich T, Shih MC, et al. Racial/ethnic variations in associations between socioeconomic factors and tooth loss. Community Dent Oral Epidemiol 2009;37(3):267–75.

53. Eke PI, Dye BA, Wei L, et al. Prevalence of periodontitis in adults in the United States: 2009 and 2010. J Dent Res 2012;91:914–20.

54. Meisel P, Reifenberger J, Haase R, et al. Women are periodontally healthier than men, but why don't they have more teeth than men? Menopause 2008;15(2):270–5.

55. Shigli K, Hebbal M, Angadi-Gangadhar S. Relative contribution of caries and periodontal disease in adult tooth loss among patients reporting to the Institute of Dental Sciences, Belgaum, India. Gerodontology 2009;26(3):214–8.

56. Russell SL, Ickovics JR, Yaffee RA. Exploring potential pathways between parity and tooth loss among American women. Am J Public Health 2008;98(7):1263–70.

57. Russell SL, Mayberry L. Pregnancy and oral health: a review and recommendations to reduce gaps in practice and research. MCN Am J Matern Child Nurs 2008;33(1):32–7.

58. Russell SL, Ickovics JR, Yaffee RA. Parity and untreated dental caries in US women. J Dent Res 2010;89(10):1091–6.

59. National Center for Health Statistics. Health, United States, 2011: with special feature on socioeconomic status and health. Hyattsville (MD). Available at: http://www.cdc.gov/nchs/fastats/lifexpec.htm. Accessed December 3, 2012.

60. National Center for Health Statistics. Health, United States, 2011: with special feature on socioeconomic status and health. Hyattsville (MD): National Center for Health Statistics; 2012. Available at: http://www.cdc.gov/nchs/fastats/lifexpec.htm. Accessed December 3, 2012.

61. Statistics Canada, CANSIM, table 102–0512. Available at: http://www.statcan.gc.ca/tables-tableaux/sum-som/l01/cst01/health72a-eng.htm. Accessed December 3, 2012.

62. Centers for Disease Control and Prevention. QuickStates: percentage of adults aged 35-44 years with no permanent tooth loss from disease, by race/ethnicity and sex. National Health and Nutrition Examination Survey, United States 1988-1994 and 1999-2004. MMWR Morb Mortal Wkly Rep 2009;58(8):205.

63. Wu B, Liang J, Plassman BL, et al. Oral health among white, black, and Mexican-American elders: an examination of edentulism and dental caries. J Public Health Dent 2011;71(4):308–17.

64. Dye BA, Tan S, Smith V, et al. Trends in oral health status: United States, 1988-1994 and 1999–2004. National Center for Health Statistics. Vital Health Stat 2007;11(248).

65. Quandt SA, Chen H, Bell RA, et al. Disparities in oral health status between older adults in a multiethnic rural community: the rural nutrition and oral health study. J Am Geriatr Soc 2009;57(8):1369–75.

66. Beltrán-Aguilar ED, Barker LK, Canto MT, et al, Centers for Disease Control and Prevention (CDC). Surveillance for dental caries, dental sealants, tooth retention, edentulism, and enamel fluorosis–United States, 1988–1994 and 1999–2002. MMWR Surveillance Summaries August 26, 2005;54(03):1–44.

67. Gooch BF, Eke PI, Malvitz DM. Public health and aging: retention of natural teeth among older adults–United States, 2002. MMWR 52(50):1226–29.
68. Centers for Disease Control and Prevention. Public Health and Aging: Retention of Natural Teeth Among Older Adults—United States, 2002. MMWR December 19, 2003;52(50):1226–122.
69. Centers for Disease Control and Prevention. Total Tooth Loss Among Persons Aged Greater Than or Equal to 65 Years – Selected States, 1995–1997. MMWR March 19, 1999;48(10):206–10.
70. Marcus SE, Drury TF, Brown LJ, et al. Tooth retention and tooth loss in the permanent dentition of adults: United States, 1988–1991. J Dent Res 1996 Feb;75 Spec No:684–95.
71. Marcus SE, Kaste LM, Brown LJ. Prevalence and demographic correlates of tooth loss among the elderly in the United States. Spec Care Dentist 1994; 14(3):123–7.
72. Hunt RJ, Beck JD, Lemke JH, et al. Edentulism and oral health problems among elderly rural Iowans: the Iowa 65+ rural health study. Am J Public Health 1985; 75(10):1177–81.
73. Gürsoy M, Pajukanta R, Sorsa T, et al. Clinical changes in periodontium during pregnancy and post-partum. J Clin Periodontol 2008;35(7):576–83.
74. Barak S, Oettinger-Barak O, Oettinger M, et al. Common oral manifestations during pregnancy: a review. Obstet Gynecol Surv 2003;58(9):624–8.
75. Laine MA. Effect of pregnancy on periodontal and dental health. Acta Odontol Scand 2002;60(5):257–64.
76. Raber-Durlacher JE, van Steenbergen TJ, Van der Velden U, et al. Experimental gingivitis during pregnancy and post-partum: clinical, endocrinological, and microbiological aspects. J Clin Periodontol 1994;21(8):549–58.
77. Kornman KS, Loesche WJ. The subgingival microbial flora during pregnancy. J Periodont Res 1980;15(2):111–22.
78. Löe H, Silness J. Periodontal disease in pregnancy. I. Prevalence and severity. Acta Odontol Scand 1963;21:533–51.
79. Michalowicz BS, Hodges JS, Novak MJ, et al. Change in periodontitis during pregnancy and the risk of pre-term birth and low birthweight. J Clin Periodontol 2009;36(4):308–14.
80. Moss KL, Ruvo AT, Offenbacher S, et al. Third molars and progression of periodontal pathology during pregnancy. J Oral Maxillofac Surg 2007;65(6): 1065–9.
81. Offenbacher S, Lin D, Strauss R, et al. Effects of periodontal therapy during pregnancy on periodontal status, biologic parameters, and pregnancy outcomes: a pilot study. J Periodontol 2006;77(12):2011–24.
82. Casamassimo PS. Maternal oral health. Dent Clin North Am 2001;45(3):469–78.
83. Steinberg BJ. Women's oral health issues. J Dent Educ 1999;63(3):271–5.
84. Christensen K, Gaist D, Jeune B, et al. A tooth per child? Lancet 1998; 352(9123):204.
85. Halling A, Bengtsson C. The number of children, use of oral contraceptives and menopausal status in relation to the number of remaining teeth and the periodontal bone height. A population study of women in Gothenburg, Sweden. Community Dent Health 1989;6(1):39–45.
86. Rundgren A, Osterberg T. Dental health and parity in three 70-year-old cohorts. Community Dent Oral Epidemiol 1987;15(3):134–6.
87. Machtei EE, Mahler D, Sanduri H, et al. The effect of menstrual cycle on periodontal health. J Periodontol 2004;75(3):408–12.

88. Shourie V, Dwarakanath CD, Prashanth GV, et al. The effect of menstrual cycle on periodontal health—a clinical and microbiological study. Oral Health Prev Dent 2012;10(2):185–92.

89. Passos JS, Vianna MI, Gomes-Filho IS, et al. Osteoporosis/ osteopenia as an independent factor associated with periodontitis in postmenopausal women: a case-control study. Osteoporos Int 2012. [Epub ahead of print].

90. Bole C, Wactawski-Wende J, Hovey KM, et al. Clinical and community risk models of incident tooth loss in postmenopausal women from the Buffalo Osteo Perio Study. Community Dent Oral Epidemiol 2010;38(6):487–97.

91. Nicopoulou-Karayianni K, Tzoutzoukos P, Mitsea A, et al. Tooth loss and osteoporosis: the OSTEODENT Study. J Clin Periodontol 2009;36(3):190–7.

92. Krall EA, Dawson-Hughes B, Hannan MT, et al. Postmenopausal estrogen replacement and tooth retention. Am J Med 1997;102(6):536–42.

93. Krall EA, Garcia RI, Dawson-Hughes B. Increased risk of tooth loss is related to bone loss at the whole body, hip, and spine. Calcif Tissue Int 1996;59(6):433–7.

94. Taguchi A, Sanada M, Suei Y, et al. Effect of estrogen use on tooth retention, oral bone height, and oral bone porosity in Japanese postmenopausal women. Menopause 2004;11(5):556–62.

95. Chrysanthakopoulos NA. Reasons for extraction of permanent teeth in Greece: a five-year follow-up study. Int Dent J 2011;61(1):19–24.

96. Trovik TA, Klock KS, Haugejorden O. Trends in reasons for tooth extractions in Norway from 1968 to 1998. Acta Odontol Scand 2000;58(2):89–96.

97. Nutrition Canada. Dental report: a report from Nutrition Canada by the Bureau of Nutritional Sciences, Food Directorate, Health Protection Branch, Department of National Health and Welfare. Ottawa: Minister of National Health and Welfare. 1977.

98. Lukacs JR. Sex differences in dental caries rates with the origin of agriculture in South Asia. Curr Anthropol 1996;37:147–53.

99. Dawes C. Salivary flow patterns and the health of hard and soft oral tissues. J Am Dent Assoc 2008;139(Suppl):18S–24S.

100. Percival RS, Challacombe SJ, Marsh PD. Flow rates of resting whole and stimulated parotid saliva in relation to age and gender. J Dent Res 1994;73(8): 1416–20.

101. Eliasson L, Birkhed D, Osterverg T, et al. Minor salivary gland secretion rates and immunoglobulin A in adults and the elderly. Eur J Oral Sci 1994;114(6):494–9.

102. Meurman JH, Tarkkila L, Tiitinen A. The menopause and oral health. Maturitas 2009;63(1):56–62.

103. Lukacs JR, Largaespada LL. Explaining sex differences in dental caries prevalence: saliva, hormones, and "life-history" etiologies. Am J Hum Biol 2006;18(4): 540–55.

104. Fairweather D, Frisancho-Kiss S, Rose NR. Sex differences in autoimmune disease from a pathological perspective. Am J Pathol 2008;173(3):600–9.

105. Whitacre CC. Sex differences in autoimmune disease. Nat Immunol 2001;2(9): 777.

106. Demmer RT, Molitor JA, Jacobs DR Jr, et al. Periodontal disease, tooth loss and incident rheumatoid arthritis: results from the First National Health and Nutrition Examination Survey and its epidemiological follow-up study. J Clin Periodontol 2011;38(11):998–1006.

107. Chen HH, Huang N, Chen YM, et al. Association between a history of periodontitis and the risk of rheumatoid arthritis: a nationwide, population-based, case-control study. Ann Rheum Dis 2012. [Epub ahead of print].

108. Ferraro M, Vieira AR. Explaining gender differences in caries: a multifactorial approach to a multifactorial disease. Int J Dent 2010;2010:649643.
109. Vieira AR, Marazita ML, Goldstein-McHenry T. Genome-wide scan finds suggestive caries loci. J Dent Res 2008;87(5):435–9.
110. Deeley K, Letra A, Rose EK, et al. Possible association of amelogenin to high caries experience in a Guatemalan-Mayan population. Caries Res 2008;42(1):8–13.
111. Patir A, Seymen F, Yildirim M, et al. Enamel formation genes are associated with high caries experience in Turkish children. Caries Res 2008;42(5):394–400.
112. Conry JP, Messer LB, Boraas JC, et al. Dental caries and treatment characteristics in human twins reared apart. Arch Oral Biol 1993;38(11):937–43.
113. Holm G. Smoking as an additional risk for tooth loss. J Periodontol 1994;65(11):996–1001.
114. Ismail AI, Burt BA, Eklund SA. Epidemiologic patterns of smoking and periodontal disease in the United States. J Am Dent Assoc 1983;106(5):617–21.
115. Eklund SA, Burt BA. Risk factors for total tooth loss in the United States; longitudinal analysis of national data. J Public Health Dent 1994;54(1):5–14.
116. Reid JL, Hammond D, Burkhalter R, et al. Tobacco use in Canada: patterns and trends, 2012 edition. Waterloo (ON): Propel Centre for Population Health Impact, University of Waterloo; 2012. Available at: http://www.tobaccoreport.ca/2012/TobaccoUseinCanada_2012.pdf. Accessed January 13, 2013.
117. Centers for Disease Control and Prevention. Vital signs: current cigarette smoking among adults aged ≥18 years—United States, 2005-2010. MMWR Morb Mortal Wkly Rep 2011;60(35):1207–12.
118. World Health Organization, Tobacco Free Initiative. WHO report on the global tobacco epidemic, 2011: warning about the dangers of tobacco. 2011. Available at: http://apps.who.int/gho/data?theme=main&vid=1805. Accessed January 13, 2013.
119. Iida H, Kumar JV, Kopycka-Kedzierawski DT, et al. Effect of tobacco smoke on the oral health of U.S. Women of childbearing age. J Public Health Dent 2009;69(4):231–41.
120. Krall EA, Dawson-Hughes B, Garvey AJ, et al. Smoking, smoking cessation, and tooth loss. J Dent Res 1997;76(10):1653–9.
121. Ahlqwist M, Bengtsson C, Hollender L, et al. Smoking habits and tooth loss in Swedish women. Community Dent Oral Epidemiol 1989;17(3):144–7.
122. US Department of Agriculture, Agricultural Research Service and US Department of Health and Human Services. Dietary Guidelines for Americans 2010. 7th edition. Washington, DC: US Government Printing Office; 2010.
123. Wardle J, Haase AM, Steptoe A, et al. Gender differences in food choice: the contribution of health beliefs and dieting. Ann Behav Med 2004;27(2):107–16.
124. Rom Korin M, Chaplin WF, Shaffer JA, et al. Men's and women's health beliefs differentially predict coronary heart disease incidence in a population-based sample. Health Educ Behav 2012. [Epub ahead of print].
125. Krall E, Hayes C, Garcia R. How dentition status and masticatory function affect nutrient intake. J Am Dent Assoc 1998;129(9):1261–9.
126. Ervin RB, Dye BA. The effect of functional dentition on Healthy Eating Index scores and nutrient intakes in a national representative sample of older adults. J Public Health Dent 2009;69(4):207–16.
127. Adegboye AR, Twetman S, Christensen LB, et al. Intake of dairy calcium and tooth loss among adult Danish men and women. Nutrition 2012;28(7–8):779–84.

128. Hung HC, Colditz G, Joshipura KJ. The association between tooth loss and the self-reported intake of selected CVD-related nutrients and foods among US women. Community Dent Oral Epidemiol 2005;33(3):167–73.
129. Wamala S, Merlo J, Boström G. Inequity in access to dental care services explains current socioeconomic disparities in oral health: the Swedish National Surveys of Public Health 2004-2005. J Epidemiol Community Health 2006; 60(12):1027–33.
130. Petersen PE, Kandelman D, Arpin S, et al. Global oral health of older people—call for public health action. Community Dent Health 2010;27(4 Suppl 2):257–67.
131. Vaidya V, Partha G, Karmakar M. Gender differences in utilization of preventive care services in the United States. J Womens Health 2012;21(2):140–5. http://dx.doi.org/10.1089/jwh.2011.2876.
132. Tomar SL, Lester A. Dental and other health care visits among U.S. adults with diabetes. Diabetes Care 2000;23(10):1505–10.
133. Janes GR, Blackman DK, Bolen JC, et al. Surveillance for use of preventive health-care services by older adults, 1995-1997. MMWR CDC Surveill Summ 1999;48(SS08):51–8.
134. Kaylor MB, Polivka BJ, Chaudry R, et al. Dental services utilization by women of childbearing age by socioeconomic status. J Community Health 2010;35(2): 190–7.
135. Payne BJ, Locker D. Relationship between dental and general health behaviors in a Canadian population. J Public Health Dent 1996;56(4):198–204.
136. Payne BJ, Locker D. Oral self-care behaviours in older dentate adults. Community Dent Oral Epidemiol 1992;20(6):376–80.
137. Broadbent JM, Thomson WM, Boyens JV, et al. Dental plaque and oral health during the first 32 years of life. J Am Dent Assoc 2011;142(4):415–26.
138. Johanson CN, Osterberg T, Steen B, et al. Prevalence and incidence of dental caries and related risk factors in 70- to 76-year-olds. Acta Odontol Scand 2009; 67(5):304–12.
139. Bertea PC, Staehelin K, Dratva J, et al. Female gender is associated with dental care and dental hygiene, but not with complete dentition in the Swiss adult population. J Public Health 2007;15(5):361–7.
140. Furuta M, Ekuni D, Irie K, et al. Sex differences in gingivitis relate to interaction of oral health behaviors in young people. J Periodontol 2011;82(4):558–65.
141. Ronis DL, Lang WP, Farghaly MM, et al. Tooth brushing, flossing, and preventive dental visits by Detroit-area residents in relation to demographic and socioeconomic factors. J Public Health Dent 1993;53(3):138–45.

Oral and Pharyngeal Cancer in Women

Athanasios I. Zavras, DMD, DDS, MS, Dr MedSc[a,b,*],
Priyaa Shanmugam, BDS, MS, DSc[c], Deepthi Shetty, BDS, MPH[a],
Therese A. Dolecek, PhD[d], Linda M. Kaste, DDS, MS, PhD[d,e]

KEYWORDS

- Mouth neoplasms • Epidemiology • Health status disparities • Risk factors
- Population groups

KEY POINTS

- Incidence rates of oral and pharyngeal cancer (OPC) are lower in women than in men.
- Incidence rates of OPC among women, at least among some subgroups and sites, are increasing.
- Among non-Hispanic White women, the incidence rates of OPC have been higher than those of cervical cancer for at least the past decade.
- Susceptibility to OPC for women versus men, given the same risk behaviors, is inconclusive, although some studies suggest that women have a greater susceptibility.
- Cancer of the oral cavity and pharynx is also a woman's disease.

DESCRIPTIVE EPIDEMIOLOGY

Oral and pharyngeal cancer (OPC) is a significant global health problem, with approximately 480,000 new cases diagnosed every year globally; of these, approximately 35,000 to 40,000 new cases occur in the United States.[1,2] Women comprise 147,000 of the new cases globally and 10,000 of the new cases in the United States. Incidence estimates for 2012 are slightly increased to 11,710 newly affected women. Based on data from the Surveillance, Epidemiology, and End Results (SEER) database (2005–2009), the median age at diagnosis is 62 years.[3] About 6% of the patients are

The authors of this article have nothing to disclose.

[a] Division of Oral Epidemiology & Biostatistics, Columbia University College of Dental Medicine, 622 West 168th Street, Suite PH17-306, New York, NY 10032, USA; [b] Department of Epidemiology, Harvard School of Public Health, 677 Huntington Avenue, Boston, MA 02115, USA; [c] Department of Oral Health Policy & Epidemiology, Harvard School of Dental Medicine, 188 Longwood Avenue, Boston, MA 02115, USA; [d] Division of Epidemiology and Biostatistics, School of Public Health, Institute for Health Research and Policy, University of Illinois at Chicago, 1747 West Roosevelt Road, Chicago, IL 60608, USA; [e] Department of Pediatric Dentistry, College of Dentistry, School of Public Health, University of Illinois at Chicago, 801 South Paulina Street, Chicago, IL 60612, USA
* Corresponding author.
E-mail address: az2256@mail.cumc.columbia.edu

between 35 and 44 years, and the incidence rate increases with increasing age. Worldwide the incidence rates vary, based on the regional prevalence of risk factors such as use of tobacco, alcohol, and/or betel quid.[4] The rates among women are lower when compared with men; however, recent trends show an increase in the incidence among women.[5] In 1950, the male to female ratio was 6:1 but by the year 2002 the gap had closed to a ratio of 2:1.[5]

For the newly diagnosed patient with OPC, the effect is detrimental to both quality of life and survival (**Table 1**). More than 79,000 women die every year globally as a result of OPC, with approximately 2400 annual female deaths in the United States.[3] Based on mortality statistics from 2005 to 2009, the age-adjusted death rate was 2.5 per 100,000 men and women per year. The average 5-year survival rate of 50% has not changed significantly in the last 3 decades.[7] Surviving the disease depends, among other factors, on the clinical stage at diagnosis. Based on SEER data from 2002 to 2008, the average 5-year survival exceeds 85% if diagnosed early, drops to 57% if the cancer presents with regional stage (spread to regional lymph nodes), and further decreases to 35% when the cancer has metastasized (distant stage).

CONTRAST BETWEEN CERVICAL CANCER AND ORAL CANCER

Cervical and oropharyngeal cancers in the United States share some risk factors and etiologic factors. The potential to decrease the incidence of cervical cancer in the

Table 1
Gender-stratified incidence, mortality, and 5-year prevalence rates based on World Health Organization GLOBOCAN 2008 data and projections

Cancer	Incidence			Mortality			5-Year Prevalence		
	N	(%)	ASR (W)	N	(%)	ASR (W)	N	(%)	Proportion
Women									
World									
Lip, oral cavity	92524	1.5	2.5	44545	1.3	1.2	209581	1.4	8.5
Nasopharynx	26589	0.4	0.8	15625	0.5	0.4	68975	0.5	2.8
Other pharynx	28034	0.5	0.8	19092	0.6	0.5	59008	0.4	2.4
United States									
Lip, oral cavity	7355	1.1	2.8	1411	0.5	0.4	23372	1.1	18.4
Nasopharynx	565	0.1	0.3	186	0.1	0.1	1640	0.1	1.3
Other pharynx	2077	0.3	0.8	784	0.3	0.3	5173	0.3	4.1
Men									
World									
Lip, oral cavity	170496	2.6	5.2	83109	2.0	2.6	401075	3.0	16.3
Nasopharynx	57852	0.9	1.7	35984	0.9	1.1	153736	1.1	6.3
Other pharynx	108588	1.6	3.4	76458	1.8	2.4	229030	1.7	9.3
United States									
Lip, oral cavity	15817	2.1	7.3	2435	0.8	1.1	52326	2.4	43.2
Nasopharynx	1352	0.2	0.7	415	0.1	0.2	4094	0.2	3.4
Other pharynx	8144	1.1	3.9	2359	0.8	1.1	21536	1.0	17.8

Incidence and mortality data for all ages; 5-year prevalence for adult population only.
Rates and proportions are per 100,000, and rates are age-standardized to the World Million Standard.[6]
Abbreviation: ASR (W), age-standardized rate (world).

United States through vaccination against human papilloma virus (HPV) has been the subject of much attention and debate in the popular and scientific press.[8,9] Taking the concept further to OPC and head and neck cancers has stimulated further discussion.[10–13]

Consequently, the authors reasoned that a contrast of incidence of cervical cancer and OPC in women in the United States would help illuminate progress to date on improving the incidence rates of squamous cell carcinomas at these 2 sites. The SEER Program (1992–2009) 13 registry research data were analyzed using SEER*Stat software version 7.1.0. Data, restricted to females, included total oral cavity and pharynx (OCP) (lip, tongue, salivary gland, floor of mouth, gum and other mouth, naso-pharynx, tonsil, oropharynx, hypopharynx, and other OCP) and cervix uteri; both with histology type ICD-O-3=8050-8084. Parameters included annual age-adjusted inci-dence rates per 100,000 standardized to the 2000 United States standard population (www.seer.cancer.gov).

Fig. 1 contrasts OPC and cervical cancers for all women. Cervical cancer decreases from nearly 8 per 100,000 women in 1992 to just below 5 per 100,000 in 2009. A less dramatic decrease is seen for OPC, from just over 5 per 100,000 in 1992 to above 4 per 100,000 in 2009. The incidence rates for the 2 cancers appear to be closing in on each other. More startling is the contrast conveyed in **Fig. 2**. Among non-Hispanic white women, the incidence rate of OPC has been higher than that for cervical cancer for almost every year since 1994, and rather distinctively so starting around 2000.

Choosing to contrast these 2 sets of cancers can be argued against, as the linkages to HPV may be incongruent and there are inherent limitations of secondary data anal-ysis. However, the comparisons help illustrate that oral cancer is a woman's cancer. Continued surveillance of HPV-associated cancers is warranted. Studies monitoring the impact of HPV vaccines suggest that within the short time since the introduction of quadrivalent HPV there is "evidence of a substantial decrease in vaccine-type HPV prevalence in the community, as well as evidence of herd protection."[14] The potential impact on OPC cancers should be included in future monitoring of the impact of HPV vaccine. In addition, traditional risk-factor monitoring and interventions should be retained.

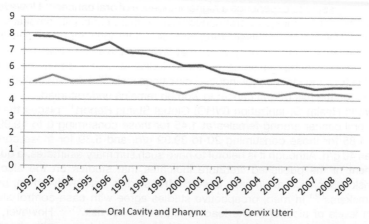

Oral Cavity and Pharynx   Cervix Uteri

Fig. 1. Cancer of the oral cavity and pharynx compared with cancer of the cervix uteri in women of all races/ethnicity, annual age-adjusted incidence per 100,000. Surveillance, Epidemiology, and End Results (SEER) data, 1992 to 2009.

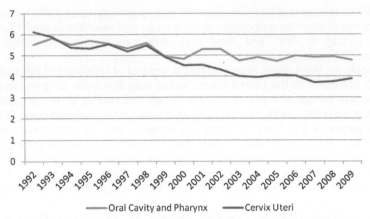

Fig. 2. Cancer of the oral cavity and pharynx compared with cancer of the cervix uteri in white non-Hispanic women, annual age-adjusted incidence per 100,000: SEER data 1992 to 2009.

ANALYTICAL EPIDEMIOLOGY: RISK FACTORS

The 2 predominant risk factors for OPC in the United States population are alcohol and tobacco consumption. More than 75% of the variation in the incidence can be explained by excessive tobacco and alcohol use; individuals exposed to the combination of high levels of both substances experience the greatest risk.[15] Other risk categories include diet, genetic predisposition, having a potentially malignant lesion such as erythroplakia, and the effect of carcinogenic HPV types, especially HPV-16 and HPV-18.

ALCOHOL AND ORAL CANCER

Excessive alcohol consumption has been consistently associated with risk of cancer, particularly cancers of the liver, digestive tract, and oral cavity.[16] In the United States, men who consume more than 2 drinks per day and women who consume more than 1 drink per day seem to experience a higher incidence of oral cancer.[17] However, most studies of the epidemiology of oral cancer involve men, especially smokers. Among nonsmokers, OPCs are relatively rare, and few published studies have included enough cases to provide meaningful information about the effect of alcohol, especially among women.[18] Although some evidence indicates that women may be more susceptible than men to alcohol-induced carcinogenesis,[19,20] the magnitude of alcohol's effect on the risk of oral cancer in women remains understudied.

The World Health Organization (WHO) Global Status Report[16] places the relative risks for oral cancer among females at 1.45 for those consuming 0 to 19.99 g/d of alcohol, 1.85 for those consuming 20 to 39.99 g/d, and 5.39 for those consuming more than 40 g/d. Although it is helpful to have such summary estimates, a qualitative assessment of the published literature indicates that studies on the alcohol-oral cancer risk association are mostly case-control studies that involve men, predominantly smokers.[3,20] In men, prospective studies agree with case-control studies in that high levels of alcohol intake lead to higher cancer risk.[21,22] However, among women the role and extent of alcohol as a risk factor for oral cancer has been inconsistent[23–26]; studies have been mostly case-control in design and have very few female participants.

Few studies have been conducted that indicate a change in the male to female ratio in higher risk for oral cancer in women. Among 67 nonsmoking and nondrinking patients (22 males and 45 females) with newly diagnosed, previously untreated oral squamous cell carcinoma (OSCC), 15 developed recurrence, 10 metastasis, and 3 both conditions during a median follow-up of 16.7 months.[27] In this study it is notable that the number of women is twice that of men. Among previously undiagnosed nonsmoking, nondrinking patients with oral cancer, 28 were mostly female (75% vs 30%, P<.001), young (median 31.5 years vs 35.5 years, P = .007) and white (89% vs 60%, P = .006).[28] A descriptive study of 172 nonsmoking, nondrinking patients reported that 45% were women, with more than half the patients being positive to HPV-16.[29]

In a recent prospective study of women in France the majority of the nonsmokers (93%) were nondrinkers, and among those who consumed alcohol the level of intake was very high (>100 g/d).[30] A large multicenter pooled case-control study of 15 studies from North America, Europe, and South America showed that overall, for men and women, the odds ratio (OR) for 3 or more drinks per day versus no drinking was 2.04 (95% confidence interval [CI] = 1.29–3.21) with a weak effect of alcohol among never smokers.[31] A case-control study in Italy found that the risk increased among nonsmoking females only for those consuming 35 or more drinks per week.[24] In the authors' study using the Nurses Health Study (NHS) I data, a prospective analysis of about 88,800 women with 26 years of follow-up found that high alcohol intake ($\geq$30 g/d or approximately 2 drinks/d) was significantly associated with an increased risk of oral cancer after adjusting for age, tobacco use, folate intake, and follow-up time.[32] This analysis also showed a significant interaction between alcohol consumption and folate intake; alcohol appears to increase risk significantly only for those with low folate intake (<350 μg/d).

Low or moderate alcohol intake does not appear to increase the risk of oral cancer, even being associated with decreased risk. The literature on the role of low or moderate consumption on the risk of developing oral cancer or on a possible threshold effect is inconsistent. Some case-control studies have observed a U-shaped relationship between the risk of oral cancer and alcohol consumption. More specifically, a U-shaped relationship has been reported in 6 of 16 case-control studies; according to these studies, drinking small amounts of alcohol seems to be protective but drinking high amounts seems to be detrimental.[20] In other studies, the existence of a U-shaped curve could not be assessed because of the low cutoff point of using fewer than 4 drinks per day. However, the U-shaped curve has been observed mostly in men, possibly because of the low samples of women in the highest consumption strata.[33] It is currently unclear as to why alcohol at lower levels may be protective against oral cancer. It is plausible that low levels of alcohol in postmenopausal women are correlated with increased insulin sensitivity and elevated estrogen levels.[34] Recently, an analysis of 74,372 women participants of the National Institutes of Health–American Association of Retired Persons cohort showed a protective effect of menopausal hormone therapy (MHT). Women who had especially received estrogen-progestin MHT had a 0.47-fold risk of developing squamous cell carcinoma of the upper aerodigestive tract (protective association).[35] However, this is a preliminary report that requires further study.

Multiple mechanisms are involved in alcohol-induced carcinogenesis, and several studies have been conducted in both humans and animals.[36] Locally in the oral cavity the ethanol in alcohol produces epithelial atrophy, which increases the penetration of carcinogens through the oral mucosa.[37] This process may occur because of either the elimination of the lipid component of the barrier present in the epithelial layer or reorganization of the cell membrane by ethanol, which increases permeability. Ethanol by itself has not been proved to be carcinogenic[38]; however, acetaldehyde, the primary metabolic product of ethanol, has been established as carcinogenic in animal experiments and possibly carcinogenic in humans as well.[39] Acetaldehyde causes DNA mutations, and interferes with DNA synthesis and repair.[40] Acetaldehyde can also be produced by oral bacteria, adding to the total circulating salivary acetaldehyde.[40] Regarding the genetics of alcohol metabolism, the production of acetaldehyde from ethanol is facilitated by alcohol dehydrogenase (ADH). Acetaldehyde is further converted to acetate by aldehyde dehydrogenase (ALDH). It is interesting that genetic polymorphisms of both ADH and ALDH are associated with an increased risk of head and neck cancers.[41]

As regards gender differences, it is currently unclear if there are differences in the effect of alcohol intake on oral cancer. Most studies have involved men, with women being grossly underrepresented among study participants. It is possible that there may be differences in susceptibility to alcohol-induced carcinogenesis, with women being more susceptible, although the evidence is inconclusive.[19,20] It is also possible that a gender effect may exist in alcohol gastric metabolism, which in turn may affect the bioavailability of acetaldehyde in the oral epithelial tissue. In men, the blood level of alcohol is higher when given intravenously than when drinking it.[42] However, women have been found to have similar blood levels of alcohol irrespective of whether the alcohol was given orally or intravenously. This finding could be due to the lower gastric metabolism of ethanol in comparison with men.[12,13] Studies on cancer of the liver have shown that liver damage is higher in females than in males at lower intake of alcohol and shorter duration of intake. Hormonal differences in men and women can also play a role in the joint effect of folate and alcohol and how they influence differences in the risk of oral cancer.[34]

As the epidemiology of oral cancer in women remains understudied, more studies are urgently needed to explore and validate biological pathways involving alcohol consumption and the risk of oral cancer among women.

TOBACCO AND ORAL CANCER

Smoking and tobacco use pose a serious risk of death and disease for women. Annually, cigarette smoking kills an estimated 173,940 women in the United States.[43] Worldwide, it is estimated that men smoke nearly 5 times as much as women, but the ratios of female to male smoking prevalence rates vary dramatically across countries. In high-income countries such as Australia, Canada, the United States, and most countries of western Europe, women smoke at nearly the same rate as men. However, in many low-income and middle-income countries women smoke much less than men. For example, in China 61% of men are reported to be current smokers, compared with only 4.2% of women. Similarly, in Argentina 34% of men are reported to be current smokers compared with 23% of women.[44] The most common form of tobacco use is smoking of manufactured cigarettes, although in some areas of the world (eg, Asia), other forms of tobacco ingestion are used such as the smoking of traditional hand-rolled flavored cigarettes referred to as beedis, use of water pipes to smoke tobacco, use of snuff, smokeless tobacco, and reverse cigarette smoking.

Prevalence of Smoking Among Women in the United States

Results from survey by the Centers for Disease Control and Prevention (CDC) in 2010 showed that more than 1 in 6 American women aged 18 years or older (17.3%) smoked cigarettes. The highest rates were seen among American Indian/Alaska

Native women (36%) followed by multiracial women (23.8%), white (19.6%), African American (17.1%), Hispanic (9%), and Asian women (4.3%). In general, the less education a woman has, the more likely it is she will smoke. For instance, women with less than a high school education are more than twice as likely as college graduates to smoke.[45]

In 2008, approximately 15% of young women aged 20 to 24 years smoked during pregnancy. Even among younger teenagers 15 to 19 years old, 13.1% smoked during pregnancy. The lowest rates were seen in mothers younger than 15 years (3.2%), between 40 and 54 years (4.6%), 35 to 39 years (4.9%), and 30 to 34 years of age (5.6%).[46]

Risks Associated with Tobacco Use Among Women

Intensity, duration, and age at smoking

Data suggest that women may be more sensitive than men to some of the harmful effects of smoking, with evidence that risk increases with the number of cigarettes smoked.

Dose response is measured in terms of intensity of smoking (cigarettes/d), duration of smoking, or pack-years. A positive significant trend was found among women who smoked cigarettes and used tobacco. Macfarlane and colleagues[25] showed that women who had 1 to 18 cigarette pack-years had a relative risk of 2.6, whereas men who had 1 to 33 cigarette pack-years had a relative risk of 1.1. Women who smoked more than 18 pack-years had a risk of 4.6, whereas men who smoked more than 33 pack-years had a risk of only 1.3. With an increase in the number of cigarettes smoked daily or an increase in daily tobacco consumption there was an increase in risk, and the trend was statistically significant. According to Hayes and colleagues,[47] the risk of developing oral cancer was higher in women than in men. Women who smoked 1 to 9 cigarettes/d had a risk of 2.2 compared with a risk of 0.9 in men. Women who smoked more than 40 cigarettes/d had a risk of 28.1, compared with a risk of only 4.9 in their male counterparts. The P trend for daily cigarette intake was .0001 for women. Hammond and Seidman[48] concluded that women who were regular smokers had a risk of 3.3 of developing cancer of the upper aerodigestive tract. As the use of tobacco in terms of g/d increased, it was associated with higher risk of oral cancer. For women who use about 1 to 7 g of tobacco per day the risk was 5.6, and when tobacco use increased to more than 8 g/d the risk was 5.9.[33] According to Blot and colleagues,[23] younger women had a higher risk of developing cancers of the aerodigestive tract. Women in the age group 17 to 24 had a risk of 3.1 and those younger than 17 had a risk of 2.9, whereas women who were 25 years and older had a risk of 2.8.

The OR increased with an increase in pack-years for women. ORs for smoking and drinking were greater in women with respect to oropharyngeal and hypopharyngeal cancers, but were similar for both men and women for oral-cavity and laryngeal cancers. For 30 to 39 pack-years, for cancer of the oral cavity the OR is 3.18, for oropharyngeal cancer the OR is 1.34, for hypopharyngeal cancer the OR is 6.62, and for laryngeal cancer the OR is 2.22.[49]

Cessation of smoking

Relative risks for former smokers were always lower than those for current smokers. Hayes and colleagues[47] showed that women who were current smokers had a risk of 4.9 compared with 3.9 for men. When risks among women were examined by years since quitting, a negative trend was seen. Women who had quit smoking for less than 2 years had a risk of 14.1 compared with women who had a risk of 8.7 who had quit smoking for about 2 to 9 years, a risk of 2.1 for those who had quit smoking for about

10 to 19 years, and a risk of only 0.8 for those who had quit smoking for more than 20 years.[50]

Type of tobacco

In the study by Hayes and colleagues,[47] women who use only other forms of tobacco had a higher risk for oral cancer in comparison with women who used cigarettes and other forms of tobacco. Consumption of black tobacco and filter-tipped cigarettes led to a higher risk of oral cancer than did consumption of blond tobacco and cigarettes without a filter. Women who used black tobacco had a risk of 6.9, compared with a risk of 6 among women who used blond tobacco. Among women who used filter-tipped cigarettes, the risk was 6.3 compared with a risk of 5.2 among women who used cigarettes without a filter.[33] For more details on the effects of tobacco on cancer risk, and especially for aerodigestive cancers, the reader is encouraged to consult the International Agency of Research on Cancer (IARC) Monograph 83, which contains many of the studies referenced in this article.

DIET AND ORAL CANCER

Dietary factors may play a role in the risk of developing oral cancer. Apart from alcohol intake, the relation between fruit and vegetable intake and a lower risk of oral cancer has been explored across the globe.[51]

A critical review of several studies by Boeing and colleagues[52] reported an inverse relation between consumption of fruits and vegetables and the risk of cancer. Most of the studies in this review reported risk that was not statistically significant or was dependent on smoking status, thus implying that the risk reduction could be associated with lifestyle or with lack of statistical control of smoking. Based on the strength of evidence, the investigators concluded that the presence of an inverse relation between consumption of fruits and vegetables and that of cancer is "probable." The preventive role of foods and nutrients in the development of oral and pharyngeal cancer was evaluated in a review that included 30 case-control studies and a few cohort studies.[53] These studies reported consistent inverse associations with fruit and vegetable consumption, β-Carotene, vitamin C, and selected flavonoids. Risk of oral cancer was also inversely associated with whole-grain cereals (not refined grains). Another review of 40 case-control studies and 6 cohort studies in Italy reported an inverse relationship between risk of oral and pharyngeal cancer and fruit and vegetable consumption. The pooled relative risk for high vegetable consumption is 0.52 for and high fruit consumption 0.55, based on 18 case-control studies.[53]

In industrialized countries, dietary factors account for approximately 30% of cancers overall and 10% to 15% of oral cancers.[54,55] In developing countries, around 60% of cancers of the oral cavity, pharynx, and esophagus are attributed to low intake of fruits and vegetables.[55] The level of carcinogenicity varies by region and depends on environmental and social factors.[54] The protective effects of fruits and vegetables on the risk for oral cancer have been explored in several studies, but the results have been inconsistent. In the previous studies, when controlling for smoking and drinking, the protective effects of fruits and vegetables were not as strong. This finding may be partly due to lower consumption of fruits and vegetables among heavy smokers and drinkers. Most of the studies have been among men and case-control in design.

Fruits and vegetables have been hypothesized to protect against head and neck cancer because they are rich in potentially anticarcinogenic compounds, including antioxidants, carotenoids, fiber, folate, flavonoids, plant sterols, phenolic acids, and vitamin C.[56] These anticarcinogenic compounds in the diet can reduce the risk of cancer by avoiding the formation of carcinogens, reducing their metabolic activation and increasing their detoxification. Some studies have reported that the anticarcinogenic effect of a diet rich in fruits, in particular, can possibly detoxify the carcinogenic effect of tobacco smoking. Evidence on the exact mechanism of action in the oral cavity is not clear, and more studies that evaluate the biological mechanism in the oral cavity are required.

Prospective studies have evaluated the protective effects of fruits and vegetables on the risk of developing oral cancer. In a large prospective study conducted in the United States, a total of 787 participants (608 men, 179 women) were diagnosed with head and neck cancer during 4 years of follow-up.[57] The investigators reported strong inverse associations with increased intake of fruits and vegetables per serving per 1000 calories per day. Results from the multivariate analyses showed the strongest protective effect for total vegetables (hazard ratio 0.89; 95% CI 0.82–0.97) in contrast to other studies that have reported stronger effects for fruits. In the European Investigation into Cancer and Nutrition study (EPIC) from 7 European countries with varying follow-up periods, 97 cases of cancer of the oral cavity, pharynx, and esophagus were identified among females.[58] The investigators found a stronger association for intake of fruits (Q5 vs Q1: 0.60; 95% CI 0.38–0.97) but not for vegetables. This result contrasts with that of the United States prospective study.[57] Two other prospective studies have been conducted, but these were among men. A study among Japanese men in Hawaii followed for 24 years reported 92 cases of cancers of the upper aerodigestive tract. The investigators reported an inverse association with longer duration of fruit intake.[59] The protective effects of fruits and vegetables on the risk of oral precancerous lesion (OPL) among United States male health professionals showed a 30% to 40% reduction in risk.[60] In this study, citrus fruits and citrus fruit juice were found to be protective for OPL risk, but no significant associations were reported for specific vegetable groups.

Meta-analyses that summarize the findings from case-control and cohort studies have found overall fruit and vegetable intake to be significantly protective.[61–63] However, in the 2 studies that included only women, the results showed a significant protective effect for higher intake of vegetables (OR 0.65; 95% CI 0.47–0.9) but not for fruits. In the studies among men (n = 2 for fruit intake, n = 3 for vegetable intake), the results were significant for vegetable intake but not for fruit intake. In a review of case-control studies, protective effects were observed in some, but about half of the studies did not show any protective effect.[64] In some of the studies the effect was observed only among men. A multinational case-control study recruited cases from hospitals and referral centers from 9 countries.[65] The study reported that higher consumption of fruits and vegetables lowered the risk for oral cancer among ever drinkers (OR 0.4; 95% CI 0.3–0.6) and ever smokers (OR 0.4; 95% CI 0.3–0.6), but not among never drinkers and never smokers. Individuals who drink and smoke may have a tendency to eat lesser amounts of fruits and vegetables. Therefore, the results observed in this study might be due to residual confounding in smoking and drinking categories.

Studies in recent years have reported an association between folate deficiency and the risk of cancer.[66,67] For example, dietary folate intake has been found to be associated with a lower risk of colorectal cancer.[68,69] In oral cancer, only a few case-control studies have considered the possible influence of folate, and their results have been inconsistent.[70–73] Similarly inconsistent are the analyses that consider the combined use of low folate and high alcohol,[73] despite the fact that a strong interaction seems to exist in colon cancer.[68,74]

Low levels of serum folate have been previously observed in patients with head and neck cancer,[75,76] but few case-control studies have been conducted to shed light on the role of folate in the possible prevention of oral cancer; most of the published studies have reported no association.[71,73,77] A recent hospital-based case-control study that included 115 female cases reported an inverse association with folate intake (OR 0.53; 95% CI 0.40–0.69) for the highest tertile of intake (≥301).[72] In this study, the combined effect of high alcohol intake (≥38 drinks/wk) and low folate intake (<236 μg/d) showed a 22-fold increase in risk. The joint association of alcohol and folate with the risk of major chronic disease has been studied in the Nurses Health Study, and a significant interaction between alcohol and folate intake has been reported in breast and colon cancers.[78] In this study, other than breast and colon cancer, risks from all other cancers including oral cancer were evaluated together as "other cancer." In prospective analyses among female NHS participants, high folate intake appears to decrease the risk of oral cancer among alcohol drinkers.[32]

The mechanism whereby low folate accentuates the association between alcohol and the risk of oral cancer is currently unclear. Folate is essential for DNA synthesis and repair, and for the methylation of biological substances, including phospholipids, DNA, and neurotransmitters.[79] DNA methylation is important in the maintenance of DNA stability and in gene expression. Alcohol interferes with several aspects of normal folate transport and metabolism including dietary folate intake, intestinal absorption, transport to tissues, folate storage in the liver, and urinary excretion.[80–82] Human and animal experiments suggest that the acute toxicity of alcohol on folate is primarily related to its influence on folate metabolism in the liver.[57] Because metabolism of acetaldehyde from ethanol occurs locally in the oral cavity,[40] cleavage of folate can occur in the microenvironment of the oral cavity,[83] deterring the positive effects of folate. Thus, by impairing folate status and metabolism, ethanol may enhance cancer risk both systemically and locally and disrupt the DNA synthesis, repair, and methylation of the squamous epithelial oral cell.[40]

Most of the studies conducted previously have been case-control studies that are more prone to recall and selection bias. Moreover, the number of female participants included in these studies was fewer. The method of dietary assessment also varies across studies. Overall, although the prospective studies reported significant protective effects with higher intake of fruits and vegetables, the results are not consistent. Recalling and quantifying dietary information is difficult.[84] In a review of studies validating methods for measuring diet, it was reported that participants' current dietary intake can influence the recall of past diet. The highest correlation between past and current diet was only among foods consumed very often. Future prospective studies that include large samples of women should be conducted to fully elucidate the role of diet in the prevention of oral cancer.

HPV AND ORAL CANCER

Excessive smoking and alcohol consumption continue to be important risk factors for oral cancer; however, in the past few years evidence from epidemiologic studies suggests that more than 25% of head and neck cancers are caused by HPV.[85]

HPV is a nonenveloped, double-stranded DNA virus that infects basal epithelium through microabrasions and tissue disruption.[86] There are more than 100 different strains and of these approximately 40 are known to infect the genital area, 50% of which are classified as high-risk types. Of the high-risk types HPV-16 and HPV-18 are found to be associated with cervical cancers globally.[86] The CDC report that about 20 million persons in the United States are currently infected with HPV.[87] HPV is spread through sexual contact, and local and systemic immune responses to HPV may be delayed until months after HPV DNA is detected at the cervix. As a result, HPV infection remains undetected.[86] Over the past years several studies have established that HPV is the most common risk factor for cervical cancer.[88] In recent years, HPV has been evaluated as a potential risk factor for head and neck OSCCs. In a worldwide systemic review of head and neck squamous cell carcinomas, investigators reported a higher prevalence of HPV-16 in OSCC.[89] HPV prevalence was found to be higher in North America than in Europe and Asia. A meta-analysis (1982–1997) on HPV as a risk factor for OSCC reported that HPV showed high prevalence in oral dysplastic and carcinomatous epithelium when compared with normal mucosa. The investigators also reported that detection of high-risk HPV was 2.8 times greater than detection of low-risk HPV.[90] Results from a review of case series of cancers of the upper aerodigestive tract showed HPV DNA in 46% of the cancers located in the oral cavity and pharynx. However, the methods used differed from study to study.[91]

A recent prospective study in Taiwan evaluated 173 patients with advanced oral cancer over a 5-year period.[92] The investigators reported higher prevalence of HPV-16 and HPV-18–related oral cancers. The presence of HPV-16 infection was significantly associated with higher distant metastases ($P = .005$) and poor survival ($P = .01$).

In a hospital nested case-control study from Johns Hopkins University on HPV infection and oropharyngeal cancer, the investigators found that the risk for OSCC increased significantly (OR 14.6; 95% CI 6.3–36.6) among those with positive oral HPV infection.[93] The study also reported that HPV was associated with oral cancer (OR 16.0; 95% CI 5.4–47.7), even among those without a history of drinking and tobacco use, which are 2 important risk factors for the disease. The results from this study emphasized that HPV-16 is a significant independent risk factor for oral cancer. In a case-control study conducted in Sao Paulo, the investigators reported that there was a higher prevalence of oncogenic subtypes of HPV among cases (74%), with higher odds (OR 25.5; 95% CI 3–222).[94] Serum antibodies against HPV-16, -18, and -31 viral capsids were detected using an immunoassay technique with polymerase chain reaction methods.[95] HPV DNA was detected in 19% of cases and 5% of controls, and the odds for HPV detection in oral cells was 2.14 (95% CI 0.4–13.0). Another case-control study in Taiwan found the prevalence of high-risk HPV types to be higher among cases of OSCC than in control lesions (11/51 vs 8/90; OR 2.8; 95% CI 1.1–7.6).[96] Prevalence of HPV was compared between 49 case and control specimens in Slovenia obtained from the same set of individuals.[97] Following amplified DNA analysis, no significant differences were found (9.1% vs 6.7%; $P = .694$).

In a population-based case-control study, infection with high-risk HPV was shown to be a strong risk factor for OSCC (OR 63; 95% CI 14–480).[98] Forty-seven (36%) of the patients with cancer had 1 or more specimens that were positive for a high-risk HPV type (81% of which were HPV-16). In a cross-sectional study, among 51 cases 42% were HPV-positive, with a higher prevalence among men than women.[99] Human immunodeficiency virus (HIV)-seronegative (n = 396) and HIV-seropositive (n = 190) subjects were compared in another cross-sectional study, which found a higher prevalence of HPV among HIV-seropositive individuals.[100] A prospective proportional hazards analysis among 253 participants reported HPV among 62% of the cases, of which 90% were high-risk types.[101] Other studies include case series with small sample sizes (10–15 cases).[102,103]

SUMMARY

OPC is a woman's disease requiring greater attention to prevention and health care. In fact, among non-Hispanic white women the incidence rate of OPC has been higher than that of cervical cancer for almost every year since 1994, and rather distinctively so starting around 2000. Research shows that women's perceptions, knowledge, and attitudes about these 2 types of cancer differ significantly. Women widely recognize the risk of cervical cancer and the need for regular screenings, but the same is not true for oral and pharyngeal cancer. Proactive screening for oral and pharyngeal cancer remains low in health care priorities, often with dire consequences. A comprehensive strategy is needed that identifies high-risk groups and targets them for preventive efforts and early discovery of OPC.

REFERENCES

1. Oral Cavity and Oropharyngeal Cancer. American Cancer Society. Available at: http://www.cancer.org/cancer/oralcavityandoropharyngealcancer/detailedguide/index. Accessed March 23, 2013
2. Oral cancer. 2012. Available at: http://www.oralcancerfoundation.org/facts/. Accessed March 20, 2013.
3. Cancer of the oral cavity and pharynx. SEER stat fact sheets. National Cancer Institute. Available at: http://seer.cancer.gov/statfacts/html/oralcav.html. Accessed March 23, 2013
4. Parkin M, Bray F, Ferlay J, et al. Global cancer statistics, 2002. CA Cancer J Clin 2005;55:74–108.
5. Cancer, Oral. Oral health Topics. American Dental Association. Available at: http://www.ada.org/2607.aspx?currentTab=2. Accessed March 23, 2013.
6. Segi M. Cancer mortality for selected sites in 24 countries (1950–57). Sendai (Japan): Department of Public Health, Tohoku University of Medicine; 1960.
7. SEER. Cancer statistics. Available at: http://seer.cancer.gov/statfacts/html/oralcav.html. Accessed March 20, 2013.
8. Abdelmutti N, Hoffman-Goetz L. Risk messages about HPV, cervical cancer, and the HPV vaccine Garasil in North American News Magazines. J Cancer Educ 2010;25:451–6.
9. Pierce Campbell CM, Menezes LJ, Paskett ED, et al. Prevention of invasive cervical cancer in the United States: past, present, and future. Cancer Epidemiol Biomarkers Prev 2012;21:1402–8.
10. Moscicki AB. Editorial HPV-associated cancers: it's not all about the cervix. Prev Med 2011;53:S3–4.
11. D'Souza G, Dempsey A. The role of HPV in head and neck cancer and review of the HPV vaccine. Prev Med 2011;53:S5–11.
12. Chaturvedi AK. Epidemiology and clinical aspects of HPV in head and neck cancers. Head Neck Pathol 2012;6:S16–24.
13. Lingen MW, Xiao W, Schmidt A, et al. Low etiologic fraction for high-risk human papillomavirus in oral cavity squamous cell carcinomas. Oral Oncol 2013;49(1): 1–8.
14. Kahn JA, Brown DR, Ding L, et al. Vaccine-type human papillomavirus and evidence of herd protection after vaccine introduction. Pediatrics 2012;130:e249.
15. Rothman K, Keller A. The effect of joint exposure to alcohol and tobacco on risk of cancer of the mouth and pharynx. J Chron Dis 1972;25:711–6.
16. WHO. Global status report on alcohol. Geneva (Switzerland): Department of Mental Health and Substance Abuse; 2004.
17. Alcohol and cancer. Amercan Cancer Society. Available at: http://www.cancer.org/acs/groups/content/@healthpromotions/documents/document/acsq-017622.pdf. Accessed March 23, 2013

18. Fioretti F, Bosetti C, Tavani A, et al. Risk factors for oral and pharyngeal cancer in never smokers. Oral Oncol 1999;35(4):375–8.

19. Blume SB. Women and alcohol. A review. JAMA 1986;256(11):1467–70.

20. Franceschi S, Bidoli E, Negri E, et al. Alcohol and cancers of the upper aerodigestive tract in men and women. Cancer Epidemiol Biomarkers Prev 1994;3(4): 299–304.

21. Cancela Mde C, Ramadas K, Fayette JM, et al. Alcohol intake and oral cavity cancer risk among men in a prospective study in Kerala, India. Community Dent Oral Epidemiol 2009;37:342–9.

22. Kato I, Nomura A, Stemmermann G, et al. Prospective study of the association of alcohol with cancer of the upper aerodigestive tract and other sites. Cancer Causes Control 1992;3(2):145–51.

23. Blot W, McLaughlin J, Winn D, et al. Smoking and drinking in relation to oral and pharyngeal cancer. Cancer Res 1988;48(11):3282–7.

24. Talamini R, La Vecchia C, Levi F, et al. Cancer of the oral cavity and pharynx in nonsmokers who drink alcohol and in nondrinkers who smoke tobacco. J Natl Cancer Inst 1998;90(24):1901–3.

25. Macfarlane GJ, Zheng T, Marshall JR, et al. Alcohol, tobacco, diet and the risk of oral cancer: a pooled analysis of three case-control studies. Eur J Cancer B Oral Oncol 1995;31(3):181–7.

26. Zavras A, Douglass C, Joshipura K, et al. Smoking and alcohol in the etiology of oral cancer: gender-specific risk profiles in the south of Greece. Oral Oncol 2001;37(1):28–35.

27. Kruse A, Bredell M, Gratz K. Oral squamous cell carcinoma in non-smoking and non-drinking patients. Head Neck Oncol 2010;2(24):1–3.

28. Harris S, Kimple R, Hayes D, et al. Never-smokers, never-drinkers: unique clinical subgroups of young patients with head and neck squamous cell cancers. Head Neck 2010;32(4):499–503.

29. Dahlstrom K, Little J, Zafereo M, et al. Squamous cell carcinoma of the head and neck in never smoker-never drinkers: a descriptive epidemiologic study. Head Neck 2008;30(1):75–84.

30. Girod A, Mosseri V, Jouffroy T, et al. Women and squamous cll carcinomas of the oral cavity and oropharynx: is there something new? J Oral Maxillofac Surg 2009;67:1914–20.

31. Hashibe M, Brennan P, Benhamou S, et al. Alcohol drinking in never users of tobacco, cigarette smoking in never drinkers, and the risk of head and neck cancer: pooled analysis in the International Head and Neck Cancer Epidemiology Consortium. J Natl Cancer Inst 2007;99(10):777–89.

32. Shanmugham J, Zavras A, Rosner B, et al. Alcohol-folate interactions in the risk of oral cancer in women: a prospective cohort study. Cancer Epidemiol Biomarkers Prev 2010;19(10):2516–24.

33. Merletti F, Boffetta P, Ciccone G, et al. Role of tobacco and alcoholic beverages in the etiology of cancer of the oral cavity/oropharynx in Torino, Italy. Cancer Res 1989;49(17):4919–24.

34. Suba Z. Gender-related hormonal risk factors for oral cancer. Pathol Oncol Res 2007;13(3):195–202.

35. Freedman N, Lacey JJ, Hollenbeck A, et al. The association of menstrual and reproductive factors with upper gastrointestinal tract cancers in the NIH-AARP cohort. Cancer 2010;116(6):1572–81.

36. Poschl G, Stickel F, Wang XD, et al. Alcohol and cancer: genetic and nutritional aspects. Proc Nutr Soc 2004;63(1):65–71.

37. Figuero Ruiz E, Carretero Pelaez MA, Cerero Lapiedra R, et al. Effects of the consumption of alcohol in the oral cavity: relationship with oral cancer. Med Oral 2004;9(1):14–23.

38. Wight AJ, Ogden GR. Possible mechanisms by which alcohol may influence the development of oral cancer–a review. Oral Oncol 1998;34(6):441–7.

39. Alcohol drinking. Biological data relevant to the evaluation of carcinogenic risk to humans. IARC Monogr Eval Carcinog Risks Hum 1988;44:101–52.

40. Seitz HK, Stickel F. Molecular mechanisms of alcohol-mediated carcinogenesis. Nat Rev Cancer 2007;7(8):599–612.

41. Brennan P, Lewis S, Hashibe M, et al. Pooled analysis of alcohol dehydrogenase genotypes and head and neck cancer: a HuGE review. Am J Epidemiol 2004; 159(1):1–16.

42. Badger T, Ronis M, Seitz HK, et al. Alcohol metabolism: role in toxicity and carcinogenesis. Alcohol Clin Exp Res 2003;27(2):336–47.

43. American Lung Association. Women and tobacco use. 2012. Available at: http://www.lung.org/stop-smoking/about-smoking/facts-figures/women-and-tobacco-use.html. Accessed March 20, 2013.

44. World Health Organization. Gender empowerment and female-to-male smoking prevalence ratios. 2011. Available at: http://www.who.int/bulletin/volumes/89/3/10-079905/en/index.html. Accessed March 20, 2013.

45. American Cancer Society. Women and smoking. 2011. Available at: http://www.cancer.org/acs/groups/cid/documents/webcontent/002986-pdf.pdf. Accessed March 20, 2013.

46. American Lung Association. Trends in tobacco use. 2011. Available at: http://www.lung.org/finding-cures/our-research/trend-reports/Tobacco-Trend-Report.pdf. Accessed March 20, 2013.

47. Hayes RB, Bravo-Otero E, Kleinman DV, et al. Tobacco and alcohol use and oral cancer in Puerto Rico. Cancer Causes Control 1999;10:27–33.

48. Hammond EC, Seidman H. Smoking and cancer in the United States. Prev Med 1980;9:169–73.

49. Lubin J, Muscat J, Gaudet M, et al. An examination of male and female odds ratios by BMI, cigarette smoking, and alcohol consumption for cancers of the oral cavity, pharynx, and larynx in pooled data from 15 case-control studies. Cancer Causes Control 2011;22:1217–31.

50. Choi SY, Kahyo H. Effect of cigarette smoking and alcohol consumption in the aetiology of cancer of the oral cavity, pharynx and larynx. Int J Epidemiol 1991;20:878–85.

51. Scully C, Bagan J. Oral squamous cell carcinoma: an overview of current understanding of aetiopathogenesis and clinical implications. Oral Dis 2009;15:388–99.

52. Boeing H, Bechthold A, Bub A, et al. Critical review: vegetables and fruits in the prevention of chronic diseases. Eur J Nutr 2012;51:637–63.

53. Garavello W, Lucenteforte E, Bosetti C, et al. The role of foods and nutrients on oral and pharyngeal cancer risk. Minerva Stomatol 2009;58(1–2):25–34.

54. Petti S. Lifestyle risk factors for oral cancer. Oral Oncol 2009;45(4–5):340–50.

55. Diet, Nutrition and the Prevention of Chronic Diseases. Report of a Joint WHO/FAO Expert Consultation Technical Report Series, No 916. Geneva (Switzerland): World Health Organization; 2003.

56. Taghavi N, Yazdi I. Type of food and risk of oral cancer. Arch Iran Med 2007; 10(2):227–32.

57. Freedman N, Park Y, Subar A, et al. Fruit and vegetable intake and head and neck cancer risk in a large United States prospective cohort study. Int J Cancer 2007;122(10):2330–6.
58. Boeing H, Dietrich T, Hoffmann K, et al. Intake of fruits and vegetables and risk of cancer of the upper aero-digestive tract: the prospective EPIC-study. Cancer Causes Control 2006;17:957–69.
59. Chyou P, Nomura A, Stemmermann G. Diet, alcohol, smoking and cancer of the upper aerodigestive tract: a prospective study among Hawaii Japanese men. Int J Cancer 1995;60(5):616–21.
60. Maserejian NN, Giovannucci E, Rosner B, et al. Prospective study of fruits and vegetables and risk of oral premalignant lesions in men. Am J Epidemiol 2006; 164(6):556–66.
61. Riboli E, Norat T. Epidemiologic evidence of the protective effect of fruit and vegetables on cancer risk. Am J Clin Nutr 2003;78(Suppl):559S–69S.
62. Pavia M, Pileggi C, Nobile C, et al. Association between fruit and vegetable consumption and oral cancer: a meta-analysis of observational studies. Am J Clin Nutr 2006;83:1126–34.
63. Sanchez MJ, Martinez C, Nieto A, et al. Oral and oropharyngeal cancer in Spain: influence of dietary patterns. Eur J Cancer Prev 2003;12(1):49–56.
64. Winn D, Ziegler R, Pickle L, et al. Diet in the etiology of oral and pharyngeal cancer among women from the Southern United States. Cancer Res 1984;44: 1216–22.
65. Kreimer AR, Randi G, Herrero R, et al. Diet and body mass, and oral and oropharyngeal squamous cell carcinomas: analysis from the IARC multinational case-control study. Int J Cancer 2006;118(9):2293–7.
66. Duthie SJ. Folic acid deficiency and cancer: mechanisms of DNA instability. Br Med Bull 1999;55:578–92.
67. Kim YI. Folate and carcinogenesis: evidence, mechanisms, and implications. J Nutr Biochem 1999;10:66–88.
68. Giovannucci E. Alcohol, one-carbon metabolism, and colorectal cancer: recent insights from molecular studies. J Nutr 2004;134:2475S–81S.
69. Terry P, Jain M, Miller AB. Dietary intake of folic acid and colorectal cancer risk in a cohort of women. Int J Cancer 2002;97:864–7.
70. Almadori G, Bussu F, Galli J. Serum folate and homocysteine levels in head and neck squamous cell carcinoma. Cancer 2002;94:1006–11.
71. De Stefani E, Ronco A, Mendilaharsu M, et al. Diet and risk of cancer of the upper aerodigestive tract. II. Nutrients. Oral Oncol 1999;35:22–6.
72. Pelucchi C, Talamini R, Negri E, et al. Folate intake and risk of oral and pharyngeal cancer. Ann Oncol 2003;14(11):1677–81.
73. Weinstein S, Gridley G, Harty L. Folate intake, serum homocysteine and methylenetetrahydrofolate reductase (MTHFR) C677T genotype are not associated with oral cancer risk in Puerto Rico. J Nutr 2002;132:762–7.
74. La Vecchia C, Negri E, Pelucchi C, et al. Dietary folate and colorectal cancer. Int J Cancer 2002;102:545–7.
75. Almadori G, Bussu F, Galli J, et al. Serum levels of folate, homocysteine, and vitamin B12 in head and neck squamous cell carcinoma and in laryngeal leukoplakia. Cancer 2005;103(2):284–92.
76. Eleftheriadou A, Chalastras T, Ferekidou E, et al. Association between squamous cell carcinoma of the head and neck and serum folate and homocysteine. Anticancer Res 2006;26(3B):2345–8.

77. McLaughlin J, Gridley G, Block G, et al. Dietary factors in oral and pharyngeal cancer. J Natl Cancer Inst 1988;80(15):1237–43.
78. Jiang R, Hu FB, Giovannucci EL, et al. Joint association of alcohol and folate intake with risk of major chronic disease in women. Am J Epidemiol 2003;158: 760–71.
79. Hamid A, Wani NA, Kaur J. New perspectives on folate transport in relation to alcoholism-induced folate malabsorption—association with epigenome stability and cancer development. FEBS J 2009;276(8):2175–91.
80. Hillman RS, Steinberg SE. The effects of alcohol on folate metabolism. Annu Rev Med 1982;33:345–54.
81. Mason JB, Choi SW. Effects of alcohol on folate metabolism: implications for carcinogenesis. Alcohol 2005;35:235–41.
82. McMartin KE, Collins TD, Shiao CQ, et al. Study of dose-dependence and urinary folate excretion produced by ethanol in humans and rats. Alcohol Clin Exp Res 1986;10:419–24.
83. Shaw S, Jayatilleke E, Herbert V, et al. Cleavage of folates during ethanol metabolism. Role of acetaldehyde/xanthine oxidase-generated superoxide. J Biochem 1989;257(1):277–80.
84. Friedenrich C, Stimani N, Riboli E. Measurement of past diet: review of previous and proposed methods. Epidemiol Rev 1992;14:177–96.
85. Joseph A, D'Souza G. Epidemiology of human papillomavirus-related head neck cancer. Otolaryngol Clin North Am 2012;45(4):739–64.
86. Wiley D, Masongsong E. Human papilloma virus: the burden of infection. Obstet Gynecol Surv 2006;61(6):S3–14.
87. Human papilloma virus and cancer. Department of Health and Human Services. Available at: http://www.cdc.gov/hpv/cancer.html. Accessed March 23, 2013
88. Munoz N, Castellsague X, Gonzalez A, et al. HPV in the etiology of human cancer. Vaccine 2006;24:S3–10.
89. Kreimer AR, Clifford GM, Boyle P, et al. Human papillomavirus types in head and neck squamous cell carcinomas worldwide: a systematic review. Cancer Epidemiol Biomarkers Prev 2005;14(2):467–75.
90. Miller CS, Johnstone BM. Human papillomavirus as a risk factor for oral squamous cell carcinoma: a meta-analysis, 1982-1997. Oral Surg Oral Med Oral Pathol Oral Radiol Endod 2001;91(6):622–35.
91. Franceschi S, Munoz N, Bosch XF, et al. Human papillomavirus and cancers of the upper aerodigestive tract: a review of epidemiological and experimental evidence. Cancer Epidemiol Biomarkers Prev 1996;5(7):567–75.
92. Lee L, Huang C, Liao C, et al. Human papilloma virus-16 infection in advanced oral cavity cancer patients is related to an increased risk of distant metastases and poor survival. PLoS One 2012;7(7):e40767.
93. D'Souza G, Kreimer AR, Viscidi R, et al. Case-control study of human papillomavirus and oropharyngeal cancer. N Engl J Med 2007;356(19):1944–56.
94. Silva C, Silva I, Cerri A, et al. Prevalence of human papillomavirus in squamous cell carcinoma of the tongue. Oral Surg Oral Med Oral Pathol Oral Radiol Endod 2007;104(4):497–500.
95. Pintos J, Black MJ, Sadeghi N, et al. Human papillomavirus infection and oral cancer: a case-control study in Montreal, Canada. Oral Oncol 2007;44(3): 242–50.
96. Luo CW, Roan CH, Liu CJ. Human papillomaviruses in oral squamous cell carcinoma and pre-cancerous lesions detected by PCR-based gene-chip array. Int J Oral Maxillofac Surg 2007;36(2):153–8.

97. Kansky AA, Seme K, Maver PJ, et al. Human papillomaviruses (HPV) in tissue specimens of oral squamous cell papillomas and normal oral mucosa. Anticancer Res 2006;26(4B):3197–201.

98. Hansson BG, Rosenquist K, Antonsson A, et al. Strong association between infection with human papillomavirus and oral and oropharyngeal squamous cell carcinoma: a population-based case-control study in southern Sweden. Acta Otolaryngol 2005;125(12):1337–44.

99. Ibieta BR, Lizano M, Fras-Mendivil M, et al. Human papilloma virus in oral squamous cell carcinoma in a Mexican population. Oral Surg Oral Med Oral Pathol Oral Radiol Endod 2005;99(3):311–5.

100. Kreimer AR, Alberg AJ, Daniel R, et al. Oral human papillomavirus infection in adults is associated with sexual behavior and HIV serostatus. J Infect Dis 2004;189(4):686–98.

101. Gillison ML, Koch WM, Capone RB, et al. Evidence for a causal association between human papillomavirus and a subset of head and neck cancers. J Natl Cancer Inst 2000;92(9):709–20.

102. Bagan JV, Jimenez Y, Murillo J, et al. Lack of association between proliferative verrucous leukoplakia and human papillomavirus infection. J Oral Maxillofac Surg 2007;65(1):46–9.

103. Koyama K, Uobe K, Tanaka A. Highly sensitive detection of HPV-DNA in paraffin sections of human oral carcinomas. J Oral Pathol Med 2007;36(1):18–24.

Interactions Between Patients and Dental Care Providers
Does Gender Matter?

Marita R. Inglehart, Dr. phil. habil.

KEYWORDS

- Patient-provider interactions • Dentists • Communication • Dental care
- Gender identity

KEY POINTS

- Research concerning the role of gender in patient-physician interactions shows that gender differences exist both in verbal and nonverbal communication and that the issue of patient-provider concordance received a lot of attention. Earlier research on the effects of being in concordant versus discordant relationships focused mainly on demographic similarity, whereas newer research argues that perceived similarities are more predictive of treatment outcomes.
- Lessons learned from the findings in the medical field are that more research is needed and that this research needs to consider that gender identity does not exist in a vacuum but is affected by a person's additional identities.
- Concerning the role of gender in communication in the dental office, research showed that perceptions of dentists and patients are influenced by gender: traditional gender stereotypes are applied to perceptions of dentists and also shape perceptions of patients.
- Pediatric dental patients prefer gender-concordant interactions with dentists and physicians. Adult dental patients in gender-concordant relationships differ in what they value about their dentist as well as in their self-perceptions from patients in gender-discordant relationships.
- The content of patient-dentist communication is affected by the fact that the prevalence of certain issues such as eating disorders, abuse, and the use of tobacco products differs for male and female patients. The process of communication is shaped by gender identities, gender stereotypes, and attitudes. Future research needs to consider the degree to which ongoing value change will shape gender roles and in turn interactions between dental patients and their providers.

INTRODUCTION

Constructive communication between a patient and a dental care provider is crucial. Such communication affects whether a patient returns for a future visit,[1–5] how the

Department of Periodontics and Oral Medicine, University of Michigan–School of Dentistry, 1011 North University, Ann Arbor, MI 48109-1078, USA
E-mail address: mri@umich.edu

Dent Clin N Am 57 (2013) 357–370
http://dx.doi.org/10.1016/j.cden.2013.02.003
0011-8532/13/$ – see front matter © 2013 Elsevier Inc. All rights reserved.

patient responds during the dental visit,[6] whether a patient makes the best possible treatment decisions,[7] and even how well the patient cooperates with treatment recommendations after the visit.[8] Numerous studies provided support for the importance of good patient-provider communication for patients' satisfaction with their provider,[9–12] for reducing patients dental fear and anxiety,[13,14] for increasing their confidence in their dentist,[15,16] and for achieving more positive treatment outcomes.[17]

One factor that crucially affects communication in general[18,19] and patient-dental care provider communication specifically[20] is the cultural background of the communication partners. Research on cross-cultural communication therefore focuses on gaining a better understanding of the dynamics of communication between persons from different cultural backgrounds. These investigations are of interest when considering interactions between patients and dental care providers and specifically when analyzing the role of gender in this context. A person's gender identity as well as gender stereotypes and attitudes clearly affect interactions and communication.[21] This situation is complicated by the fact that patients' and providers' gender is not the only significant cultural factor that will shape their communication. Other characteristics such as their socioeconomic, educational, and ethnic/racial background; sexual orientation; ability status; and religious denomination clearly affect the way patients and dentists and dental hygienists interact with each other. Although addressing the effects of this complex constellation of factors on patient-provider interactions would go beyond the scope of this article, it is important to keep this issue in mind when considering the role of gender in this context.

The first objective of this article is to consider the role of patients' and medical care providers' gender in their interactions in general (Part 1). Questions addressed in this section focus on whether gender concordance matters in medical settings and whether there are gender differences in verbal and nonverbal communication. Part 2 then analyzes how gender matters in interactions in the dental office. This analysis begins with the simple question how male and female patients differ in their use of dental care services and the reasons they have for seeking dental care. The next section focuses on gaining a better understanding of how patients perceive male versus female dentists and how dentists perceive male and female patients with different types of dental issues such as missing frontal incisors or malocclusion. Having a better understanding of the mutual perceptions will set the stage to explore if male and female pediatric and adult dental patients have gender preferences for their dentist and if so, if these gender concordance considerations affect patients' responses to gender-consistent versus gender-inconsistent interactions. The final section of this article focuses on gender differences in patient-dental care provider interactions in general and specifically when communicating (1) about abuse and intimate partner violence and (2) with a patient who does not have a heterosexual orientation. The discussion and conclusion part addresses how the growing numbers of female dentists might affect dentists' professional activities and community involvement and how dental and dental hygiene education as well as oral health-related research needs to become involved in exploring these issues.

PART 1: PATIENT-PROVIDER INTERACTIONS AND GENDER: GENERAL CONSIDERATIONS

Disparities in health and health care are no longer seen solely as a function of structural factors.[22,23] Instead, attention has increasingly begun to move to analyzing how patient characteristics such as race and gender and the patient-doctor relationship are related to health care disparities.[24,25] An earlier paradigm shift to focusing on patient-centered care brought additional attention to the role of such factors as gender and race. One aspect of the patient-centered interaction style is whether the patient and the provider are in "concordance," meaning that they share the same characteristic.[26] For example, gender concordance refers to a situation in which both the patient and the provider have the same gender.[27] One interesting question is whether gender concordance has positive effects on patients' responses to their interactions with their medical care providers.

Does Gender Concordance Matter?

Early studies exploring whether concordance matters in patient-physician relationships focused on one hand on the type of concordance, mainly on whether the relationship was for example race or gender concordant, and on the other hand on the consequences of concordant relationships. Some studies on the effects of race-concordant interactions showed positive effects such as increased patient satisfaction, trust, use of health care services, and joint decision making,[26,28–30] whereas others found no significant effects[31,32] or concluded that the evidence was inconclusive.[33] More recent studies therefore moved away from defining concordance in terms of demographic characteristics to considering more subjective factors such as perceived similarity[27] or informational versus interactional concordance.[34]

Research on the meaning of perceived similarity showed that this concept consisted of 2 separate aspects, namely, (1) perceived similarity related to personal matters such as similar beliefs and values and (2) perceived similarity concerning social characteristics.[27] The data showed that the degree of personal similarity (together with physicians' patient-centered communication) was associated with higher ratings of trust, satisfaction, and intention to adhere.[27]

Coran and colleagues[34] approached unraveling the relevance of concordance in a slightly different way. The investigators differentiated perceptions of similarity as being related either to information or to the interaction per se. The investigators defined informational concordance as the extent to which physicians and patients agreed about patient information such as self-rated health and pain, whereas interactional concordance referred to the degree to which patients and physicians agreed on interaction characteristics such as the patients' level of trust. It was shown that both discordances were associated with patients' dissatisfaction with their physician.

The move from defining concordance as a similarity between patients' and providers' demographic characteristics to an assessment of perceptions of similarities[27] or to a determination of similarities in perceptions of informational and interactional aspects raises an interesting question. This question is whether male and female patients and providers differ in their verbal and nonverbal communication. If such differences can be identified, they might shape perceptions of similarities, which in turn might affect patient satisfaction, trust, and cooperation with treatment recommendations.

Gender Differences in Communication Between Patients and Providers

Gender differences in verbal communication

As the percentage of female physicians increased,[35] an interest seemed to arise in exploring whether male and female physicians differ in their interactions with their patients. Research in medical settings found several significant differences in the communication of male and female physicians as well as that of female and male patients.

Concerning physicians, research showed that female physicians had longer patient visits with more verbal exchanges.[36,37] Female physicians also emphasized different aspects of care, paid more attention to psychosocial issues,[38–41] and valued empathy more than their male colleagues.[42]

Concerning gender differences in patients' communication style, research showed that female patients received more information with less medical jargon,[43] asked more questions, presented more symptoms, and gave more information in their medical history.[44]

Gender differences in nonverbal communication

In addition to verbal communication, nonverbal communication plays an important role. Research showed that women differed in several aspects of nonverbal communication from men such as in smiling, facial expressiveness, and touching.[45] Women also showed more back-channel responses such as nodding and responding with "I see" and so forth compared with men.

However, when Sandhu and colleagues[46] conducted a systematic review of the impact of gender dyads on doctor-patient communication in 2009, they concluded that the evidence base was too small and that further research is needed.

Lessons Learned from Medical Research

What lessons can dental clinicians and researchers learn from the findings reported from medical research?

First, it is quite obvious that male and female physicians and patients differ in their verbal and nonverbal communication from their counterparts. However, as Sandhu and colleagues[46] pointed out, more research is needed.

Second, analyzing the communication of male and female providers independent of the gender of their patients might not result in a sufficient understanding of the complexity of these issues. Studying the dynamics of gender-concordant and gender-discordant dyads and considering not only demographic concordance but also perceived similarities might result in a more comprehensive understanding.

Third, analyzing the role of gender in patient-provider interactions without considering physicians' and patients' intersecting identities might further limit our understanding of the complexity of these issues.

PART 2: COMMUNICATION IN THE DENTAL OFFICE: HOW DOES GENDER MATTER?
Male and Female Dental Patients: General Considerations

Before analyzing the gender effects in patient-provider interactions in dental offices, it is to be noted that national statistics show that women in the United States have been slightly more likely than men to report a dental visit during the past year.[47] Research also showed that women were more likely to engage in oral-health-related behavior such as tooth brushing.[48–52] In addition, differences in esthetic concerns related to oral health might exist already in young children[53] and oral health issues such as malocclusion might be perceived by others differently depending on the patient's gender.[54]

Differences in the prevalence of specific issues related to oral health might shape the content of communication in dental offices. For example, eating disorders are much more prevalent among women,[55] whereas the use of tobacco products is more common among men.[56] However, both issues need to be addressed in oral health education.

Overall, it might be important to understand how male and female dentists are perceived by their patients and how patients with different oral health issues are perceived by others, because these stereotypes might shape expectations for interactions. Next, it will be interesting to explore whether pediatric and adult dental patients have preferences for male versus female dentists and whether these preferences are a function of their own gender. Once patients interact during a dental visit, it will be interesting to analyze if gender affects these interactions. Finally, 2 issues related to gender, domestic violence and the role of patients' sexual orientation in patient-provider interactions, are also discussed.

How Does Gender Matter in Perceptions of Dentists and Patients?

Perceptions of male and female dentists

In 2008, Smith and Dundes[57] assessed whether traditional gender stereotypes are applied to dentists. Traditionally, women tended to be characterized as more caring, submissive, and expressive than men, whereas men tended to be perceived as more competitive, assertive, and competent than women.[58,59] The investigators therefore asked college and noncollege students whether certain traits were more characteristic of male dentists, female dentists, or neither gender.[57] It was found that female dentists were perceived as more likely to make patients relaxed and to take more time to discuss issues than their male colleagues. On the other hand, male dentists were perceived as more likely to expect patients to endure pain without complaints, being more devoted to their career than their family, and as more likely to be attracted to the power of their profession than their female colleagues. In consideration of these findings, the investigators suggested to encourage dental students to consider how these preconceived stereotypes might affect their own patients' perceptions and thus influence their rapport and communication with their patients.

Perceptions of male and female dental patients

One question is whether patients with different oral health issues are perceived differently as a function of their gender. Olsen and Inglehart[54] explored this question in 2 contexts. In their first study, they assessed how adults perceived persons with normal occlusion or with different malocclusions (open bite, deep bite, under bite, overjet, crowding, and spacing). Specifically they explored how occlusion affected others' perceptions of male and female target persons' attractiveness, intelligence, personality, and the desire to interact in personal and professional settings with these persons. Overall, they found that persons with normal occlusion were rated as most attractive, intelligent, agreeable, and extraverted, whereas persons with an under bite were rated as least attractive, intelligent, and extraverted. Female targets were rated more positively than male targets.

In a second study, the investigators studied observers' perceptions of male and female persons with normal occlusion versus those with a missing frontal incisor or with malocclusion and their willingness to potentially interact with these persons.[60] Overall, **Table 1** shows that persons with normal occlusion were evaluated as more attractive and intelligent, having a more positive personality and being more desirable to interact with than persons with a missing incisor or malocclusions. A female with a missing incisor was rated as least attractive, least intelligent, least conscientious and agreeable, and least extraverted. The only category in which males with a missing incisor received more negative responses than females with missing incisors was concerning behavioral intentions to interact with the depicted person in personal (eg, as a neighbor or friend) or professional settings (eg, as a colleague).

Based on the results of these studies, it can be concluded that missing a frontal incisor or having a malocclusion negatively affects how others perceive a person and how much they want to interact with the person. In addition, it was quite obvious that women with missing frontal incisors would be most critically evaluated. Although these 2 studies included dental patients as respondents and did not ask dental care

Table 1
Ratings of male and female target persons with normal occlusion, occlusion with missing incisor, and malocclusions

Characteristic[a]	Photo Gender	Normal Occlusion	Missing Incisor	Malocclusion	P (gender) P (o by g)[b]
Attractiveness	Male	5.19	4.11	4.61	.298
	Female	5.68	3.59	5.07	.005
Intelligence	Male	5.35	4.59	4.89	.199
	Female	5.51	4.43	5.29	.039
Personality factors					
Conscientiousness	Male	4.82	4.56	4.81	<.001
	Female	5.58	4.57	5.30	.011
Agreeableness	Male	4.17	3.13	3.89	.339
	Female	4.58	2.71	4.19	.004
Neuroticism	Male	2.63	3.04	2.82	.065
	Female	2.36	3.04	2.54	.463
Lack of openness	Male	3.55	3.92	3.67	.172
	Female	3.29	4.07	3.37	.136
Extraversion	Male	5.27	4.94	4.78	.026
	Female	5.15	4.24	4.85	.007
Behavioral intention					
Index: desire to interact	Male	4.45	3.47	4.11	<.001
	Female	5.05	3.82	4.84	.305

[a] The scores ranged from "1" = "lowest expression" to "7" = "highest expression" of the characteristic.
[b] "P (gender)" refers to the significance of the main effect of "gender"; "P (o by g)" refers to the significance of the interaction effect between the 2 variables "occlusion status (with the 3 conditions "normal occlusion," "malcocclusion" and "missing incisor") and "gender."
   Data from Olsen JA, Inglehart MR. Occlusion and person perception: an experimental exploration. Comm Dent Oral Epid, in press.

providers for their perceptions and evaluations of the photographs, one might wonder whether dentists and dental hygienists respond in similar ways to patients, or even more harshly. It would be interesting to explore this question in future research.

Gender Concordance in the Dental Office

Given the findings that dental care providers' as well as patients' gender matter, one interesting question is whether pediatric and adult dental patients have clear preferences for male versus female providers and whether such preferences are affected by the patients' gender.

Does gender concordance matter to pediatric dental patients?
Pediatric dental patients' negative experiences during dental treatment can have long-term consequences such as dental fear and avoidance of future treatment.[61–63] Understanding the factors that affect the communication between a child patient and dental care provider is therefore important. The first impressions of providers based on their gender might affect a child and could contribute to creating good or bad rapport with the pediatric patient. Research showed that children as young as 3 years were well aware of their own gender identity.[64–66] In addition, even young children's gender identity affected their preferences for other children, toys, or activities already in young children[67] and these younger children already have very specific

gender stereotypes.[68,69] By the time they go to preschool, they have a clear notion of which behavior is typical for a woman and which is typical for a man.[70] Research also showed that children are not able to ignore gender information.[71]

Given these findings, Redwine[72] explored children's positive and negative choices of male versus female adults as their doctors, dentists, and teachers and especially whether the depicted persons' and their own gender mattered. She collected data from 184 pediatric dental patients between 4 and 8 years of age (mean = 6.05 years) before a regularly scheduled dental appointment. The children were presented with photographs of male and female adults and were asked to choose the person they wanted as their dentist, their doctor, and their teacher. The results showed that female children preferred female dentists, doctors, and teachers, whereas male children preferred male dentists and doctors, but female teachers. Based on these findings it can be concluded that children between 4 and 8 years of age prefer health care providers of their own gender.

Does gender concordance matter to adult dental patients?

Although gender concordance was preferred by patients in some medical settings,[73,74] data in dental settings are not as clear.[75,76]

One recent study by Berger and Inglehart[77] analyzed dental-visit-related attitudes and self-perceptions of 297 dental patients and 291 dental students in gender-consistent versus gender-inconsistent relationships. Compared with patients in gender-discordant relationships, patients in gender-consistent relationships were younger and valued more that their dentist had the same gender and ethnic/racial background, had a family, and was relatively young and attractive; they also perceived themselves as more intelligent, more attractive, and more physically fit than patients in gender-discordant relationships. These findings raise the question whether age-related changes need to be considered in future research studies of gender issues in patient-provider interactions.

Gender and Patient-Dental Care Provider Interactions: Special Issues

While research concerning the role of gender in patient-dental care provider interactions is scarce,[57] an increased understanding of how gender stereotypes affect perceptions of patients and providers and their behavior is much needed. Given the growing number of female dentists in the United States,[78] as well as in other industrialized countries such as Germany,[79] it is crucial to prepare future providers for their professional lives in gender-integrated settings. The fact that female dentists will head up dental offices will affect not only patient-provider interactions[80] and its outcomes[12] but also the interactions between dentists and staff members.[81]

In addition, 2 gender-related communication issues deserve special attention because they are likely to cause communication challenges and breakdowns and are widely neglected in dental offices.

The role of patients' sexual orientation in patient-provider interactions

The first issue is that dentists and dental hygienists have persons with nonheterosexual orientations among their patients.[82] Recent research documented that substantial numbers of adults in the United States self-identified as gay, lesbian, or bisexual and that the number of same sex couples living together is increasing.[83,84] According to the US Census in the year 2000, 601,209 lesbian and gay couples and thus over 1.2 million US adults reported to live together in an unmarried partner relationship in the United States, which represents about 0.4% of the overall US population.[83] These lesbian and gay couples lived in 99.3% of US counties, and only 22 of the 3219 counties in the United States did not report any gay or lesbian couple.[84] It is crucial to gain a better understanding of how culturally sensitive care can be provided to lesbian, gay, bisexual, and transgender (LGBT) patients. In 2001, the Gay and Lesbian Medical Association published a companion document to Healthy People 2010 describing concerns that health care providers should be aware of when treating sexual minorities.[85] Access to care is a problem for sexual minorities, as it is for other minority groups in the United States. However, sexual minorities often face an additional barrier because they cannot get health insurance through their partners. In addition, this document described health disparity issues for patients from LGBT backgrounds in the areas of nutrition, weight, consumption of alcohol, use of tobacco products, and domestic violence. For example, Ridner and colleagues[86] found that the smoking rates of self-identified lesbian or bisexual women in college was 4.9 times higher than the rates of heterosexual women and that these self-identified students were 10.7 times more likely to drink alcohol compared with students who did not self-identify as being lesbian or bisexual. Given that the use of tobacco products and the consumption of alcohol are related to patients' oral health, it is important for dental care providers to be aware of the high prevalence of these health-related issues in their patients from LGBT backgrounds.

One problem that providers might face when they interact with patients from LGBT backgrounds is that many of these patients do not disclose their sexual orientation to their health care providers.[87] Homophobia is still a problem that causes many LGBT patients to not disclose their sexual orientation to their health care providers out of fear of discrimination or substandard care.[88] However, not disclosing can have an adverse psychological impact on a patient-provider interaction, and "coming out" to a health care provider can make the patient feel more like a "whole" person.[89] Cultural competency is an important tool to create a supportive relationship between health care providers and patients.[10] For example, McKelvey and colleagues[90] reported that medical and nursing students who had less knowledge about sexual minorities (and sex in general) had the worst attitudes toward sexual minorities and topics relating to sexual minorities.

Communication about abuse

One second specific issue that is directly related to patient-dental care provider communication and gender is the issue of encountering patients who were abused.[91] Every year, an estimated 5.3 million adult women in the United States are victims of intimate partner violence/abuse (IPV/A).[92] Dentists and dental hygienists may be the first providers who encounter these patients[92] because they focus on the head, neck, and facial region during routine examinations and oral cancer screenings. Head, neck, and facial injuries are by far the most common IPV/A-related injuries.[93–96] The American Dental Association has recognized that dentists have an opportunity to identify and discuss IPV/A and has therefore called dentists to start recognizing and responding to evidence of IPV/A.[97] In addition, a survey with battered women found that victims of IPV/A would like their dentists to address suspected abuse,[87] and other investigators reported that these patients wanted to receive brochures, informational pamphlets, and referrals to women's groups and other agencies.[88]

Despite these facts, dentists rarely screen patients for abuse and fail to intervene when abuse is suspected.[98,99] Love and colleagues[100] reported, for example, that 87% of dentists stated that they never screened new patients for IPV/A, 85% did not screen for abuse at checkups, and only 39% indicated that they often or always screen for IPV/A when injuries have occurred to the face or neck. Of the 30% practitioners who suspected abuse, only 3% reported the case to the authorities.[98] In addition, Tilden and colleagues[101] found that only 26% of dental hygienists discussed abuse with patients when they saw potential signs of domestic violence. A survey of battered women who sought dental care reported that 87% of women who presented at the dental office with physical injuries due to abuse were not asked about the injuries or about IPV/A issues.[87] Gaining a clear understanding of how to detect abuse in patients and how to address it with the patients is therefore crucial.

PART 3: SUMMARY

Successful patient-provider communication is crucial for assuring that a patient receives the best possible care. Understanding the ways in which the gender of the provider and the patient affect this communication is important. Unfortunately, the first conclusion at the end of this article has to be to point out that there is a lack of research concerning these issues in the dental literature. Future research is much needed. This research has to consider that a person's gender does not exist in a vacuum but is tightly interwoven with the person's personal, social, and cultural characteristics. Understanding the complexity of cross-cultural communication issues is therefore important.

A second conclusion is that dentists and dental hygienists need to be better educated about gender-related issues in communication both during their predoc-toral/undergraduate education and during continuing education courses.

The final conclusion focuses on the fact that increasing numbers of dentists will be women in the future. A recent national survey concerning leadership issues and the role of gender showed encouraging findings.[102] The data from 135 female and 458 male dentists showed that women were more positive toward taking a leadership role in organized dentistry and in supporting community-based efforts through volunteering and organizing community events compared with men. Women also placed higher value on taking on a leadership role in their community, on a state and national level, and rated the importance of taking a leadership role in their own practice as higher than men. Women also felt better prepared by their predoctoral dental education for leadership roles than male practitioners. Given the change in the percentage of female practitioners in dentistry, the question arises how this change will affect the culture of this profession and the image that the profession has. Engaging women leaders in shaping the future of the profession needs to include raising awareness for the need to prepare all dental care providers to become successful communicators in an increasingly more diverse world.

REFERENCES

1. Dixon GS, Thompson WM, Kruger E. The West Coast Study. I: self-reported dental health and the use of dental services. N Z Dent J 1999;95(420): 38–43.
2. Sergi HG, Klages U, Zentner A. Pain and discomfort during orthodontic treatment: causative factors and effects on compliance. Am J Orthod Dentofacial Orthop 1998;114:684–91.
3. Polat O, Karaman AI. Pain control during fixed orthodontic appliance therapy. Angle Orthod 2005;75(2):210–5.
4. Polat O, Karaman AI, Durmus E. Effects of preoperative ibuprofen and naproxen sodium on orthodontic pain. Angle Orthod 2005;75(5):791–6.
5. Wang SJ, Briskie D, Hu J, et al. Illustrated information for parent education - parent and patient responses. Pediatr Dent 2010;32(4):295–303.

6. Kloostra PK, Eber RM, Wang H, et al. Surgical vs. non-surgical periodontal treatment – psychosocial factors and treatment outcomes. J Periodontol 2006;77(7): 1253–60.
7. Patel AM, Richards RS, Wang H, et al. Surgical or non-surgical periodontal treatment? Factors affecting patient decision making. J Periodontol 2006;77(4): 678–83.
8. Inglehart MR, Widmalm SE, Syriac PJ. Occlusal splints and quality of life – does the quality of the patient-provider relationship matter? Oral Health Prev Dent, in press.
9. Kim JS, Boynton JR, Inglehart MR. Parents' presence in the operatory during their child's dental visit: a person-environmental fit analysis of parents' responses. Pediatr Dent 2012;34(5):337–43.
10. Okullo I, Astrom AN, Haugejorden O. Influence of perceived provider performance on satisfaction with oral health care among adolescents. Community Dent Oral Epidemiol 2004;32(6):447–55.
11. Shouten BC, Eijkman MA, Hoogstraten J. Dentists' and patients' communicative behavior and their satisfaction with the dental encounter. Community Dent Health 2003;20(1):11–5.
12. Sondell K, Soderfeldt B, Palmqvist S. Dentist-patient communication and patient satisfaction in prosthetic dentistry. Int J Prosthodont 2002;15(1):28–37.
13. Hottel TL, Hardigan OC. Improvement in the interpersonal communication skills of dental students. J Dent Educ 2005;69(2):281–4.
14. Corah N, O'Shea R, Bissell G. The dentist-patient relationship: perceptions by patients of dentist behavior in relation to satisfaction and anxiety. J Am Dent Assoc 1985;111:443–6.
15. Corah N, O'Shea R, Bissell G, et al. The dentist-patient relationship: perceived dentist behaviors that reduce patient anxiety and increase satisfaction. J Am Dent Assoc 1988;116:73–6.
16. Van der Molen HT, Klaver AA, Duyx MP. Effectiveness of a communication skills training programme for the management of dental anxiety. Br Dent J 2004;196: 101–7.
17. Carey JA, Madill A, Manogue M. Communication skills in dental education: a systematic research review. Eur J Dent Educ 2010;14(2):69–78.
18. Warren TL. Cross-cultural communication: perspectives in theory and practice. Amityville (NY): Baywood Publishing Company; 2006.
19. Norales FO. Cross-cultural communication: concepts, cases and challenges. Amherst (NY): Cambria Press; 2006.
20. Inglehart MR, Tedesco L. Increasing orthodontic patient cooperation in the 21st century: the role of cross-cultural communication issues. In: McNamara JA, Trotman CA, editors. Creating the compliant patient. Craniofacial Growth Series, Center for Human Growth and Development. Ann Arbor (MI): University of Michigan; 1997. p. 181–93.
21. Ashmore RD, Del Boca FK, editors. The social psychology of female-male relations. A critical analysis of central concepts. Orlando (FL): Academic Press; 1986.
22. Ackerson LK, Viswanath K. The social context of interpersonal communication and health. J Health Commun 2009;14:5–17.
23. Shim JK. Cultural health capital: a theoretical approach to understanding health care interactions and the dynamics of unequal treatment. J Health Soc Behav 2010;51:1–15.
24. Schulman KA, Berlin JA, Harless W, et al. The effect of race and sex on physicians' recommendations of cardiac catheterization. N Engl J Med 1999;340: 618–26.

25. Thornton RL, Powe NR, Roter D, et al. Patient-physician social concordance, medical visit communication and patients' perceptions of health care quality. Patient Educ Couns 2011;85:e201–8.
26. Cooper LA, Roter DL, Johnson RL, et al. Patient-centered communication, ratings of care, and concordance of patient and physician race. Ann Intern Med 2003;139(11):907–15.
27. Street RL, O'Malley KJ, Cooper LA. Understanding concordance in patient-physician relationships: personal and ethnic dimensions of shared identity. Ann Fam Med 2008;6(3):198–205.
28. LaVeist TA, Nuru-Jeter A. Is doctor-patient race concordance associated with greater satisfaction with care? J Health Soc Behav 2002;43(3):296–306.
29. LaVeist TA, Nuru-Jeter A, Jones KE. The association of doctor-patient race concordance with health service utilization. J Public Health Policy 2003; 24(3–4):312–23.
30. King WD, Wong MD, Shapiro MF, et al. Does racial concordance between HIV-positive patients and their physicians affect the time to receipt of protease inhibitors? J Gen Intern Med 2004;19(11):1146–53.
31. Beach MC, Roter DL, Wang NY, et al. Are physicians' attitudes of respect accurately perceived by patients and associated with more positive communication behaviors? Patient Educ Couns 2006;62(3):347–54.
32. Lasser KE, Mintzer IL, Lambert A, et al. Missed appointment rates in primary care: the importance of site of care. J Health Care Poor Underserved 2005;16(3):475–86.
33. Meghani SH, Brooks JM, Gipson-Jones T, et al. Patient-provider race-concordance: does it matter in improving minority patients' health outcomes? Ethn Health 2009;14:107–30.
34. Coran JJ, Koropeckyj-Cox T, Arnold CL. Are physicians and patients in agreement? Exploring dyadic concordance. Health Educ Behav 2013;20(10):1–9.
35. Ross S. The feminization of medicine. Am Med Assoc J Ethics 2003;5. Available at: http://virtualmentor.ama-assn.org/2003/09/msoc1-0309.html. Accessed February 15, 2013.
36. Meeuwesen L, Schaap C, Van der Staak C. Verbal analysis of doctor-patient communication. J R Soc Med 1991;32:1143–50.
37. Roter D, Lipkin M, Korsgaard A. Sex differences in patients' and physicians' communication during primary care medical visits. Med Care 1991;20: 1083–93.
38. Bertakis KD, Franks P, Azari R. Effects of physician gender on patient satisfaction. J Am Med Womens Assoc 2003;58:69–75.
39. Maheux B, Dufort F, Beland F, et al. Female medical practitioners: more preventive and patient oriented. Med Care 1990;28:87–92.
40. Roter DL, Hall JA, Aoki Y. Physician gender effects in medical communication: a meta-analytic review. JAMA 2002;288:756–64.
41. Roter DL, Hall JA. Physician gender and patient-centered communication: a critical review of the empirical research. Annu Rev Public Health 2004;25: 497–519.
42. Barnsley J, William AP, Cockerill R, et al. Physician characteristics and the physician-patient relationship. Impact of sex, year of graduation, and specialty. Can Fam Physician 1999;45:935–42.
43. Waitzkin H. Information giving in medical care. J Health Soc Behav 1985;26: 81–101.
44. Elderkin-Thompson V, Waitzkin H. Differences in clinical communication by gender. J Gen Intern Med 1999;14:112–20.

45. Hall JA, Irish JT, Roter DL, et al. Gender in medical encounters: an analysis of physician and patient communication in primary care setting. Health Psychol 1994;13:384–92.
46. Sandhu H, Adams A, Singleton L, et al. The impact of gender dyads on doctor-patient communication: a systematic review. Patient Educ Couns 2009;76: 348–55.
47. Centers for Disease Control. Health, United States, 2011. Table 98 (page 1 of 2). Dental visits in the past year, by selected characteristics: United States, selected years 1997–2010. Available at: http://www.cdc.gov/nchs/data/hus/hus11.pdf. Accessed February 15, 2013.
48. Bertea PC, Staehelin K, Dratva J, et al. Female gender is associated with dental care and dental hygiene, but not with complete dentition in the Swiss adult population. J Public Health 2007;15:361–7.
49. Al-Omari QD, Hamasha AA. Gender-specific oral health attitudes and behavior among dental students in Jordan. J Contemp Dent Pract 2005;6(1):107–14.
50. Fukai K, Takesu Y, Maki Y. Gender differences in oral health behavior and general health habits in an adult population. Bull Tokyo Dent Coll 1999;40(4): 187–93.
51. Nanakorn S, Osaka R, Chusilp K, et al. Gender differences in health-related practices among university students in northeast Thailand. Asia Pac J Public Health 1999;11(1):10–5.
52. Sakki TK, Knuuttila ML, Anttila SS. Lifestyle, gender and occupational status as determinants of dental health behavior. J Clin Periodontol 1998;25(7): 566–70.
53. Christopherson EA, Briskie D, Inglehart MR. Objective, subjective, and self-assessment of preadolescent orthodontic treatment need - a function of age, gender, and ethnic/racial background? J Public Health Dent 2009;69(1):9–17.
54. Olsen JA, Inglehart MR. Malocclusions and perceptions of attractiveness, intelligence and personality, and behavioral intentions: an experimental exploration. Am J Orthod Dentofacial Orthop 2011;140(5):669–79.
55. Johansson AK, Norring C, Unell L, et al. Eating disorders and oral health: a matched case-control study. Eur J Oral Sci 2012;120(2):61–8.
56. Hitchman SC, Fong GT. Gender empowerment and female-to-male smoking prevalence ratios. Bull World Health Organ 2011;89:195–202.
57. Smith MK, Dundes L. The implications of gender stereotypes for the dentist-patient relationship. J Dent Educ 2008;72(5):562–70.
58. Hutson-Comeaux SL, Kelly JR. Gender stereotypes of emotional reactions: how we judge an emotion as valid. Sex Roles 2002;47:1–10.
59. Maccoby EE. Gender and relationships: a developmental account. Am Psychol 1990;45:513–20.
60. Olsen JA, Inglehart MR. Occlusion and person perception: an experimental exploration. Comm Dent Oral Epid, in press.
61. Chapman HR, Kirby-Turner NC. Dental fear in children - a proposed model. Br Dent J 1999;187:408–12.
62. Locker D, Liddell A, Dempster L, et al. Age of onset of dental anxiety. J Dent Res 1999;78:790–6.
63. Inglehart MR, George S, Feigal RJ. Dental fear in pediatric patients – challenges and opportunities for dental care providers. J Dent Hyg 2003;12(3): 11–5.
64. Frable DE. Gender, racial, ethnic, sexual, and class identities. Annu Rev Psychol 1997;48:139–62.

65. Hollander SZ. Socialization influences on the acquisition of gender constancy. Israel: Dissertation Yeshiva University; 2001 (See also: Dissertation Abstracts International: Section B: The Sciences & Engineering; Vol. 62(7-B) Feb 2002, US: Univ. Microfilms International; 2002, 3400.).
66. Cross W. Shades of African American: diversity in African-American identity. Philadelphia: Temple Univ. Press; 1991.
67. Campbell A, Shirley L, Heywood C. Infants' visual preferences for sex-congruent babies, children, toys, and activities: a longitudinal study. Br J Dev Psychol 2000;18:479–98.
68. Riley PJ. The influence of gender on occupational aspirations of kindergarten children. J Vocat Behav 1981;19(2):244–50.
69. Cann A, Palmer S. Children's assumptions about the generalizability of sex-typed abilities. Sex Roles 1986;15(9–10):551–6.
70. Sandberg DE, Meyer-Bahlburg HF, Ehrhardt AA. The prevalence of gender-atypical behavior in elementary school children. J Am Acad Child Adolesc Psychiatry 1993;32(2):306–14.
71. Fagot BI, Leinbach MD, O'Boyle C. Gender labeling, gender stereotyping, and parenting behaviors. Developmental Psychology 1992;28(2):225–30.
72. Redwine E. The effects of children's age, gender and ethnicity on their preference of male or female health care providers from different ethnic groups. A thesis submitted in partial fulfillment for the degree of Master of Science (Pediatric Dentistry). Ann Arbor (MI): University of Michigan. School of Dentistry; 1998.
73. Fennema K, Meyer DL, Owen N. Sex of physician: patients' preferences and stereotypes. J Fam Pract 1990;30:441–6.
74. Schmittdiel J, Grumbach K, Selby J, et al. Effect of physician and patient gender concordances on patient satisfaction and preventive care practices. J Gen Intern Med 2000;15:761–9.
75. Newton JT, Davenport-Jones L, Idle M, et al. Patients' perceptions of general dental practitioners: the influence of ethnicity and sex of dentist. Soc Behav Personal 2001;29(6):601–6.
76. Bare LC, Dundes L. Strategies for combating dental anxiety. J Dent Educ 2004; 68(11):1172–7.
77. Berger ER, Inglehart MR. Patient-provider relationships - Does gender and attractiveness consistency matter? AADR Meeting. Tampa, March 21–24, 2012.
78. Woolfolk MW, Price SS. Efforts to increase student diversity in allied, predoctoral, and advanced dental programs in the United States: a historical perspective. J Dent Educ 2012;76(1):51–64.
79. Gross D, Schaefer G. "Feminization" in German dentistry. Career paths and opportunities – a gender comparison. Womens Stud Forum 2011;34:130–9.
80. Adair SM, Schafer TE, Waller JL, et al. Age and gender differences in the use of behavior management techniques by pediatric dentists. Pediatr Dent 2007; 29(5):403–8.
81. Gorter RC, Bleeker JC, Freeman R. Dental nurses on perceived differences in their dentist's communication and interaction style. Br Dent J 2006;201:159–64.
82. Anderson JI, Patterson AN, Temple HJ, et al. Lesbian, gay, bisexual, and transgender (LGBT) issues in dental school environments: dental student leaders' perceptions. J Dent Educ 2009;73(1):105–18.
83. Laumann EO, Gagnon JH, Michael RT, et al. The social organization of sexuality: sexual practices in the United States. Chicago: University of Chicago; 1994.
84. Smith DM, Gates GJ. Gay and lesbian families in the United States: same-sex unmarried partner households. Human Rights Campaign Report; 2001.

85. Gay and Lesbian Medical Association and LGBT health experts. Healthy People 2010 Companion Document for Lesbian, Gay, Bisexual, and Transgender (LGBT) Health. San Francisco (CA): Gay and Lesbian Medical Association; 2001.
86. Ridner SL, Frost K, LaHoie AS. Health information and risk behaviors among lesbian, gay, and bisexual college students. J Am Acad Nurse Pract 2006; 18(8):374–8.
87. Fikar C, Keith L. Information needs of gay, lesbian, bisexual, and transgendered health care professionals: results of an internet survey. J Med Libr Assoc 2004; 92(1):56–65.
88. Dinkel S, Patzel B, McGuire M, et al. Measures of homophobia among nursing students and faculty: a Midwestern perspective. Int J Nurs Educ Scholarsh 2007;4(1):art.24.
89. Cant B. Exploring the implications for health professionals of men coming out as gay in healthcare settings. Health Soc Care Community 2005;14(1):9–16.
90. McKelvey RS, Webb JA, Baldassar LV, et al. Sex knowledge and sexual attitudes among medical and nursing students. Aust N Z J Psychiatry 1999;33: 260–6.
91. Sheridan RA, Inglehart MR. Intimate partner violence/abuse – Faculty and students' perspectives. AADR Meeting. Tampa, March 21–24, 2012.
92. Available at: http://www.michigan.gov/dhs/0,00.html,7-124-5460_7261-15005–, 1607. Accessed February 15, 2013.
93. Tjaden P, Thoennes N. Extent, nature and consequences of intimate partner violence: findings from the National Violence against Women Survey. Atlanta (GA): National Institute of Justice and the Centers of Disease Control and Prevention; 2000.
94. Perciaccante JV, Ochs HA, Dodson TB. Head, neck, and facial injuries as markers of domestic violence in women. J Oral Maxillofac Surg 1999;57(7): 760–2 [discussion: 762–3].
95. Le BT, Dierks EJ, Ueeck BA, et al. Maxillofacial injuries associated with domestic violence. J Oral Maxillofac Surg 2001;59(11):1277–83 [discussion: 1283–4].
96. Meskin LH. If not us, then who? J Am Dent Assoc 1994;125(1):10–2.
97. Muelleman RL, Lenaghan PA, Pakieser RA. Battered women: injury locations and types. Ann Emerg Med 1996;28(5):486–92.
98. Statement 99h-1996. Policy statement: expansion of ADA efforts to educate dental professionals in recognizing and reporting abuse and neglect. American Dental Association transactions. Chicago: American Dental Association; 1996. p. 684.
99. McDowell JD, Kassebaum DK, Fryer GE Jr. Recognizing and reporting victims of domestic violence: a survey of dental practitioners. Spec Care Dentist 1994; 14(2):49–53.
100. Love C, Gerbert B, Caspers N, et al. Dentists' attitudes and behaviors regarding domestic violence: the need for an effective response. J Am Dent Assoc 2001; 132:85–93.
101. Tilden VP, Schmidt TA, Limandri BJ, et al. Factors that influence clinicians' assessment and management of family violence. Am J Public Health 1994; 84(4):628–33.
102. Forest A, Taichman R, Inglehart MR. Leadership-related attitudes and values among dentists – Does gender matter? IADR/AADR Meeting. Seattle, March 20–24, 2013.

Emerging Topics for Dentists as Primary Care Providers

Linda M. Kaste, DDS, MS, PhD[a,b,]*, Jocelyn R. Wilder, MPH, MS[b],
Leslie R. Halpern, MD, DDD, PhD, MPH[c]

KEYWORDS

- Primary health care • Papillomavirus vaccines • Sex education • Human milk
- Interdisciplinary communication

KEY POINTS

- Sex and gender health aspects are components of the emerging role of the oral health care provider as a primary health care provider. However, many of these have not yet been well researched in the oral health arena.
- Human papilloma virus vaccine, now a recommended vaccine for 11- to 12-year-old boys and girls, is a topic that patients and parents of adolescents are likely to expect oral health care providers to offer advice about because of oral cancer implications.
- Patients of sexual minority orientations may have disproportionate risks for oral diseases. Included in these concerns are tobacco and alcohol usage.
- Nursing and medicine are pursuing inclusion of sexual minorities in their respective curricula. Dentistry should consider these models in dental education.

INTRODUCTION

The most recent strategic plan of the National Institutes of Health Office of Research on Women's Health (ORWH)[1] has the vastness of women's health research whittled down to 6 goals (**Box 1**). This ORWH strategic plan approach is significantly different than from its 2 predecessors. The 2020 plan does not place disease-specific emphasis, instead "it encompasses disease-specific research in a broader vision of women's health that can benefit both women and men by increasing our

The authors have nothing to disclose.
[a] Department of Pediatric Dentistry, College of Dentistry, University of Illinois at Chicago, 801 S Paulina Street, MC 850, Rm 563A, Chicago, IL 60612, USA; [b] Division of Epidemiology and Biostatistcs, School of Public Health, University of Illinois at Chicago, 1603 W Taylor Street, MC 923, 9th Floor, Chicago, IL 60612, USA; [c] Oral and Maxillofacial Surgery, Meharry Medical College, School of Dentistry, 1005 DB Todd Jr. Boulevard, Nashville, TN 37208, USA
* Corresponding author. Department of Pediatric Dentistry, College of Dentistry, University of Illinois at Chicago, 801 S Paulina Street, MC 850, Rm 563A, Chicago, IL 60612.
E-mail address: kaste@uic.edu

Box 1
Goals from *Moving into the Future with new Dimensions and Strategies: A Vision for 2020 for Women's Health Research*

1. Increase sex differences research in basic science studies

2. Incorporate findings of sex/gender differences in the design and application of new technologies, medical devices, and therapeutic drugs

3. Actualize personalized prevention, diagnostics, and therapeutics for girls and women

4. Create strategic alliances and partnerships to maximize the domestic and global impact of women's health and wellness research

5. Develop and implement new communication and social networking technologies to increase understanding and appreciation of women's health and wellness research

6. Employ innovative strategies to build a well-trained, diverse, and vigorous women's health research workforce

Data from ORWH, NIH, USDHHS. Moving into the future with new dimensions and strategies: a vision for 2020 for Women's Health Research: strategic plan. vol. 1. 2010. Available at: http://orwh.od.nih.gob/research/strategocplan/ORWH_StrategicPlan2020_Vol1.pdf. Accessed January 30, 2013.

understanding of the role of sex/gender factors in differential disease risk, vulnerability, progression, and outcome, as well as the effects of being female on health."[1] Hence, within the strategic plan, there is no specific section on oral health or dentistry. The report is stratified by the cross-cutting interdisciplinary themes that contribute to the establishment of the 6 goals. This article discusses this collaborative momentum in the context of the inclusion of dentistry in an evolving definition of primary health care with emerging health topics.

A patient's visit to the dentist is a valuable moment to improve oral and overall health, reinforce positive health messaging, and educate on health promotion and disease prevention. In the United States, most of the population, even among the adult population, report being seen by either their physician or dentist in the past year.[2] A readily acceptable role in dentistry exists to reinforce the negative effects of sugar-sweetened beverages, as an example of bridging primary health care. Guidance on such beverages could abate dental caries,[3] as well as help to address the caloric-related factors of obesity.[4]

There are other oral and general health topics for which interdisciplinary links are becoming more transparent and more familiar to the dental workforce. The reader is referred to previous articles in this issue.

However, there are emerging topics that are less familiar in dentistry. Several of these topics are presented in this article to help raise awareness, if needed, of areas to be encountered in dental life-long-learning as the science bases are evolving. The topics chosen for this article complement the accompanying articles in this special issue. Our chosen topics are not comprehensive lists of emerging topics in women's oral health related to the dentist's role as a primary health care provider. We have selected topics ones that general dentists need to be familiar with as partners in interdisciplinary health care, including the dentist as a discussant with adolescent patients and their parents about the human papilloma virus (HPV) vaccine; sexual health distinctions between minority groups and heterosexuals; and whether human milk microbiome may provide insight into preventing early childhood caries.

HPV VACCINE

As a result of increasing knowledge of the relationship between oral cancer and HPV, a dentist is on the front line to educate adult and child patients about high-risk behaviors and the HPV vaccine. The dentist may actually be able to reach patients, such as adolescents, who are not seen frequently by physicians or nurse practitioners. A sample of adolescents from the Child Health Assessment and Monitoring Program (CHAMP) found that 14% of male and 20% of female adolescents had not received a preventive checkup in the past 12 months.[5]

Although the HPV vaccine is recommended by the Centers for Disease Control, the American Academy of Pediatrics, and the American Academy of Family Physicians for all children aged 11 to 12 years (www.cdc.gov/vaccines/teens), it is still new and not well known. A particular concern is whether parents are aware of the recommendation for boys.[6] As the vaccine is given in 3 separate visits to a health care provider, alternative settings (nonphysician visits) are being suggested.[7] Some parents are actually more comfortable with alternative settings.[8] Perhaps an alternative location of the future could be the dental office?

In addition, physicians may need help in getting vaccination messages across to parents and their adolescent children. Seventeen percent of parents indicated that they were not aware of the HPV vaccine being available for their child's sex.[5] This was that case for more than one-quarter (27%) of the parents of boys indicating that they did not receive a recommendation from their physician, compared with 14% for the parents of girls.[5] It is estimated that between 10% and 30% of girls aged 11 to 17 years received the vaccine a year after it was licensed for use in girls compared with 2% of the boys aged 11 to 17 years a year after it was licensed for use in boys.[5] Is this an opportunity for dentists to further serve their patients?

Collaborations between health care providers and the parents of adolescents to improve the health status of adolescents is seen as feasible and is being proposed as an indirect way for preparing parents to talk with their children in addition to the direct communication between the health care provider and the adolescent.[9] This model seems transferrable to the dental health care provider. Northridge and colleagues[10] describe their view of the role of the dentist with regard to HPV and oropharyngeal cancer, with the expectations of dental profession transitions, yet the need to appropriately respond to patients currently.

SEXUAL MINORITIES

General health planning is recognizing that health differences may exist between sexual minorities and heterosexuals. A lesbian, gay, bisexual, and transgender (LGBT) companion document was generated for *Healthy People 2010*.[11] *Healthy People 2020* has LGBT as a recognized subpopulation of concern, but the associated materials have not yet been publically shared.

An aspect of health and wellness among sexual minorities that readily translates to oral health risk is disproportionate risk behaviors. Behaviors that have been documented include smoking tobacco,[12,13] hazardous drinking of alcohol,[12,14] and intimate partner violence.[15]

Another topic for which dentists may develop a helpful role is eating disorders, with special attention to sexual minorities. National estimates for high school students show astounding rates of practices linked to oral health consequences (see the article by Kim and colleagues in this issue) that raise concern by race/ethnicity and sexual orientation.[16] Among girls, the highest number of self-reports of purging was by lesbian Latinas (26.7%). However, among boys, 2 groups reported purging rates higher than 30%: African American bisexuals (35.3%) and bisexuals of other ethnicity (30.4%).[16]

In January 2013, the US Centers for Disease Control and Prevention released data on victimization by sexual orientation.[15] Reporting information achieved via the 2010 National Intimate Partner and Sexual Violence Survey (NISVS), the data show that bisexual women encounter higher rates of rape and sexual violence by any perpetrator than either lesbian or heterosexual women. Bisexual women also encounter higher rates of rape and physical violence by an intimate partner than either lesbian or heterosexual women. Intimate partner violence and sexual violence were reported by lesbian women and gay men at rates equal to or higher than for heterosexuals. See the article by Halpern in this issue for further insight into oral health care provider awareness of intimate partner violence.

Recent educational perspectives have been provided on health care professional sex education for nursing and medicine. The nursing education review by Lim and Bernstein[17] provides interesting insight into concerns for the aging LGBT patient and specifically identifies a 2011 Institute of Medicine consensus report that provides insight into the historical development of health professional treatment of nonheterosexual people.[18] A recent article discusses medical education's view on "sexuality education"[19] and getting beyond reproductive health topics into healthy sexuality as a component of optimal health care. Selected elements from a medical school curricular perspective[19] that may be of value to dentistry are shown in **Box 2**.

Box 2
Selected components on human sexuality from medical school curricula for consideration for dental school curricula

Attitudes

1. Self-awareness and reflection on personal beliefs, values, and attitudes toward sex and how they may influence care of the patient

2. Awareness of the variability of normal sexual expression (gender identity, sexual orientation, and so forth)

3. Awareness of ethical issues in sex and relationships

Knowledge

1. Knowledge of the biology of sexual development at the molecular and organism level

2. Reproductive biology

3. Sexually transmitted infections

4. Impact of medical illnesses and their treatments on sexual function

5. Sexuality in special populations (adolescents, aged, disabled)

6. Sociological issues (ethnicity, race, culture, religion, sexual orientation, and economic status)

7. Lesbian/gay/bisexual/transgender sexuality and sexual health care for these populations

8. Sexual abuse and violence

Skills

1. Sexual history taking

2. Comfort with sexual language and terminology in a fashion understandable to patients

Adapted from Shindel AW, Parish SJ. Sexuality education in North American Medical Schools: current status and future directions. J Sex Med 2013;10:3–18.

HUMAN MILK MICROBIOME

Technological advances have enabled examination of human interactions of the digestive system microbiota, diet and nutrition, and immune response.[20] Building from that understanding, recent animal and human research began looking at milk, directly from the mother's breast to the offspring, in a new direction. Might there be a suggestion from this work that could help prevent dental caries, especially in young children? The recognition that mother's milk contributes to an infant's immune response seems well established. However, the perspective that the mother's milk may establish the commensal gut microbiota is being explored. A pathway of maternal gut and oral commensal bacteria through lactation presented to offspring via milk was demonstrated for rhesus monkeys.[21] This work has now been augmented by human studies; the human milk microbiome is seen to differ over the course of lactation, by maternal weight, and by mode of delivery.[22] Further work relating to the oral health status of the mother to the bacteria present in her milk is clearly needed.

SUMMARY

The information presented is only the tip of the iceberg for the emerging gatekeeper role of the oral health care provider in the overall health and well-being of patients. This overview adds to our understanding of successful oral health involvement in inter-disciplinary sets of core competencies for health care providers. Oral diseases are part of the bigger systemic health picture. Building beyond women's health as repro-ductive health topics into healthy sexuality as a component of optimal health care will need to include competency at the individual learner, educational institution, and health system levels.

REFERENCES

1. ORWH, NIH, USDHHS. Moving into the future with new dimensions and strategies: a vision for 2020 for Women's Health Research: strategic plan. vol. 1. 2010. Available at: http://orwh.od.nih.gob/research/strategocplan/ORWH_StrategicPlan 2020_Vol1.pdf. Accessed January 30, 2013.
2. US Department of Health and Human Services. Summary health statistics for U.S. adults: National Health Interview Survey, 2011. Vital and Health Statistics, Series 10, No. 256. Hyattsville (MD): CDC National Center for Health Statistics; 2012.
3. Harris R, Gamboa A, Dailey Y, et al. One-to-one dietary interventions undertaken in a dental setting to change dietary behaviour. Cochrane Database Syst Rev 2012;(3):CD006540. http://dx.doi.org/10.1002/14651858.CD006540.pub2.
4. Morenga LT, Mallar S, Mann J. Dietary sugars and body weight: systematic review and meta-analyses of randomized controlled trials and cohort studies. BMJ 2012;345:e7492. http://dx.doi.org/10.1136/bmj.e7492.
5. Gilkey MB, Moss JL, McRee AL, et al. Do correlates of HPV vaccine initiation differ between adolescent boys and girls? Vaccine 2012;30:5928–34.
6. Reiter PL, McRee AL, Kadis JA, et al. HPV vaccine and adolescent males. Vaccine 2011;29:5595–602.
7. Reiter PL, McRee AL, Pepper JK, et al. Improving human papillomavirus vaccine delivery: a national study of parents and their adolescent sons. J Adolesc Health 2012;51:32–7.
8. McRee AL, Reiter PL, Pepper JK, et al. Correlates of comfort with alternative settings for HPV vaccine delivery. Hum Vaccin Immunother 2013;9(2). [Epub ahead of print].

9. Ford CA, Davenport AF, Meier A, et al. Partnerships between parents and health care professionals to improve adolescent health. J Adolesc Health 2011; 49:53–7.

10. Northridge ME, Manji N, Piamonte RT, et al. HPV, oropharyngeal cancer, and the role of the dentist: a professional ethnical approach. J Health Care Poor Underserved 2012;23:47–57.

11. Gay and Lesbian Medical Association (GMLA). Healthy people 2010: a companion document for LGBT health. San Francisco (CA): GMLA; 2001.

12. Herrick AL, Matthews AK, Garofalo R. Health risk behaviors in an urban sample of young women who have sex with women. J Lesbian Stud 2010;14:80–92.

13. Matthews AK, Hotton A, DuBois S, et al. Demographic, psychosocial, and contextual correlates of tobacco use in sexual minority women. Res Nurs Health 2011; 34:141–52.

14. Hughes TL, Szalacha LA, Johnson TP, et al. Sexual victimization and hazardous drinking among heterosexual and sexual minority women. Addict Behav 2010;35: 1152–6.

15. Walters ML, Chen L, Breiding MJ. The National Intimate Partner and Sexual Violence Survey (NISVS): 2010 findings on victimization by sexual orientation. Atlanta (GA): National Center for Injury Prevention and Control, Centers for Disease Control and Prevention; 2013.

16. Austin SB, Nelson LA, Birkett MA, et al. Eating disorder symptoms and obesity at the intersections of gender, ethnicity, and sexual orientation in US high school students. Am J Public Health 2013;103:e16–22.

17. Lim FA, Bernstein I. Promoting awareness of LGBT issues in aging in a baccalaureate nursing program. Nurs Educ Perspect 2012;33(3):170–5.

18. Institute of Medicine. The health of lesbian, gay, bisexual, and transgender people: building a foundation for better understanding. Washington, DC: National Academy Press; 2011.

19. Shindel AW, Parish SJ. Sexuality education in North American Medical Schools: current status and future directions. J Sex Med 2013;10:3–18.

20. Kau AL, Ahern PP, Griffin NW, et al. Human nutrition, the gut microbiome and the immune system. Nature 2011;16:327–36.

21. Jin L, Hinde K, Tao L. Species diversity and relative abundance of lactic acid bacteria in the milk of rhesus monkeys (Macaca mulatta). J Med Primatol 2011; 40:52–8.

22. Cabrera-Rubio R, Collado MC, Laitinen K, et al. The human milk microbiome changes over lactation and is shaped by maternal weight and mode of delivery. Am J Clin Nutr 2012;96:544–51.

Index

Note: Page numbers of article titles are in **boldface** type.

A

Abuse, violence and. See *Violence, and abuse*.
Age, risk factors for caries and, 303
Alcohol, consumption of, and oral cancer, 342–344
Anesthetic agents, side effects of, genotypes linked to, 248

B

Baby bottle tooth decay, 304
Behavioral factors, risk factors for caries and, 304
Biofilm, dental, risk facters for caries ralated to, 305
Breast cancer, 189–190

C

Cancer, oral and pharyngeal. See *Oral and pharyngeal cancer*.
Cardiovascular disease, and adult women, 187–188
    association with oral health, 214
Caries, description of, 302
    during pregnancy, 202
    factors protecting against, 305
    prevalence and incidence of, in United States, 305–306
        worldwide, 306–307
    prevalence and risk assessment of, impact of gender on, **301–315**
    risk factors for, 301–302
        related to dental biofilm, 305
        related to diet, 304
        related to host, 302–304
Cariogenic food consumption, and dietary behaviors, 212–213
Central sensitivity syndrome, 239, 240
Cervical cancer, and oral cancer, risk factors for, and contrast between, 340–342
Child abuse, 283
Condylar resorption, idiopathic, and temporomandibular disorders, 238–239
Craniofacial anomalies, gender differences in, 267–269

D

Dental care, and oral health, during pregnancy, 185–186, **195–210**
    during pregnancy, future directions in, 206
Dental care providers, and patients, communication about abuse, 364–365
        interactions between, **357–376**
            gender and, 358–360

Dent Clin N Am 57 (2013) 377–382
http://dx.doi.org/10.1016/S0011-8532(13)00021-9
0011-8532/13/$ – see front matter © 2013 Elsevier Inc. All rights reserved.

Moving?

Make sure your subscription moves with you!

To notify us of your new address, find your **Clinics Account Number** (located on your mailing label above your name), and contact customer service at:

Email: journalscustomerservice-usa@elsevier.com

800-654-2452 (subscribers in the U.S. & Canada)
314-447-8871 (subscribers outside of the U.S. & Canada)

Fax number: 314-447-8029

Elsevier Health Sciences Division
Subscription Customer Service
3251 Riverport Lane
Maryland Heights, MO 63043

*To ensure uninterrupted delivery of your subscription, please notify us at least 4 weeks in advance of move.

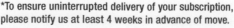

Moving?

Make sure your subscription moves with you!

To notify us of your new address, find your **Clinics Account Number** (located on your mailing label above your name), and contact customer service at:

Email: journalscustomerservice-usa@elsevier.com

800-654-2452 (subscribers in the U.S. & Canada)
314-447-8871 (subscribers outside of the U.S. & Canada)

Fax number: 314-447-8029

Elsevier Health Sciences Division
Subscription Customer Service
3251 Riverport Lane
Maryland Heights, MO 63043

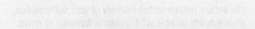

Printed and bound by CPI Group (UK) Ltd, Croydon, CR0 4YY

03/10/2024

01040441-0005